The Politics of Nursing Knowledge

Anne Marie Rafferty

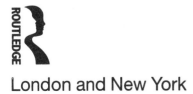

London and New York

*For my mother, Bridget Rafferty
and the memory of my father,
Michael Smith Rafferty*

First published 1996
by Routledge
11 New Fetter Lane, London EC4P 4EE

Simultaneously published in the USA and Canada
by Routledge
29 West 35th Street, New York, NY 10001

Typeset in Times by Routledge
Printed and bound in Great Britain by Mackays of Chatham
PLC, Chatham, Kent

British Library Cataloguing in Publication Data
A catalogue record for this book is available from the British
Library

Library of Congress Cataloguing in Publication Data
Rafferty, Anne Marie.
The politics of nursing knowledge/Anne Marie Rafferty.
Includes bibliographical references and index.
1. Nursing – Study and teaching – Government policy – Great
Britain. 2. Nurses – Education – Political aspects – Great Britain.
3. Professional socialization – Great Britain. 4. Occupational
prestige – Great Britain. 5. Nurses – Social conditions – Great
Britain. I. Title.
[DNLM: 1. Education, Nursing – organization & administra-
tion – Great Britain. 2. Education, Nursing – history – Great
Britain. 3. Nursing – trends – Great Britain. 4. Social Conditions
– Great Britain.   WY 18 R137p 1996]
RT81.G7R34   1996
610.73'071'141–dc20

ISBN 0–415–11491–8 (hbk)
ISBN 0–415–11492–6 (pbk)

The Politics of Nursing Knowledge

The entry of nursing into higher education has raised a number of questions about its academic identity and future. *The Politics of Nursing Knowledge* puts into context the historical factors which have shaped the development of nurse education and lays the foundations for an historical sociology of nursing knowledge.

Based on substantial new research and drawing on government and professional records, *The Politics of Nursing Knowledge* looks at how nurse education has been shaped by wider social attitudes towards gender and class. In a critical reappraisal of Florence Nightingale's vision of nursing, Anne Marie Rafferty explores the implications of Nightingale's belief that nursing training should be regarded as an education of character rather than an intellectual discipline. Analysing the relationship between nursing and associated professions, the author traces the evolution of training and policy-making from the origins of hospital reform in the 1860s to the start of the National Health Service (NHS) in 1948.

Examining the contemporary issues affecting nursing, *The Politics of Nursing Knowledge* questions the extent to which the notion of a 'profession' is compatible with the career patterns and lifestyle opportunities of the majority of nurses, who are women. Looking to the future of nursing as an academic discipline, the final chapter asks whether an intellectually self-confident culture can emerge or whether the contradictions of professionalism and the health care system will prevent nursing from achieving its full potential.

Anne Marie Rafferty is Director of the Centre for Policy in Nursing Research, London School of Hygiene and Tropical Medicine, and Research Associate at the Wellcome Unit for the History of Medicine, University of Oxford.

Contents

Acknowledgements

I have accumulated many debts in the course of producing this book. Many friends and colleagues have contributed to it in visible and invisible ways; my heartfelt thanks to all of them. Dr Charles Webster was an inspiring supervisor who launched me into the research upon which the book is based and who has been a most generous and unfailing source of advice, encouragement, expertise and humour. Professor Pamela Gillies has been a tower of strength and fellow traveller along the path taken by this book, and I am deeply in her debt forever. Colleagues at the Wellcome Unit for the History of Medicine in Oxford provided a haven of friendship, facilities and a model community of scholarship. Josephine Guy was a friend and critic of style and substance. I am especially grateful to Richard Smith, Elizabeth Peretz, Anne Summers and Professor Michael Dols, who sadly died before I could thank him. Professor Robert Dingwall shared his insights and interest in nursing so generously with me. Elizabeth Rafferty provided immeasurable support when all seemed bleak and beyond. The research upon which this thesis is based could not have been begun without a Department of Health nursing research studentship. The Wellcome Trust generously continued the support of the research and I am deeply grateful to them. No historical research can be completed without the thoughtful consideration of librarians and archivists. I am deeply grateful to librarians of the Bodleian and Radcliffe Science Libraries, Radcliffe Infirmary, Oxford, the Royal College of Nursing, London, and the University of Nottingham. Susan McGann, archivist at the Royal College of Nursing, has been unstinting in her support and friendship. The staff of the Public Record Office were efficient and very helpful in their retrieval of files consulted at Kew. Many thanks to

Edwina Welham and Alison Poyner at Routledge for their patience and perseverance.

Colleagues from Oxcept, John Radcliffe Hospital, the Department of Nursing Studies Department, University of Nottingham, and the University of Pennsylvania, where I spent an academic year as a Harkness Fellow, have given me more than collegial support. In particular I should like to thank Wendy Green and Jill Buckledee from Oxcept, and Professor Jane Robinson and Mark Avis from Nottingham. Professors Linda Aiken and Joan Lynaugh from the University of Pennsylvania were exemplary role models and mentors for me in the USA. Joan Lynaugh's enthusiasm for this work and her leadership of the International Council of Nurses (ICN) Centennial Project, in which I have had the privilege of participating, have been inspirational. Throughout the period of writing this book I have also benefited from the scholarly and social support of the ICN History Collective, which I have found a model of collaborative exchange and research. Latterly I have been privileged to work with excellent colleagues at the London School of Hygiene and Tropical Medicine. Jenny Stanley has helped to prepare this manuscript with her usual skill and efficiency. Lara Marks, Jo-Ann Crawford and Aylish Wood have provided shelter and sustenance during my research trips.

My family have spurred me on, especially my mother, Bridget Rafferty, with her 'faith'. The stories of her own nursing experiences have kindled my imagination and form part of the written and unwritten history of this study. Special thanks also go to Katie McCaughey and Danny and Peter Rafferty for their support and sustenance. Last but not least, a great debt of gratitude is due to my father, Michael Rafferty, for his constant confidence and encouragement throughout our adventures and misadventures. We miss his sense of values, humour and humanity immeasurably.

Abbreviations

AHM	Association of Hospital Matrons
BHA	British Hospitals Association
BMA	British Medical Association
BNA	British Nurses' Association
CAB	Cabinet Committee
CMB	Central Midwives Board
COHSE	Confederation of Health Services Employees
ED	Board of Education
EMS	Emergency Medical Service
GMC	General Medical Council
GNC	General Nursing Council
GPDST	Girls' Public Day Schools Trust
ICN	International Council of Nurses
ICW	International Council of Women
LAB	Ministry of Labour and National Service
LCC	London County Council
MH	Ministry of Health
NALGO	National Association of Local Government Officers
NAPSS	National Association for the Promotion of Social Science
NAWU	National Asylum Workers Union
NHS	National Health Service
NPFN	National Pension Fund for Nurses
NUCO	National Union of County Officers
PRO	Public Record Office
PUTN	Professional Union of Trained Nurses
RBNA	Royal British Nurses' Association
RCN	Royal College of Nursing
RMN	Registered Mental Nurse

RMPA	Royal Medico-Psychological Association
RRC	Royal Red Cross
SMA	Socialist Medical Association
SRN	State Registered Nurse
SSRN	Society for the State Registration of Nurses
T	Treasury
TB	Tuberculosis
TUC	Trades Union Congress
VAD	Voluntary Aid Detachment
WSPU	Women's Social and Political Union

Introduction

Education lies at the centre of professional work and expertise and therefore occupies a pivotal position in the shaping of occupational culture and the politics of nursing. Far from being a value-neutral and disinterested activity, education represents a powerful vehicle for socialisation and the transmission of culture. But nursing education has been characterised by the inculcation of moral values and virtues rather than intellectual prowess. Indeed 'virtue' has been at the 'heart' of nursing education since it began to be codified in the mid-nineteenth century. So close has this connection been that early nurse education could be described as training in virtue itself. But if nurses have benefited from association with virtue, they have also been burdened with it too. The construction of nursing as an essentially, if not essentialist, 'moral' metier has undermined attempts by nurses to acquire access to the prestigious centres of learning and institutions through which social privilege and rewards are distributed. The result has been that a self-confident intellectual culture in nursing has been slow to develop and nurses' capacity to innovate and exercise leadership has been severely curbed. The dilemma for nurses, as Reverby rightly points out, has been the order to care in a society which refuses to value caring.[1] But it is a dilemma which extends beyond the value and character of caring; it derives from a deep anti-intellectual prejudice attached to women's work in general, and to the gendering of skill more particularly.

This book developed out of a long-standing interest in trying to understand the intellectual and social subordination of nurses. As a student nurse I had been puzzled and intrigued by the boundaries that seemed to be drawn between nursing and medical knowledge and practice as promulgated in the classroom and the sometimes chaotic conditions of the clinical environment. From the perspective of the perplexed student trying to locate and test the limits of a clinical role (and doubtless the patience of many a ward sister), the invisible lines that separated medicine from nursing appeared not only fluid but arbitrary divisions – until, that is, one tried to challenge those boundaries, and then one found just how rigid and fixed they could be. I knew that the knowledge base of nursing had changed; my mother had trained as a nurse and I had been enthralled by her stories of fever nursing in the 1930s, her wartime escapades and clinical experiences. Like many children with a taste for the ghoulish, I developed a morbid fascination with the more graphic images of pathology contained in the surgical and medical textbooks that were tucked away in discreet spots in the house. I devoured it, like any 'illicit' literature, for its sensationalist portrayal of the monstrous and the macabre. Through my mother's stories, and subsequently as a student of nursing and health care history, I became gripped by the attempt to understand the manner in which knowledge in nursing could shift in shape and size. To be sure, patients were no longer treated with anti-toxins for diphtheria and intravenous infusions were no longer considered a major technology managed by doctors, but what had occurred in clinical cultures and the social relations between nursing and medical staff? How pliable were these? Moreover, I found it intriguing to think that my mother, now so strong, intelligent, wise and with such a well-developed critical sensibility, could have deferred so naturally to the authoritarian regimes of hospital life in the 1930s and 1940s. How could a culture of learning develop when it seemed there was so little to inspire beyond the humdrum of ward activity, the rare encouraging remark or the occasional beacon in the form of sister tutor? But what are the factors that have shaped the opportunities for nurse education at the beginning of and towards the end of the twentieth century? What is the relationship between power, authority, knowledge and practice?

This book has two main objectives: first, to identify the pressures that have shaped nursing education and policy-making in England and Wales between 1860 and 1948; and second, to consider the role that ideas about the educability of nurses and the status of nursing have played in this genesis and genealogy of nursing knowledge. The argument of the book can be summarised as follows. Throughout the period under discussion, nursing education in England and Wales proved a chronic problem, for which there was no single solution and little evidence of obvious movement towards achieving the intellectual and social aspirations of nurse leaders. Instead, nursing education fluctuated in public importance during episodes of crisis and reflected the wider problems of adjusting the supply of female labour to the changing demands for welfare. Historians of nursing have tended to underestimate the importance of welfare policy in explaining reform. Rather they are prone to explain reform in terms of the agency and initiative of nurse leaders. Examination of government policy, however, reveals the limited extent to which internal reform within nursing could be achieved without government support and, at times, government initiative. The relationship between government and nursing was, nevertheless, not an easy one, and a central argument of this book is that education policy was the product of conflict, rather than consensus between groups equal in power. It is in the context of convergence between government and occupational priorities that the formation and implementation of nurse education policy in Britain can best be understood.

As the vector and vehicle of occupational culture and closure, education assumes totemic significance for professionals and analysts alike. A number of studies have explored the institutional politics associated with the development of nurse training. The theme of occupational dilution provided the organising principle for Brian Abel-Smith's pioneering review of the 'high politics' of general nursing in England between 1800 and 1948. Abel-Smith's work predates that of sociologists such as Davies, who in the late 1970s applied insights from the Weberian and Marxist sociology of the study of the professions to nursing in Britain.[2] Excluded from both Abel-Smith's and Davies's accounts, however, was any detailed consideration of the intellectual origins of training and in-depth treatment of the pluralist politics which shaped curricular content and controversies. Maggs, in a cross-sectional comparative analysis of British hospital nurses, examined the social origins of recruits to a sample of provincial, metropolitan, Poor Law and voluntary hospitals from 1881–1914. He concluded that the calibre of recruits and training fell short of that aspired to by reformers. By examining career histories alongside work culture and literary portrayals of nurses in the Victorian novel, Maggs shows how expanding work opportunities for women had a crucial impact upon the supply of nursing labour into hospitals. Summers delineates the complex motives of reformers who advocated the hospital as the focus for nursing reform in the mid-nineteenth century.[3] In particular, she explains the social and ideological pressures which drove the crusade against the domiciliary nurse and propelled the career profile of hospital nursing in an upward direction.

Dingwall, Rafferty and Webster address the tension between proletarianisation and professionalisation as expressed in the division between specialist segments of the occupation, rank and file and leadership interests. They focus particularly upon the interactions between pressure groups, the state and their impact upon policy formation.[4] In the USA, Rosenberg's, Reverby's and Melosh's analyses of the forces shaping the 'culture', as well as the construction of caring as women's work, remain unparalleled.[5] Where Rosenberg plots the trajectory of nursing work and training against the 'hospitalisation' of disease in the late nineteenth century, Reverby refracts nursing work through a women's history and labour process lens. Both Rosenberg and Reverby explore the shifting economic and ideological demands which shaped nursing work between 1850 and 1945. Both explore the subterranean theme of nursing as human 'capital', servicing the interests of social elites. Less well elaborated, however, is the specific role that knowledge and work culture play in the social stratification of occupations within health care. Melosh shares common ground with Rosenberg's and Reverby's analyses of the 'institutionalisation' of nursing. However, her concern lies more directly in analysing nursing work and organisational culture as a case study in the social construction of skill, and the implications that this has for different models of occupational development. As a critic of the hospital, Melosh locates the 'golden age' of nurses' autonomy in the public health nursing movement of the inter-war period.[6]

Chapter 1 argues that methods of labour supervision were imported into hospitals from the commercial world in the mid-nineteenth century. Patients' and nurses' roles can therefore be understood as an extension of those prevailing in the industrial workplace. Nurses provided an important source of mediation between the poor and the philanthropic classes. Improving the moral conduct of nurses was perceived as an important adjunct to reforming the moral condition of the working classes. In this sense nurses became the objects as well as the subjects of reform. The key to reforming the 'character' of nurses was training. The hospital provided the ideal location to administer the discipline necessary to realise the new order of health care. Here it was the moral rather than the technical attributes of contemporary nurses which were singled out for criticism by reformers. The caricature of Sarah Gamp came to symbolise the deficiencies of contemporary nursing.[7] Such criticisms, however, can be seen as part of the wider campaign to reform working-class morals, and nowhere was this more apparent than in the attack on drunkenness in nurses. The campaign to reform nursing in the mid-nineteenth century was therefore less an attempt to redefine nursing work than to reconstruct the class basis of the occupation.

The prime exponent of 'character' training for nurses was Florence Nightingale. Recent scholarship has exposed the deficiencies and modest impact of the Nightingale School's achievements upon the codification of practice.[8] Rarely, however, has there been any attempt to explain the social and intellectual provenance of Nightingale's ideas on training. Chapter 2 argues that the hospital, as conceived by Nightingale, was a microcosm of society, reflecting and reproducing contemporary methods of educational provision for girls and women. Nurse training as 'character' building consolidated rather than challenged authority relations in society at large, and the elevation of 'moral' rather than intellectual skills reinforced essentialist notions of womanhood.

Nurse reformers who were committed to a professional model for nursing distanced themselves from character training. For them it epitomised the general anti-intellectualism which was used to justify the exclusion of women from professional work. These 'new' nurses, then, adopted an alternative strategy, appropriating a technical and scientific discourse from medicine. However, the application to nursing of a medical model of training organisation generated conflict between radical nurses, doctors and administrators. These tensions were most dramatically played out in the registration debate. Chapter 3 traces the cross-currents of controversy between the Nightingale anti-registrationist and the Bedford Fenwick-led pro-registrationist lobbies. The registrationist challenge to medical authority, and the perceived disruption of the probationer's loyalty to her training hospital, were bitterly resented by anti-registrationist nurses, doctors and administrators. It was the implied analogy between nursing and medical registration or licensure which lay at the heart of the controversy between pro- and anti-registrationists.

British nurses were not alone in organising for registration. Chapter 4 examines the extent to which the registration question in Britain was shaped by international influences, in particular contact between British and American nurses. Relations between the leading pro-registrationist organisation in Britain and Mrs Bedford Fenwick broke down, leading her to look to America for intellectual and moral support to carry registration forward. The achievement of registration in different states of America and British dominions was used as a precedent for arguing for the benefits of registration for British nurses. There has been little additional work extending Davies's pioneering comparative analysis of professional power in British and American nursing. Davies argues that although the motives and strategies of nurse leaders were remarkably similar, important distinctions of social structure separated the two contexts.[9] The passing of the Nurses' Registration Act in England and Wales, however, also has to be understood in the context of the Ministry of Health's plans to reconstruct the health services. It was fortuitous that governmental and occupational objectives coincided, but each was working to a different agenda. The nature of these agendas and the fragility of the consensus forged between the organisations concerned is discussed in Chapter 5.

As a step towards the establishment of an elected General Nursing Council (GNC), a Caretaker Council was established in 1920. Differences which had divided the registrationist factions before the passing of the Nurses' Registration Act resurfaced in the early work of the provisional Caretaker Council. Clashes between its moderate and radical members led to a crisis, and its eventual collapse marks the first of a series of defeats for the radical view of nurse education, according to which standards for recruitment and training should be established independent of the resource base of the hospital. Chapter 5 examines the forces which precipitated the downfall of Mrs Bedford Fenwick and the extinction of her elitist vision of training for nurses.

The regulating authority in nursing education, the GNC, was hampered in its efforts by problems associated with adjusting the supply of female labour to the changing demands for welfare in the inter-war period. Failure to exert sufficient 'quality' control over recruitment forced organisations in both countries to concentrate upon selection and activity analysis as the key to regulating the flow of labour. Selection and 'efficiency' techniques borrowed from educational and industrial psychology were applied to nursing. Chapter 6 discusses the response of nurse leaders, officials and pressure groups to the intensifying demographic crisis affecting the nursing labour market in the 1930s. Education was consistently perceived as the solution to labour market problems in nursing. Labour supply and regulation provoked the first of several national investigations into nurse training and conditions in both countries. I consider the work of the Lancet Commission (1930–2) against the background of the deepening crisis in the economic and labour market conditions of the 1920s and 1930s.

Although conditions eased in the mid-1930s, recruitment problems in nursing re-emerged towards the end of the decade as employment opportunities for women expanded with the economic recovery. Under the twin pressures of trade union organisation and industrial protest by nurses, the government instituted the first official investigation into nursing training and services under the chairmanship of the Earl of Athlone in 1938. Chapter 7 examines the pressures shaping the content, methods and objectives of nurse education policy-making in the late 1930s.

Recurrent crises in recruitment throughout the war and preparations for the National Health Service (NHS) elevated nursing, of necessity, into an issue of the highest national importance. Nursing services and education occupied a central and sensitive position in the early politics of the National Health Service. Experts applied their social scientific research skills to unravelling the recruitment riddle and produced one of the most radical critiques of nursing education, arguing for state-funded programmes supporting full student status for recruits. Chapter 8 considers the manner in which, notwithstanding the importance of nursing in the calculus of care, the history of the early NHS revealed that the traditional relationship between nursing service and education remained intact: long-term goals were sacrificed to short-term contingencies.

One of the key theoretical assumptions of this book is that organisational change and the reform of nurse education occurred by analogy; leaders borrowed ideas and strategies for policy-making from sources of authority that they admired or regarded as successful. Part of that transfer of ideas is evident in the intellectual and social exchange that occurred between nurse leaders throughout the international nursing world. The cognitive strategies which nurses have adopted in order to obtain professional 'uplift' have been characterised by two main approaches: the 'assimilationist' and the 'separatist'. In the former, nurses learn the language of education and research used by the 'established' disciplines, and articulate nursing problems through methods 'owned' by these disciplines. The latter, separatist strategy involves creating and claiming a new language, one which reflects the cultural specificity of nursing – that is, its 'difference' and distance from other disciplines. These strategies are not unique to nurses; they are typical of many marginal groups struggling to establish their identity in an environment where they are parvenus. Nurses have utilised both these strategies in legitimising their claims to knowledge and expertise. In doing so, they have, at different times, sought the proxy patronage of medicine and social science to authorise claims to specialised knowledge, and to elaborate the academic basis of nursing expertise. Although nurses may have been the passive recipients of knowledge and work 'passed down' by others, they have also attempted to take control of that knowledge through research and curriculum development. The conclusion of this book argues that the rise of academic nursing has been accompanied by a series of dilemmas for nursing as a discipline. These derive from the crisis of authority experienced in the intellectual identity of nursing as an academic subject, a crisis that nursing shares with other disciplines periodically.[10] Treating nursing education as a cultural resource allows the status and value of different forms of knowledge, and the exclusionary devices used to police cognitive and social privilege, to be examined. This book attempts, in particular, to cast some light on the role of education in creating and sustaining the power relations underpinning the politics of knowledge in the health care division of labour.

Chapter 1

Reformatory rhetoric

INTRODUCTION

The campaign to reform nursing which began in the mid-nineteenth century was less an attempt to redefine nursing work than one to reform the nurse's character and skills through reconstructing the class basis of the occupation. Moral rather than technical attributes of nurses were singled out for criticism. Indeed the attack upon Sarah Gamp and her contemporaries can be seen as an extension of the wider campaign to reform working-class morals. To understand why Mrs Gamp and her co-workers provided such a convenient and powerful symbol for reform, we have first to appreciate the nature of her success and the consequent threat which she and her counterparts posed to reformers. There were three major interest groups who conspired to squeeze Sarah Gamp and her like out of the health care market: medical practitioners, religious sisterhoods and nurses keen to expand employment opportunities for educated women.[1] As this chapter will show, an examination of the discredited features of Sarah Gamp helps to explain the emergence of a consensus between these groups of reformers. This chapter considers the allegations made against nurses and the interests of the various participants in the discourse of denigration.

MEDICAL MANOEUVRES

Anne Summers has attempted to explain the reasons why it was that the hospital nurse, rather than her arguably more skilful domiciliary counterpart, became the focus for reformed nursing.[2] Maggs and Summers maintain that reformers used the caricature of Sarah Gamp as a convenient symbol with which to criticise the alleged deficiencies of contemporary nursing.[3] Sarah Gamp was, of course, the notorious character in Charles Dickens's novel *Martin Chuzzlewit* (1844). Mrs Gamp is introduced in Chapter 19 as a 'female functionary, a nurse and watcher, and performer of nameless offices about the persons of the dead'.[4] Summers cites Dr Edward Sieveking's injunction to illustrate reformers' antipathy to Mrs Gamp and those she represented:

> let it cease to be a disgrace to be called a nurse; let the terms of nurse and gin-drinker no longer be convertible; let us banish the Mrs Gamps to the utmost of our power; and substitute for them clean, intelligent, well-spoken, Christian attendants upon the sick.[5]

At a time when therapeutic competence depended more on placebos than on clinical efficacy, Mrs Gamp and her like posed a considerable threat to medical authority. Not only did she have a clientele of her own, which by-passed medical referral systems, she also held strong views on remedies and treatment. When these were combined with a potential to provide a comprehensive range of services from 'watching' (basic nursing care) to laying out the dead and attending lying-in women, the domiciliary nurse was a veritable general practitioner.[6]

The available evidence suggests that Dickens's portrayal of Mrs Gamp was a faithful reflection of some of the working lives of women who worked independently in the homes of their patients.[7] Until the numbers of hospital beds expanded significantly towards the end of the nineteenth century, the home remained the dominant location where paid work for the care of the sick, both serious and more minor, was conducted for all classes.[8] Yet the domiciliary nurse has left few traces of her existence beyond scattered diaries and novels.[9] Although direct reference to competition for patients does not feature prominently in the medical literature of the time, the relative invisibility of the domiciliary nurse may in part reflect medical perceptions of her social value, rather than the absence of competition. Training provided the means of bringing nurses under medical control and defusing conflicts of authority between doctors and nurses of the old order.[10]

SCAPEGOAT AND SUCCESS

What medical men objected to was the independence and unsupervised nature of much of the work of the domiciliary nurse. In his guide on the domestic management of the sick room Thompson laments the dearth of properly instructed nurses, who, he claims, rely upon 'imperfect experience and accident' as the basis for their practice.[11] Malpractice was especially common, it was alleged, among those who 'with the usual temerity of ignorance, presume to oppose their own opinions to those of the physician'.[12] Hospital training was identified as the solution both to neglect and to the obstinate opposition to medical orders. Moreover, such training would also provide an antidote to incompetence: 'we should no longer hear of doses of medicines being given hazardous to life; or of patients poisoned by topical applications administered as internal medicines'.[13] Textbooks on nursing written by doctors exhorted nurses to follow medical instructions without deviation. The influence of such literature obviously presupposed high levels of literacy among nurses and, unsurprisingly, literacy became a common stipulation of a trained nurse's qualifications. Whilst doctors may have taken particular exception to nurses' resistance to their authority, their complaints can also be understood as a smokescreen for their own clinical failure. It is tempting to see Sarah Gamp's appeal to polemicists in terms of her easy conversion into a scapegoat for doctors' therapeutic frustrations and inability to answer back.

CONFIDENCE AND CURE

Institutionalising training therefore provided a means of simultaneously supervising labour and socialising the nurse into conformity with medical orders; that is, it eroded the domiciliary nurse's contractual, economic and personal independence with patients. The domestic and hence private and privileged nature of the nurse–patient relationship posed a threat to medical authority. Medical insecurity is aptly illustrated by Thompson's insistence that nurses should avoid any discussion with the patient which might undermine confidence in the physician or medical attendant.[14] The slightest suggestion that the disease was not progressing favourably towards a cure was to be avoided:

> all whisperings, consultations, exchanges of looks, denoting anxiety for his fate, as well as all expressions of commiseration respecting his condition, should be carefully refrained from by every attendant in the sick room.[15]

Medical vulnerability was further increased by the sensitivity of doctors to market forces. If confidence were lost in one medical attendant's competence, another could be procured in his place: paying patients called the tune and the prescriptive medical literature advised physicians to accommodate the invalid's whims.[16] Significantly, however, as medical practice became academically and scientifically more self-confident, 'toadying' to the patient came to be ridiculed as the hallmark of the 'quack'.[17]

QUALMS OF QUACKERY

Education has generally been identified as the key to fulfilling professionalising ambitions for many groups of workers, including doctors and nurses.[18] In the nineteenth century it provided the means for inculcating nurses with the rationalist ethos and values of scientific medicine, thus facilitating their compliance with medical orders. At the same time it was widely believed that the better informed the nurse – that is, the better 'educated' according to current medical norms – the less likely she was to be the victim of the 'low' prejudices associated with Sarah Gamp. Doctors could thus assert their claims to superiority over nurses by exploiting simultaneously their moral, social, educational and gender differences. They did so at a time when 'regular' practitioners of medicine were also coming under pressure for space in the health care market from 'irregular' male medical practitioners – that is, from 'quacks'. When unable to differentiate themselves from the latter groups on the grounds of therapeutic efficacy, medical men could invoke educational qualifications as an alternative means of legitimation. Appeals to 'enlightenment' values and to liberal university education were thus asserted by regular practitioners as the benchmark of their professionalism. In a series of binary oppositions the so-called 'brotherhood of science' was contrasted with the sectarianism and superstition of quacks; ethical motives were contrasted with base material motives; and the rationalism of regular practitioners of medicine with the unwarranted pretension of quacks.[19] Significantly, charges levelled against 'quacks' by regular practitioners were identical to those levelled against the domiciliary nurse. Indeed so close are the parallels that the denigration of the domiciliary nurse can also be understood as an extension of the wider medical campaign to stamp out quackery. But the domiciliary nurse's representation of a particular form of female independence and power, as well as her social identification with working-class culture, posed the major threat to authority, obedience, control and reform of the 'lower orders'. Medical men sought some means of neutralising and subordinating this threat.

Along with doctors, philanthropists also had an interest in nurses as useful vehicles in their Christianising mission, in that nursing appeared to legitimise their access to the poor. Both groups, doctors and philanthropists, although driven by different motives, perceived the advantages that training would have in inculcating obedience, self-discipline and control in nurses and the working classes. The nurse provided access to groups otherwise immune from the influence of the so-called 'higher' professions. In particular, religious reformers stressed the moral benefit of nurses as embodiments of Christian virtue. In this way an unlikely partnership between medical science and spirituality emerged to create a powerful catalyst for reform.

TEMPERANCE AND TEMPTATION

As I have suggested, the attack on Sarah Gamp can be seen as part of a wider attack on working-class morals. Nowhere was this more apparent than in the attack on drunkenness in nurses launched by the evangelical and temperance movements.[20] The National Association for the Promotion of Social Science (NAPSS) provided a unified focus for a number of organisations interested in remedying social policy problems.[21] Poverty was perceived as an impediment to the moral development of the individual, and social amelioration policies were promoted to generate self-reliance, industry, thrift, cleanliness and rationality among the 'lower orders'. Although members of the Association acknowledged the complexity of social problems, there was a definite tendency to view these as monocausal and ultimately reducible to the demon drink. As the great subverter of character, drink had to be eliminated if character was to be fortified against temptation.

The notion of character building became pivotal to those educational reform campaigns associated with temperance, evangelical Christian and social scientific movements. A number of commentators from these groups found a common forum in societies such as the Epidemiological Society, or the NAPSS.[22] Florence Nightingale delivered papers to the Epidemiological Society, as did Dr Edward Sieveking. Both contributed to the proceedings and meetings of the NAPSS, along with such figures as Louisa Twining, William Farr, Frances Cobbe, Emily Davies and Mary Carpenter.[23] The NAPSS was divided into a number of different sections and provided a platform for reform in a number of spheres: law, education and public health, and prisons. Modelled on the British Association for the Advancement of Science, Smith argues that the NAPSS neither assumed the mantle of positivist sociology nor inquired systematically into social structures.[24] Its *raison d'être* was more intimately concerned with providing a campaigning rostrum for mobilising public opinion and moving government towards legislative action.[25] No comprehensive analysis of the Association's achievements exists in spite of its influence upon protective legislation in the 1860s and 1870s. Smith suggests this may in part be attributed to the fact that the Association fizzled out in the 1880s, as its lobbying tactics of direct state intervention became increasingly unpopular and its founding generation began to fall away. Moreover its reputation may have been terminally injured by the imprisonment of its initial leader, George Woodyatt Hastings, son of the British Medical Association's founder, for fraud in 1892.[26]

Reform of nurse training in this context can be understood as part of the wider social scientific movement aimed at the relief of social evils, in which poverty and crime were conflated with disease as threats to social stability.[27] Sieveking had been arguing from the mid-1850s that nurses could do much to obviate the pauperising effects of disease in 'deserving' labourers and mechanics.[28] Although not to be regarded as a *deus ex machina*, a system which involved nurses working in the dwellings of the poor could relieve a large amount of destructive misery whilst simultaneously effecting a corresponding diminution in the poor rates.[29] The call for reform of nurse training therefore emerged from interest groups and individuals associated with organisations devoted to the solution of current large-scale social problems.[30] The correlation between the alleged moral weakness of pre-reform nurses and the 'labouring classes' is illustrated by attitudes of reformers and their supporters towards nurses and drink.

Debate about the role of intoxicants was conducted through medico-literary portraits by novelists such as Dickens and Wilkie Collins. Furthermore, Barfoot notes that Wilkie Collins prided himself on the authenticity of, for example, medical details included in his narrative.[31] Such literature may well have been used as an alternative reform weapon for temperance campaigners. The much-publicised association between nurses, nostrums and alcohol was also institutionalised within the reward regimes of nursing itself. Alcohol was distributed and imbibed as a routine part of nurses' diet and patients' treatment. Indeed so common was the practice that one nurse wrote a pamphlet on the possibility of discharging her duty without resorting to intoxicating drinks.[32]

Surprisingly, though, very little has been written on the subject of nurses and drink, apart from an attention to reformers' propaganda against the old-style nurse. The link between nurses, nursing care and alcohol in the nineteenth century was nevertheless a natural one. One contemporary abstainer offers an interesting portrayal of the use of alcohol by her fellow hospital nurses. Her account begins with a description of the challenge she received from other nurses to practise abstention after entering hospital. It was predicted that, at most, she could last six weeks without succumbing. The author recounts she was the only probationer, out of a total of thirty in a large London teaching hospital, who did not imbibe, of whom twelve were ladies.[33] A pint and a half of porter was issued as a routine part of the nurse's diet. After some months of agitation, she found it was possible to have milk as a substitute.

Alcohol and stimulants were used in a variety of ways by nurses. Generally they would be employed as a coping mechanism for unpleasant or physically demanding tasks. Often the sister would ask the surgeons to order the nurses a glass of wine in serious surgical cases where wound smells were particularly overpowering. Stimulants would also be used for energy during long hours of work or when there was little time for meals. Moreover alcohol was thought to protect against infections such as typhus, scarlet fever and diphtheria.[34] These benefits, however, were counterbalanced by a number of drawbacks, one of which was the inducement to callous behaviour.

Cruelty was unpardonable in a nurse and alcohol was considered as one of its most frequent causes. The health and evenness of temper in abstainers were considered to be much more stable than in even moderate drinkers.[35] The anonymous author of the tract rejected the use of alcohol by nurses in any circumstances; a little 'spirits' was even denied for district nurses laying out the dead. Much more prudent was the drinking of milk, which set an example to the poor, especially where drink was the 'bane' of the household.[36]

Alcohol was, however, consumed by virtually all groups in society throughout the first half of the nineteenth century. The widespread use of alcohol across all social classes has been attributed, by Harrison, to a number of factors. First, it was used as a thirst quencher at a time when water was either unsafe or scarce.[37] Intoxicants were also believed to impart physical stamina and were dispensed by employers where any extra physical effort was required.

But industrialisation created pressure to reduce the consumption of alcohol. As investment in expensive technology increased, stricter regulation and time-keeping practices were implemented, and these reduced opportunities for drunkenness.[38]

A number of points of contact emerged between the Temperance Movement and nursing. Specific social links were forged through the Male Nurses' Temperance Society, a significant part of whose work was concerned with caring for alcoholic patients and those suffering from delirium tremens.[39] Exposure to the effects of alcohol arguably heightened male nurses' sensitivity to such problems. Alternatively, they may have perceived the status gains to be derived from association with a respectable social movement. Female nurses were not blind to the effects of intemperance in hospital patients and commented upon the large numbers of patients who suffered from *delirium tremens* shortly after admission to hospital.[40] In some cases the effects could be lethal. One nurse described the case of a typhoid patient whose nursing required him to lie flat on his back; he was inconsolably restless and although he had a special nurse he struggled into a sitting posture and slipped out of bed. His accidental death was attributed to the restlessness induced by *delirium tremens*.[41] Temperance, on the other hand, was thought to improve a patient's chances of recovery; consequently the drinking habits of patients was the subject of one of the first questions asked by clerks taking case histories after admission.[42] Excessive drinking was thought to impoverish the blood, predisposing an individual towards blood poisoning after surgery.[43] Intemperance was viewed as problematic for women too, albeit on a lesser scale than that for men. It was identified as one of the main causes of accidents in children.[44]

Thompson bemoaned nurses' predilection for stimulants. His rancour against stimulants was only surpassed by his railing against snuff-taking by nurses.[45] Alcohol was used here not only as a restorative agent by nurses but to maintain alertness during protracted periods of duty. Medical uses of alcohol included analgesia and the relief of psychological as well as physiological strain; it was prescribed routinely as part of treatment regimes. Dr John Brown, perhaps the most celebrated advocate of stimulants, advocated alcohol prescription as a core element in his medical teaching and treatment.[46] The use of alcohol as therapy was challenged both during Brown's career and later in the 1870s when Lallemann and Perrin published their refutation of Liebig's theory that alcohol was metabolised to produce heat. This did not lead automatically to alcohol becoming discredited as a potent therapeutic agent, nor was its therapeutic reputation dented for the lack of evidence of any beneficial properties. As late as 1934 the National Temperance League was still waging a campaign against medical uses of alcohol. The cost of consumption in London General Hospitals alone exceeded £5,000 per annum.[47] Much to the chagrin of temperance campaigners, there seemed to be no dramatic decline in consumption rates. Alcohol persisted in being perceived positively as a source of vigour and 'healthy' corpulence. Even as late as the 1920s the Treasury were considering applications for government grant relief on the duty paid on spirits used for medical and surgical purposes.[48]

Importantly, the association between drinking and criminality led temperance and social reformers to draw a distinction being the respectable working class and what was pessimistically referred to as the 'residuum'. Stedman Jones explains that the residuum was regarded as dangerous, not only due to its degenerate nature but because it threatened to contaminate the classes immediately above it.[49] The conflation of the lower orders with social threat is encapsulated in Chevalier's study of crime in early nineteenth-century Paris.[50] A similar collapsing of categories is evident in the utterances of social commentators in Britain. They too expressed themselves in an emotive and politically resonant vocabulary involving terms such as 'underclass' to refer to the lowest social stratum.[51] Christian charity was perceived by reformers as a stabilising force, a social buffer mopping up disquiet and social distress. In their diagnoses of social ills, reformers rarely questioned the prevailing social order. The function of charity was to produce 'unanimity' at a time when, it was argued, attempts were being made to 'destroy all subordination . . . , and to overturn all institutions both human and divine'.[52] The belief that the social order was divinely ordained provided a powerful vindication of the status quo.

'MANUFACTURING' MORALITY

Disease was viewed as an expression of moral as well as physical welfare, and the most efficient means of providing for its formal supervision was considered to be institutional. Architecturally, hospitals were teleologically tailored to provide a disciplinary system based on continuous observation.[53] Hospitals shared certain 'sur-veillance' features and functions with other institutions such as schools and factories.[54] Medical men and religious reformers had a common interest in subjecting the nurse to constant supervision: patients' beds were arranged to facilitate supervision by nurses who in turn were overseen by their superiors.[55] Rules and regulations similar to those of the factory were applied to institutions such as schools, prisons and hospitals, with penalties imposed for breach of the rules.[56]

The hospital provided the major repository of clinical and educational material, with the capacity to train the numbers of women required for the care of the sick. Armstrong has applied Foucault's theory on the function of disciplinary systems to the development of clinical observation and medical control in hospitals.[57] The nurse can be construed as an extension of the doctor's eyes and ears; observation became one of her main functions. A system for the collection of data was introduced by those who controlled her. But her task was limited to the collection of information, whereas the province of the doctor was interpretation and analysis. Hence there was what amounted to an intellectual division of health care labour in which the nurse's role was the inferior one. This division exemplifies the 'mind–manual' dichotomy which Braverman argues characterises social differentiation in the subordination of labour in general.[58]

The organisation of labour in the hospital was also determined by the hospital–factory analogy alluded to earlier. This analogy was most forcibly expressed in the application of the term 'firm' to the visiting physicians and to house surgeons responsible for the general surgical and medical work of a group of hospital wards.[59] Time was strictly controlled and certain forms of behaviour, such as cursing, swearing and rude or indecent behaviour, were prohibited. The sexes were strictly segregated and no forms of gambling, dice or drinking were allowed. However, the detailed restrictions on nurses' and servants' activities were significantly fewer than those imposed on patients.[60] This is not surprising when one considers that the admissions policy to voluntary hospitals was regulated by a ticket system, through which local tradesmen, in their capacity as governors, could recommend their employees for treatment and so more easily monitor their welfare. Patients' roles developed as an extension of those prevailing in the workplace and involved similar forms of discipline.[61]

Although women did not work as managers in industry, they could be recruited to supervise patients in hospitals where there was already a tradition of employing female labour. They themselves were not immune from scrutiny. A system developed in which nurses as sisters were simultaneously supervisors and supervisees. Sisters were to be recruited from a class accustomed to the disciplining of female labour, in particular domestic labour.[62] The privileged status of doctors was represented by their exemption from rules of conduct. The emphasis in nurse education on moral and character training can be explained by means of an analogy between the probationer in the hospital and the skilled apprentice in the factory. The moral emphasis in nurse training developed as both a response to and an effect of industrialisation. Nurses were the targets as well as the agents of reform. Criticisms of existing nurses related to their moral character, and represented an indirect attack upon their social origins. The first wave of the campaign to reform nurses can be seen as an extension of that to create a class of deferential and disciplined labour. In other words, reconstructing the class basis of the occupation implied recruiting the respectable working class.

DICKENSIAN DICHOTOMY

The claim by contemporaries that 'pre-reform' nurses were uniformly socially disreputable has been challenged by Summers, who argues that nurses were more socially heterogeneous than historians of nursing are apt to admit. She suggests that the prominence of disparaging accounts reflects the propagandist status of the literature produced by the stakeholders of health care. The silence of nurses in this discourse reflects a bias towards the preservation of evidence by those classes whose culture is mediated through the written rather than the spoken word.[63] Nursing work was a predominantly oral rather than a written culture. There may always be the temptation for reformers to exaggerate or perpetuate negative views of the past.

Mrs Higgins, a member of the NAPSS, described nurses for the destitute in the county districts as lazy, dirty drunkards, given to profligate habits. In one case an old couple, one blind and the other paralytic, were nursed by a woman herself afflicted with cancer. Her advanced condition precipitated her demise and her substitute was little better, having one arm withered and being of an 'indifferent character'. The semi-invalid status of such nurses suggests they could scarcely be capable of physically taxing and demanding work. One very 'good' nurse in the parish was generally drunk and died from cholera in 1854.[64] The high-risk nature of the work, especially from infectious disease, suggests that nursing was more likely to attract women who were driven into the occupation for economic reasons, and at an age when it was considered they might be less susceptible to infection.

If the validity of the vilification campaign against pre-reform nurses needs to be questioned, what can we conclude about the motives of the reformers who caricatured nurses in this way? Caricatures generally exaggerate the weakest feature of an individual; as a form of literary portraiture, they possibly derive their potency from the distillation of features identified as unattractive. Dickens's comic creation of Mrs Gamp was not, however, intended to ridicule the domiciliary nurse, in that Mrs Gamp was alleged to have an original in real life.[65] While Dickens was working on *Martin Chuzzlewit* he heard through his heiress friend, the reformer Angela Burdett-Coutts, of an eccentric nurse who took care of her companion Hannah Meredith.[66] Certain features of the nurse – her yellow night cap, her predilection for snuff and spirits – are replicated in the representation of Mrs Gamp.[67] Arguably Mrs Gamp's function was as a stereotype, one which reformers used to distance themselves from the 'old' order of health care. Sarah Gamp and her counterpart, the 'new nurse', came to symbolise the discrepancy between the 'old' and the 'new' order in health care.

The 'new' nurse embodied the ideal attributes of the emerging order of health care: enlightenment, rationality, science, Christian purity, innocence, virtue, youth, freshness, gentleness, hygiene, sobriety, gentility and intelligent obedience. The 'old' nurse represented the antithesis of the new: ignorance, superstition, moral laxity, corruption, coarseness, advanced age, dogmatism, prejudice, presumption, dirt and drunkenness. Regardless of the evidence, this polarity was rigidly maintained in order to prevent compromise with tradition. Thus, through these binary oppositions, a powerful ideological wedge was driven between the present and the past. Such dichotomies reveal much about the deployment of cultural symbols and metaphors. Jordonova suggests the power of the dichotomy rests not simply in the clarity of contrast but in the dialectical relationship between the oppositional members of each pair.[68] Oppositional pairs have been characterised as a means of exploring the parameters of change without necessarily upsetting the social order. Like archetypes, they provide a coherence and cohesion in the face of threatening social disruptions and change.[69]

MOTHERS 'SUPERIOR'

By mid-century there was a further group staking a claim to a place in the nursing market, namely the religious sisterhoods. They differentiated themselves not (obviously) on the basis of gender, but on the basis of class and of the special status conferred on them by their spirituality. The forces which precipitated the entry of the sisterhoods into secular institutions derived from a curious blend of pragmatics and piety. A certain degree of entrepreneurial sensitivity was evident in the response of the sisterhoods to patients' concerns about the social gulf between themselves and the nurse. The justification for the employment of sisterhoods was not only from considerations of efficiency – that is, with regard to the division of labour which derived from a hierarchical pattern of recruitment; it was also religious. It was also hoped that the sisterhood would improve the moral climate of the hospital. The hierarchy was divided into those who did and those who did not take religious vows and those who were paid and unpaid. Thus there was a dual hierarchical system in operation based on converging spiritual and social criteria. Probationers and nurses were paid, trained for private and domestic work, and supervised by sisters. Sisters in turn paid for their own board and visited the sick poor in their homes. This did not necessarily mean that such services were necessarily cheaper. Reform occurred at a cost which was economic as well as organisational.[70] Only sisters and heads of houses were expected to undertake pastoral duties. The early religious nursing institutions capitalised upon this anxiety by providing reliable character references for paying patients to assuage fears of vulnerability associated with intimate ministrations by social 'inferiors'.[71]

Religious, medical and 'consumer' interests then conspired to marginalise Mrs Gamp and those she represented from the care of the sick. This was achieved by undermining the paying public's confidence in the 'old-style' nurse and curtailing her independence by placing her under hospital supervision and control. Reformers indulged in a form of ideological warfare which denigrated the character of the domiciliary nurse and extolled the virtue(s) of the 'new' nurse as a symbol of the new moral order of the hospital. The new hospital-trained nurse's reliability, sobriety, skill, diligence, discipline and efficiency contrasted with the Gamps she supplanted.[72] Reconstructing the order of health care presupposed reforming the characters of nurses themselves, for which training was the key. Reformulating the 'character' of nurses created the necessary social distance between the new nurses and the Gamps.[73] The proposals of Florence Nightingale, as the pre-eminent exponent of 'character' training for nurses, represented continuity with, rather than a radical break from, the past. The content and character of Miss Nightingale's views on training therefore require careful consideration.

Chapter 2

The character of training and training of character

INTRODUCTION

I have argued that the factory provided the organisational model for the development of the hospital and, by extension, the moral code for nurse training. Employers in factories conceived their task as one in which the habits, spirit and culture of a recalcitrant workforce had to be broken in order to mould labour to the mechanical demands of automation; defiance was to be replaced by unquestioning obedience to the 'machine' of disciplinary order.[1] This analogy between hospital and factory would suggest that nurse training schools found their closest comparison in factory schools and the development of technical education. However, although some provision was made for girls in Mechanics Institutes, nurse training schools tended to be modelled more closely on the girls' public school.[2] As a result they shared the strengths and weaknesses of that sector.

Quantifying and qualifying the achievements and deficiencies of educational provision for girls and women has been the objective of some feminist historians. General histories of education in the nineteenth century have concentrated more upon the experience of the middle classes rather than working classes and more on men than on women.[3] Working-class women seem to have been particularly neglected.[4] In particular, accounts exaggerate the role of a minority of middle-class women, who fought for, and benefited from, entry into higher education.[5] From the point of view of the history of nursing, this is a significant omission, for research has demonstrated that the majority of hospital nurses were recruited from the 'artisan class'.[6] In this chapter I argue that the hospital can be considered as a microcosm of society in general: that is, that the content and conduct of the programme in nurse training proposed by Florence

Nightingale mirrored the gender and class constraints which characterised contemporary attitudes towards the education of girls and women.

Florence Nightingale dominates the historiography of nursing and nurse training. Her reputation as the progenitor of 'modern' nursing has cast a long shadow over reform initiatives which predated or were contemporaneous with her own activities. Recent research has, however, provided a welcome corrective to an otherwise hagiographical record, subjecting Florence Nightingale's achievements in military and secular nursing to critical scrutiny and evaluation.[7] Nursing reform in civilian hospitals was the product of a complex set of pressures in which doctors, administrators and nurses perceived the benefits of reforming nurse training in various ways.

For doctors the hospital came to be construed as a 'museum' of clinical material and held a central position in medical education. The increasing sophistication of scientific knowledge in medical practice has been invoked as the stimulus to creating the demand for a competent observer to supervise and observe patients in doctors' absence.[8] Although this surveillance function came to be invested in the nurse, little is known of the process by which medical theory and practice 'translated' into nursing theory and practice, or of the detailed dialectic between nursing and medical practice, and in the absence of further research this thesis remains tendentious. Indeed, few studies have concentrated on the detailed experiences of medical education and practice, let alone the implications for nursing, and most of these, with the exception of Irvine Loudon's, have tended to concentrate on the 'high' politics of medical reform rather than the theory and practice of clinical teaching.[9] There is a sense in which economic considerations were important pressures in nurse training. Doctors were only ever intermittently present in hospital wards; indeed they undertook private work to compensate for what were honorary appointments with voluntary hospitals. To the extent that nursing work was perceived as providing the continuity in patient supervision and observation necessary to offset the effects of the periodic presence of medical staff, nurse training can be considered as driven by 'economic' as much as 'epistemological' concerns. The hospital was not only a catalyst for medical careers but a stage upon which new social roles and hierarchies between doctors, nurses and patients were negotiated.[10] As a microcosm of society, the hospital was constrained in the range and repertoire of relationships it could import and export.

INVESTING IN CARE

I have argued that the reform of nursing was an attempt to improve the calibre of recruits gradually rather than reconstruct the division of labour radically. Developing existing arrangements created minimal disruption to established labour relations. Nursing work was acceptable as a form of employment since it merely extended woman's domestic role into the public domain. Anne Summers has argued that the relations between women and their servants provided the template for transferring middle-class power structures to society at large – that is, 'ladies' were supposed to exercise moral supervision over female members of the lower classes, teaching them cleanliness, discipline and respect for their employers' way of life.[11]

From a managerial point of view, women were perceived as less assertive and more biddable and compliant than men. Hence an appropriation of the domestic hierarchy into the workplace made managerial and economic sense.[12] From the medical standpoint, promoting the reform of nursing, and with it the development of a subordinate stratum of labour, was less threatening than expanding recruitment to the ranks of dressers and clerks, the junior levels of the medical hierarchy. Such a strategy carried the danger that the entry gate into the medical profession could be widened at a time when protection was being sought against the entry of women into the professions.[13] Reforming nursing had other advantages. Hospitals were commonly regarded as places to be feared rather than revered. Statistical studies revealed the pernicious effects of nosocomial infection. Indeed the hospital was so closely associated with infection that the term 'hospitalism' was used to denote morbidity and mortality associated with hospital-borne fever.[14] The stigma attached to workhouse infirmaries was in fact merely the most extreme form of an opprobrium attached to institutions more generally.[15] Administrators perceived nurses as allies in rehabilitating the reputations and economic viability of the institutions which they managed.[16] Philanthropists impelled by the spirit of Protestant evangelism evolved a new code of ethics in which women were upheld as exemplars of moral excellence. The home became elevated to a sanctuary in the struggle against sin, and its institutional analogue, the hospital, was invested with similar expectations. In a world of squalor and congestion, the home provided a refuge from the moral maladies of society, and the hospital provided a space in which to effect the moral regeneration of its inmates.

Women were represented in the didactic literature of the period as moral supremacists, saviours of a society threatened with corruption, materialism and irreligion.[17] This domestic ideology was not without its selective applications; in practice it referred only to women who could afford not to be economically active.[18] The doctrine of domesticity was predicated upon a middle-class lifestyle with which few 'working' women could identify.[19]

TRAINING CHARACTER

The occupational roles emerging in the new hospital division of labour required definition. Training provided one means of institutionalising a stable and hierarchically arranged social order. The reform of nursing hinged upon the adaptation of character and attitudes to the new routine and disciplined order of the hospital. Thus the 'reformed' nurse had to absorb a new culture, a new set of norms and regulations; the old culture of 'casual' and supernumerary work was to be replaced with regularity and routine.[20] The characteristics of the new labour-force were partly dictated by fixed working hours; women with family responsibilities were automatically excluded in favour of more younger and also more pliable souls.[21]

Although Florence Nightingale was by no means the earliest exponent of training for nurses, she is indubitably its most famous.[22] Her reputation as the codifier of nursing practice remains largely intact in spite of recent critical evaluations of her contribution to training.[23] Like that of other 'heroic' characters, Florence Nightingale's status seems to have discouraged active investigation, and surprisingly little attention has been paid by researchers to tracing the genesis and genealogy of her ideas on training.[24] Her views were disseminated widely and rapidly became canonical. Florence Nightingale was the major authority to which authors of later nursing texts referred, and she was possibly the most influential 'expert witness' ever consulted on nursing matters. From her domestic domain she steered the diplomatic course of nursing through, amongst other issues, the divisive registration debate, succeeding in her objective of avoiding public involvement in the controversy.

MORAL MATTERS

Monica Baly has argued that Florence Nightingale regarded nurse training not as an 'educational' but as a 'moral' process, involving the development of character and self-control rather than 'mere' academic training.[25] Such a view presupposes that 'education' could indeed be separated from 'morality' and that such a dichotomy was one acknowledged by most Victorians. In fact this was far from being the case, for character training had long been important to those keen to use education to inculcate notions of citizenship; it formed the backbone of the public school educational system and underpinned theories of liberal education.[26] In this respect Florence Nightingale's 'moral' theory was consistent with the emphasis in contemporary educational theory on the development of personal characteristics as well as habits of thought. Her view of nurse training as a moral process can be explained further in terms of her 'organic' view of hospital structure and function. First, Rosenberg argues, she perceived the hospital as a 'moral' universe in which the microcosmic body interacted dynamically with the macrocosmic environment.[27] This 'holistic' approach to disease aetiology and pathology broke down distinctions between the physical and the moral, the mind and the body. Control of disease implied control of the 'environment,' and this was interpreted widely to include the physical and spiritual, the hospital and the external environment. Nursing was concerned with regulating that environment by placing the body in the best circumstances for nature to act upon it. The correlation between the moral order of the hospital and the moral order of society was axiomatic to Florence Nightingale: she perceived cleanliness as being literally next to Godliness. In her view filth and contamination represented states of moral distance from God which required intervention. The laws of God were revealed in nature as were the laws governing health and disease. It was thus one's Christian duty to observe and respond to such laws.

BODY POLITIC

It is tempting to regard this 'holistic' approach to physiology in terms of some metaphorical compensation for the social fragmentation associated with urbanisation. Accordingly, differentiated bodily parts would be unified in a harmonious and integrated physiological system which derived from an organismic view of how society should function. Within such a scheme the microcosm of the individual and the external social environment or macrocosm would be perfectly harmonised.[28] Florence Nightingale was sensitive to the correlation between poverty and disease but her initial solutions were more individualistic than state-interventionist. If a person failed to obey the dictates of God inherent within the organisation of his body, they could only expect disease. If a hospital were contaminated by filth, administrative irresponsibility and immorality, fevers and infections were inevitable.[29] Florence Nightingale's reference to the nursing care of patients is usually made in the context of her views on contagion. Charles Rosenberg attributes Florence Nightingale's denial of the specific nature of disease, and her commitment to the 'zymotic' theory of aetiology and transmission, to her particular brand of social activism and the influence of William Farr. The idea that disease could be induced by a specific contagion undermined Miss Nightingale's belief that disorder, filth and contaminated atmosphere were responsible for disease.[30] To accept the material as well as the metaphysical reality of contagion denied the need for nursing intervention and indeed hospitals more generally.[31] Farr, a close acquaintance of Miss Nightingale, was a medical statistician and the Compiler of Abstracts in the Registrar-General's Office. His classification of epidemic and infectious diseases as 'zymotic' were authoritative from the 1840s and held sway as the orthodoxy until challenged by contagionists.[32]

PEDAGOGY AND PROPRIETY

Florence Nightingale's views on training can be understood not only in the context of the functions of hospitals and the aetiology of disease, but also in terms of her perceptions of the role and status of women.[33] For example, the importance she attached to self-control and discipline relates to the attempt to ensure decorous conduct between men and women of different social classes in the new social environment of the hospital. Moral injunctions to regulate relations between doctors and nurses were also applied to relations between male patients and female nurses, especially where intimate ministrations were involved. For example, 'good' character was essential for the nurse to gain the respect of male patients. In the words of Florence Nightingale, a nurse should first and foremost, however, be a 'good woman', that is, she must be: 'Chaste, in the sense of the Sermon on the Mount; a good nurse should be the Sermon on the Mount' in herself.[34] 'Immodest carelessness' was one of the key impediments to the performance of the proper duties of the nurse. The gendered nature of the hospital as moral universe can be seen in the representation of men who were to act as moral sensors, finely tuned to detect the merest hint of moral laxity in women. Such views legitimised the right of men to supervise and superintend the behaviour of women. Hence the double standard attaching to female behaviour: women were simultaneously morally culpable and the superior partners in the coupling of science with sensitivity.

The need to provide clear guidelines on behaviour and social conventions in new public spaces can be seen in the importance attached to propriety and to rules of conduct in training manuals, which points to a pressing need to regulate relations between social groups of different status. The 'ethical' basis of many nursing texts reflects the more widespread preoccupation with rules of conduct as enshrined in the many etiquette texts of the period.[35] Indeed the term 'ethics' was often used interchangeably with 'etiquette' in manuals outlining the 'conduct' of clinical and social relations.[36] Nursing textbooks of the period were not only technical manuals but pedagogical tools outlining the social niceties to be observed in dealings with patients and doctors.[37] They provided a means of settling demarcation disputes between doctors and nurses. A good, intelligent and obedient nurse could always gain the confidence of the medical man by understanding clearly the dividing line between her duties and his. But if she presumed or interfered in matters beyond that line, she would be sure to lose such confidence.[38] Boundaries were not immutable, however; if a nurse could prove herself 'worthy' she could be trusted to do things not strictly within her province. A willing and obedient nurse could be of immense service to a hard-pressed house-surgeon. For example, although it was strictly speaking the house-surgeon's duty to deal with cases of postoperative anuria or dysuria, the vigilant and experienced nurse could be allowed to intervene provided she was fully appraised of and was consistent in her attention to such duties.[39]

As I have suggested, textbooks provided an important tool for mapping authority relations in the workplace. Yet it is unclear, without systematic evaluation, how far they were successful in delineating a differentiating division of labour between different occupational groups. As late as 1916 a textbook on operative technique addressed itself to nurses, dressers and house-surgeons alike.[40] The emphasis on self-control and discipline was also for practical reasons – for example, the suppression of feelings of revulsion or repugnance at unpleasant sights and smells. As one contemporary noted: 'a nurse has to undertake many disagreeable, many hard tasks. . . . In speaking of the work a nurse has to do, it is then impossible to gild or slur over the unpleasantness of those kept usually hidden.'[41] Similarly, challenging those who were deluded and delirious was believed to exacerbate their emotional instability and therefore be detrimental to their recovery.

MOEURS AND MORALE

The perceived correlation between social class, moral rectitude and the self-control associated with 'civilised' behaviour condensed into a notion of 'moral' training which in turn fulfilled a variety of objectives. Not only did it legitimise gentrification of the occupation, it also provided a psycho-social theory of nursing care. The nurse's proximity to patients meant that she was in an ideal position to influence the moral welfare of those in her care: control of others implied control of oneself. A parallel to the role of the nurse in this context might be drawn with that of the elementary schoolteacher, whose task it was to combat the temptations capable of corrupting a child's mind. Accordingly, the teacher was expected to function *in loco parentis* as a moral substitute and force in the promotion of 'civilised' and 'civilising' behaviour. The symmetry between the family and school was prominent in the minds of some educational reformers, who considered the ideal school should reflect the harmony of a well-regulated family: 'it should be a sort of extended household'.[42] The relationship between pupil and teacher was analogous to that between patient and nurse, both teacher and nurse being expected to exercise some form of moral stewardship over their charges.

However, the recruitment of 'ladies' to nursing was not perceived by Florence Nightingale as a universal solution to the problem of strengthening the moral 'fibre' of patients. She was adamant that women accustomed to hard work should form the fundamental basis of the workforce. The entry of ladies with fanciful notions of acting as ministering angels, 'moving about your wards in a very becoming hospital dress and followed wherever you go by loving looks, and murmured blessings, from grateful patients', was generally deprecated by the architects of nurse training.[43] What was required instead was an appreciation of the fact that nursing was hard work in which one might become a 'worn and sorely-harassed woman'. The demand for ladies to occupy positions of superintendence was admittedly great, but the prime qualification for this office was a practical acquaintance with every detail of nurses' work; this involved personal knowledge and experience of that work. Thus, it was argued, super-ficial knowledge was likely to bring discredit upon ladies intent upon nursing. Nothing less than a full and thorough experience was what superintendence required.[44]

The importance of the 'moral' status of nurses was reinforced by the perception of illness itself as a moral teacher.[45] The sick room was a site for spiritual as well as physical struggle. However, it did not necessarily follow that religious attendance was universally wel-comed. Some recipients of care were sceptical of the value of the clergy as a source of solace. Harriet Martineau, social critic and correspondent of Florence Nightingale, argued:

> The archangel of consolation is the friend who, at a fitting moment, reminds me of my high calling, not the clergyman, making his studied visit, not the zealous watcher for souls, who fears for mine on the grounds of difficulties of doctrine, nor the meddler, who takes charge of my spiritual relations whether I will it or not.[46]

Anti-religious sentiment and hostility could also be directed towards health missioners as bearers of bibles and balms. Bible visiting to the homes of the poor, for example, carried its own characteristic hazards. Mrs Ranyard, founder of Bible Nurses, reported the case of one of her Bible women being drenched in a bucket of excrement![47]

TESTING TEMPERAMENT

Psychological attributes such as devotion and sympathy were re-garded as powerful variables in the emotional equation of care. Together they were regarded as important forces capable of touching even the most 'callous and resistant spirit'. One medical commentator noted: 'the elderly and the stony-heart of the rough man' could not help but be moved by the winning qualities of a nurse's charms.[48] (It is worth noting in passing that no explanation is given for why the elderly, in particular, were perceived as lacking in emotion.) The nurse's emotional characteristics were particularly important in chronic illness, where demoralisation and selfishness were seen to be the inevitable sequelae of long-term sickness. Painful conditions in particular could sour the spirit. Harriet Martineau, drawing upon her own experience, remarked:

> when extreme pain seizes on us, down go our spirits, fathoms deep

and though the soul may yet be submissive and ever willing, the sickening question arise... there is no word but despair which expresses the feeling.[49]

Excess of any kind, even in kindness, sympathy and attention, could depress the spirits; the antidote was self-restraint and control. It was precisely this ideology which underpinned the middle-class preoccupation with moderation and self-discipline. The 'irksome and fagging' nature of nursing in the family meant that the work itself was a test of character and tolerance. Hence the 'good' nurse was one with the 'most untiring patience, the calmest temper, rapid perception, stamina, a strong but well-directed will, and a strong but tender hand'.[50] She could also be relied upon to act with consideration and discretion in relation to family matters, keep her counsel and provide a competent substitute where the mother of the household had fallen ill. Psycho-social and diplomatic skills were especially necessary where the patient's state of mind had been altered:

> one patient may be calm when greatly suffering, desirous of giving as little trouble as possible.... Another will be heavy almost unconscious, and often you will have to watch and use your quickness of perception.... A third person may be rendered extremely fretful and irritable, constantly desiring something new, or different and never pleased, continually complaining querulously of inattention awkwardness... a fourth invalid may be delirious, though not violent when properly managed; your courage and firmness must be unbending, your mind active, your hand steady and unshaken.[51]

Complaints of a groundless and unreasonable nature were often the greatest test of a nurse's temper. The ability to resist the temptation to respond impulsively or fancifully could be developed by training and practice. A 'surly and unthankful spirit' required a soft rather than sharp reaction.[52] Rational control of the passions and cultivation of the intellect were fundamental to the physical and mental health of an individual.[53] Training in self-command and resistance to impulse underlined the contemporary notions of mental health. Temperament was a 'master to be obeyed rather than a rebel to be overcome'.[54]

'TRUE' EDUCATION AND EDUCATION FOR TRUTH

Commentators on nursing education hoped that the spread of cheap and accessible forms of instruction would contribute to the improvement of the nurse's character and qualifications. Every nurse, it was believed, should be able to write a plain and legible hand.[55] While it was not considered essential that a nurse should be learned in natural philosophy or physic, she was nevertheless expected to have a 'common-sense understanding of much that pertains to it'.[56] By mid-century, nurses could be expected to have a modicum of educational ability and preparation. One anonymous medical commentator noted: 'It is gratifying to think that the blessings of a plain education have so far extended in the present day, that nurses may at last be expected to read.'[57] Above all else, one of the chief prerequisites of the nurse was considered to be an ample supply of common sense. Respecting the truth was also paramount. Indulging the lazy mind was only surpassed in its iniquity by the conceited mind, which denied the need for inquiry. Truthful reporting and reliable observation, monitoring patients' symptoms and conditions were all critical to clinical decision-making. Such qualities were crucial in the nurse, since the doctor was only sporadically present at the bedside and completely dependent upon the nurse for accurate information.

Three main kinds of reporting error were identified as contributing to medical negligence. These were deficiency, excess and perversion. Thus in observing clinical conditions the nurse was instructed to avoid magnifying or exaggerating, diminishing or omitting details of the patients' condition. To this end a small notebook or set of tablets was recommended to record observations or directions of clinical importance.[58] Acute, empirical observation was regarded as a necessary safeguard against the temptation by the nurse to substitute her own opinion for the 'facts'.[59] Gossiping to patients about their previous experiences with similar cases, especially those which had resulted in failure, or weighing up patients' chances of recovery were prohibited by medical men. The royal road to 'good' nursing practice was paved with a healthy respect for the 'truth' and the recognition on the part of the nurse of her own ignorance.[60] Notwithstanding these warnings, it was manual dexterity rather than intelligence that was the prerequisite for practice. A clumsy nurse, especially in surgical nursing, could be worse than useless.[61]

'BUILDING' CHARACTER

Although Florence Nightingale considered that the development of nurse training should proceed slowly and experimentally, 'system' in such matters was nevertheless essential. Without it, Florence Nightingale warned, the average nurse probationers would degenerate into 'conceited ward drudges…they potter and cobble about their patients, and make not much progress in real nursing, that is obeying the physician's and surgeon's orders intelligently and perfectly'.[62] It is ironic, in view of Miss Nightingale's ambivalent attitude towards doctors and theirs towards her, that the most concise statement of her views on training should have appeared in a medical publication.[63] Yet medical men were by no means unanimous in their support of her views; in particular, her writings on sanitary subjects met with a cool reception. In a lecture to the Ladies Sanitary Association in 1883, a physician sympathetic to Miss Nightingale's views recounted that her writings were condemned by a large number of medical men as 'rash assertions'.[64] The author attributed this evaluation to medical men's unfamiliarity with the prevention of disease – in turn the result of the exclusion of this topic from medical teaching.

Florence Nightingale did not write a nursing textbook for probationers involved in hospital care; her teachings originated in the domestic context and required extrapolation from the home to the hospital environment.[65] Teaching of probationers at St Thomas's, Miss Nightingale's flagship training project, was left in the hands of medical instructors such as Mr John Whitfield and Mr John Croft, together with Mary Crossland, the home-sister.[66] Hence Florence Nightingale's prescriptions for practice cannot be taken at face value as the record of practical achievement at St Thomas's. The chequered career of the Nightingale Fund's experiment is graphically illustrated by Baly's calculation that, of the 188 names entered onto the official register of the Fund during its first ten years, sixty-six did not complete their training year. Of this latter group three died during training (two of typhoid, one of scarlet fever) and seven resigned. Of the 122 remaining, sixty-one were dismissed for misconduct. Five of these were discharged for insobriety, the remainder on grounds of ill-health.[67] Since Florence Nightingale neither practised as a nurse nor taught after her return from the Crimea, any control exercised was exerted from a distance. Her reputation as a systematiser of training appears to have been dependent less upon the volume of her literary output than on her public status. At the same time, few maxims on the training of nurses however captured the public imagination as fully as those produced by the heroine of the Crimea.

SCHOOLING IN HEALTH

Florence Nightingale conceived of the nurse training school as a 'normal' school and wrote of a tripartite division of labour in the staffing of the training school. The trained 'home-sister' or class mistress would teach and drill the probationers in the medical instructors' lectures. She would also give singing and Bible classes and liaise with ward sisters on probationers' progress. Ward sisters would be responsible for the ward instruction of the nurses, and medical instructors for lecturing in nursing aspects of medicine and surgery, prescribing reading and examining the work of probationers orally and in written form. Baly has referred to this as the 'tripod' of nurse training, a strategy which was reinforced by probationers taking case notes and keeping diaries.[68]

Moral supervision and the moral welfare of probationers constituted a crucial element within this structure and Florence Nightingale suggested that hospitals be built with such matters in mind. Nurses, she recommended, should be assigned to self-contained wards to discourage gossiping and consorting with medical students, and to prevent mischief associated with movement between wards. Supervision was to be provided from a single vantage point, and the whole establishment was so constructed that the probationers' dining rooms and day rooms, the dormitories, the matron's residence and office converged in such a way that the probationers could be 'under the matron's immediate hourly inspection and control'.[69] The correlation with Bentham's panopticon is striking here, although such thinking was common amongst reformers interested in the psycho-social dynamics of institutional architecture.[70] Hospitals were regarded by Miss Nightingale as lawless and corrupting places requiring strict supervision and discipline to prevent misconduct.[71] Furthermore, hospitals were often built in morally insalubrious and shady areas. The nurses' home provided the necessary level of moral tutelage to assuage the fears of anxious parents allowing their daughters to live away from home. The home-sister's watchful eye ensured that pastoral were combined with tutorial duties. This brand of pastoral 'morality' was not, however, borrowed from a branch of religion. The interdenominational disputes and personal rivalries to which Miss Nightingale had been exposed and had experienced in the

Crimea had left her with an enduring scepticism of religious involvement in nursing, especially those evangelically inclined.[72] Her tirades against the 'saintly detachment', prudishness and 'squabbling' of nuns were stinging and caustic. In particular, she singled out the prudishness of sisters, arguing that it undermined the practice of ensuring thorough bodily hygiene. Training was not to be based on religious precepts, but nor was it to be exclusively concerned with moulding 'character'; intelligent observation, reporting and practical skill were also important.

'Technical' training, according to Florence Nightingale, referred to the organisational aspects of that training. Nurses were to be rotated through a selection of male and female medical and surgical and children's wards. They were to learn ward management by taking charge during the head-nurse's dinner hour and nurses' recreation hours. They were also to take 'special' duty care of certain patients such as lithotomy and tracheotomy cases when sufficiently advanced in their training.[73] Theoretical competence was also required, including keeping a diary of ward duties, noting what had been learned, taking careful notes of cases, lectures, reading and illustrations of cases nursed in the wards.[74] Understanding the case and why the patient required nursing in a particular way was crucial to efficient nursing. 'Skill' in nursing was multi-factorial and multi-purpose; it embraced a range of attributes from those concerned with 'character' to the psycho-motor and intellectual. A nurse's 'qualifications' were expected to be correspondingly broad. To facilitate learning, Miss Nightingale suggested that probationers should keep diaries of 'cases'. This was criticised by Mr Whitfield, apothecary to St Thomas's, on the grounds that it threatened to trespass on medical territory as well as making excessive intellectual demands upon probationers. According to Mr Whitfield, Miss Nightingale's standards of training exceeded the intellectual calibre of probationers.[75]

Although the accent in Miss Nightingale's writing on training may be considered a product of wider social attitudes towards educational provision for women, her own views had not always been so conventional. Elaine Showalter argues that the traditional representation of Florence Nightingale as a 'failed' feminist underestimates the radicalism of her earlier thinking on the social constraints impinging upon women's lives.[76] Susan Reverby's comment that, unlike other feminists, Miss Nightingale concentrated upon the duties and responsibilities of the nurse to the exclusion of 'rights' arguably reflects current concerns of American political culture rather than those of nineteenth-century British health care.[77] Both Showalter and Reverby illustrate the means by which historical characters are susceptible to being 'claimed' to serve the causes of their sponsors.[78] Miss Nightingale's denunciation of the petty restrictions upon women's lives appeared as an essay, *Cassandra*, originally intended as a novel but later published as an appendix to *Suggestions for Thought*.[79] Her impatience with the boundaries of social freedom for women was fully expressed here. She had amongst her friends and acquaintances protagonists in various pro-feminist campaigns, including John Stuart Mill and Barbara Leigh-Smith Bodichon, as well as leaders of the movements to extend access to the medical profession to women and to protect women against the worst excesses of the Contagious Diseases Act.[80] As mentor and reader of *Suggestions*, Benjamin Jowett, Master of Balliol College and Professor of Greek at Oxford University, recommended toning down the text of *Cassandra*.[81] Only a few copies of *Suggestions* were published in 1860.[82] *Cassandra* was published only years after Miss Nightingale's death, in 1928.[83]

Age and maturity seemed to have mellowed Florence Nightingale's youthful rebellion against the restrictions imposed upon the exercise of a woman's intellect.[84] Her attitude towards women's education became less 'liberal' than even that of some of her male contemporaries, such as Jowett, with whom she corresponded on this and related matters.[85] Jowett and Miss Nightingale were introduced in 1860 when the poet Arthur Clough asked Jowett to comment upon an anonymous manuscript, which turned out to be *Suggestions for Thought*. Clough was acting as Miss Nightingale's secretary after her return from the Crimea. Jowett agreed to review the manuscript and thus began a friendship which stretched over thirty years.

Jowett was a keen supporter of extending university entrance, particularly that at Oxford, to women. Reform of women's property rights was more important to Miss Nightingale than either education or suffrage, although by 1877 she had signed a petition urging the admission of women to medical degrees at the University of London.[86] In addition she exchanged a series of letters with John Stuart Mill on the subject of women's suffrage, but initially she refused to join the National Society for Women's Suffrage, founded in 1867, with which he was associated. However, she reconsidered her decision, joined the Society in 1868, and subscribed to its funds.[87] It is not clear whether this gesture represented a genuine shift of opinion or a mark of deference for her friend Elizabeth Blackwell, the first female physician in England and campaigner for medical degrees for women.[88]

KNOWING BY 'HEART'

The roots of education as character training can also be located in wider perceptions of women as repositories of virtue and guardians of morality in the home and family. The cult of domesticity celebrated by Victorians transformed the home into a sanctuary sealed off from the sullying sins of the secular world. In a world of squalor and congestion, the home provided a refuge from the moral maladies of society. Women as moral supremacists were represented in the medical and popular literature of the period as the saviours of a society threatened with immorality, materialism and irreligion.[89] Education provided the means of inculcating women with the values of wifely and maternal duties, and a vehicle for combating the moral decadence of working-class behaviour. Just as women were praised for their management of the moral condition of society, they were also blamed for its failure.[90]

The domestic ideology derived from the 'separate spheres' theory of a gendered division of labour, in which men's and women's roles were deemed separate but complimentary.[91] Separation of the two spheres was considered crucial to social 'progress' and stability. Separate spheres for the sexes was justified as a 'natural' division of labour based on biological characteristics and capabilities. In the case of woman, her social functions were defined by her reproductive capabilities, which justified her confinement to wifely, child-rearing and caring duties.[92] Women were held responsible for the moral and physical welfare of children, the family and ultimately the nation, but lacked the authority to determine the conditions under which their duties might be properly discharged.[93] Men, as physically and constitutionally stronger, were duty bound to protect the 'weaker sex' legally and politically. If women benefited from their role as the physical and moral regenerators of society, they were also burdened with the responsibilities that attached to the role.

The middle classes assumed working-class women would have to earn their own living and that the appropriate place to do that was as their servants. Their own supremacy depended upon the exploitation and subordination of others.[94] Deprived of equal rights, women were forced to seek intercession through men. Women's intellectual capacity was considered to be inferior to men's but compensated for by moral superiority. Woman's heart was metaphorically and materially the source of her subordination and supremacy.

The domestic ideology was not without its contradictions and selective applications. In practice it referred only to women who could afford not to be economically active: the doctrine of domesticity was predicated on a middle-class, leisured lifestyle with which few 'working' women could identify.[95] The distinction between the world of paid work and family life may have been too crude to accommodate the experience of single and married, rural and urban women.[96] Indeed the balance between the benefits and the disadvantages of industrialisation for family life is the subject of debate among historians.[97] Pinchbeck argues women gained by the transference of manufacture from the home to the family, as 'now the home was no longer a workshop, free from dust, oil and offensive smells which accompanied domestic production, many women could devote themselves and their energies to their children'.[98]

The contradictions inherent within the domestic ideology did little to undermine its power. For both working- and middle-class girls from the mid-nineteenth century towards its end, there was considerable opposition to improving the intellectual content of educational provision.[99] The employment pattern for many working women demanded domestic rather than literacy skills for successful performance.[100] Education as character training eliminated the need to improve the intellectual quality in girls' education. Carol Dyhouse has argued that even the small minority of parents who sought a 'sound' education for their daughters in one of the late nineteenth-century foundations such as the Girls' Public Day Schools (GPDT) Trust were reluctant to encourage the development of intellectual aspirations for their daughters with the same enthusiasm as they did for their sons.[101] Essentialist assumptions concerning the talents and skills of women informed curricular content. Gender stereotyping determined the pattern of attainment and provision in girls' education, besides excluding girls from the more prestigious subjects which formed the basis of the public school education and career opportunities for boys. Girls were generally considered to be more receptive to religious knowledge, but there were conflicting opinions on fluency of writing, reading, spelling, grammar, history and geography. Arithmetic was singled out as the 'weak' point in women teachers, and both it and grammar were said to be taught in a manner merely 'empirical'. 'Empirical' here was used presumably to denote the experience of the teacher concerned rather than the rigours of strict precept.[102]

QUALIFYING CHARACTER

As I have suggested, the qualifications of a nurse came to be defined in terms of character rather than intellect. A good nurse could not be turned out from bad material. As well as being sober, truthful and upright, with a fair amount of education and plenty of sound common sense, a nurse was expected to be a good disciplinarian, firm yet gentle in her manner, eager to learn and devoted to her work.[103] The 'slightest stain on her character should exclude a woman from being raised to the high office of the nurse. Her manner should convey the impression that it is in the sickroom where she finds her appointed field of sacrifice and sacred duty.'[104] The nurse, like the teacher, was portrayed by reformers as an agent of socialisation and 'civilisation'. To this end training schools in both cases attempted to 'elevate' their incumbents, in the hope that their resulting social influence could be passed on to patients and pupils alike. What was especially important in this context was the notion that nurses and teachers, especially those originally from the same class as their charges, should cease to identify with working-class culture, so disparaged in the polemic of pedagogy. Together the classroom and the ward became foci for new forms of moral and spiritual stewardship.

CONCLUSION

The mid-Victorian period has been characterised as a one of moral crisis in which women were expected to perform as the barometers and bearers of moral standards. Nurse training as 'character' training legitimised rather than challenged established authority relations within the hospital, and facilitated their transfer from the home to the hospital environment and vice versa.[105] 'Character' rather than theory or intellectual talents became the touchstone of nursing skill and qualifications. Religion, convention and finally science endorsed the stratification of skills along class and gender lines. The debate surrounding female education intensified as the domestic ideology came to be challenged by feminists towards the latter part of the nineteenth century. Not all agreed with the role prescribed for nurses by Florence Nightingale. Imbued with the spirit of suffragism and the desire to carve out independent careers for educated women, the 'new' nurses that emerged from the first wave of nursing reform strove for freedom and mobility in the health care market. They were not satisfied with the place allotted to them by the stakeholders and statesmen of health care; they strove to define their own occupational turf and territory.

Expanding employment opportunities for women provided an entrée into the public arena from which they had hitherto been excluded. In their bid for professional status the 'new' nurses looked towards medicine for a model to emulate. However, assuming the mantle of medicine meant identifying more closely with medical norms, values and practice. This presented the nursing elite with an important dilemma: how could a subordinate group such as nurses improve their independence by emulating their 'superiors'? This strategy of imitation on the part of nurse reformers contrasted with the 'gendered' strategy adopted by the women seeking entry into the medical profession.[106] Perhaps being socially more homogeneous, women in medicine perceived their gender as a strength and the best means to improve their market potential. Female nurses had to contend with the dual disadvantage of class and gender inequalities in asserting their claims to professionalism. The emphasis on 'character' training reinforced the anti-intellectualism which justified the exclusion of women from professional work. Nurse reformers committed to a professional model for nursing consequently distanced themselves from character training by adopting a strategy based on a technical and scientific approach derived from medicine. The implications of applying a medical model of training to further the autonomy of nurses, and the tensions this generated during the course of the registration debate, form the subject of the next chapter.

Chapter 3

Registration revisited

INTRODUCTION

In the present chapter I argue that the emphasis in training objectives shifted in the last forty years of the nineteenth century from an essentialist view of moral and character training to a professional model based on science. The sequence of this transition reflected the changing ambitions of nurse reformers, who considered training first as an extension of the girls' private, domestic academy in which moral, civil and Christian virtues took precedence over technical considerations and science.[1] The girls' domestic academy model originated with Florence Nightingale, the professional model with Mrs Ethel Bedford Fenwick.[2] Ironically however, the new feminist-inspired nursing elite, which emerged from the first wave of nursing reform, looked to medicine for inspiration and patronage in developing a professional model of education for nurses. Attempts to realise their aspirations generated tensions between themselves and more conservatively minded stakeholders of health care – administrative elites and some sections of the medical profession. Interestingly, rather than aligning themselves with fellow feminists keen to create schools for middle-class girls imbued with scholarly and meritocratic values, the professionalisers of nursing adopted a gendered model of educational provision borrowed from medicine.[3] The contradictions inherent in this model were most dramatically played out during the nurses' registration debate. This chapter traces the conflicts in that debate between the 'new' nurses, hospital managers and doctors. I begin with the origins of the registration movement in the late 1880s and end with the Nurses' Registration Act in 1919. I argue that an implicit analogy between nursing and medical registration was the fulcrum for the registration debate, and that the debate itself provides an early case study in the gendered politics of professionalisation.

Interestingly, despite the status of medicine as the archetypal profession, only rarely have historians or sociologists of the professions compared its professionalising strategies with those of nursing. This chapter considers the parallel between the two. Given the totemic significance of occupational licensing for the claim to professionalism, it is perhaps surprising that so few detailed studies have been conducted on the medical registration campaign.[4] Instead, medical historiography has tended to be dominated by accounts of the progress of 'science', the Whiggish appeal of which has tended in turn to reinforce medicine's claims to professionalism and to underwrite those to professional status and social success.[5] Nursing, by contrast, has had to resort to factors other than the 'epistemological privilege' of science in order to assert its claims to professionalism in the registration campaign, which is seen in Britain as a watershed.[6] Accounts of it, though, tend to have too triumphalist a tone, and more recent critical scholarship has provided a more tempered assessment of the achievements of the Act.[7]

Brian Abel-Smith has characterised the movement for registration as a 'battle'.[8] It was not, however, a single-issue contest but a protracted struggle involving a series of skirmishes and issues stretching over a thirty-year period. Part of the complexity of the debate derives from the different meanings attached to the term 'registration' by the organisations concerned. Registration schemes evolved from being voluntary and 'private' to being national and backed by state and statute. Such a progression was characteristic of a wider trend towards the process of professionalisation in the late nineteenth century – the granting of state-backed credentials for other occupations such as architecture, dentistry, teaching and accountancy.[9]

The earliest published suggestion supporting registration for nurses was made in 1874. It was not by a nurse but by Sir Henry Acland, Regius Professor of Medicine at the University of Oxford, in the preface to Florence Lees's *Handbook for Hospital Sisters*.[10] No precise details were given concerning the form that registration might take, but it was implied that medical registration could serve as a precedent. It is not clear how Sir Henry came to write the preface to the *Handbook for Hospital Sisters*, but it is conceivable that it may have been through a request from Florence Nightingale, with whom Sir Henry corresponded on a range of matters including nurses' registration. They first discussed the registration issue in the context of the registration of women doctors, and the implications this might have for differentiation between medical and nursing theory and practice. Nurses' registration was thus first debated in camera by one of its staunchest antagonists, Florence Nightingale, before it ever reached the public agenda.

LABOURING DIVISIONS

In her response to a request from Sir Henry Acland for her opinion on the education of medical women, Florence Nightingale recommended a thorough training for both sexes but considered medical women to be particularly suited to maternal and child health work.[11] She insisted that a sharp distinction be drawn between nursing and medicine:

> nursing and medicine must never be mixed up. It spoils both, keep medicine and nursing perfectly distinct. Do not let a nurse fancy herself a doctor. If you have medical women let them be as entirely distinct from nurses as medical men are . . . a smattering of nursing does a doctor good. A smattering of medicine does a nurse harm.[12]

Miss Nightingale argued that the less knowledge of medicine a hospital matron had the better, 'first because it did not improve her sanitary practice' and secondly because it would make her either miserable or intolerable to the doctor: 'miserable because in the inevitable diversity between doctors' opinions and practices she would fancy that she knew what was wrong'.[13] Here, Florence Nightingale is echoing earlier anxieties about the effect that nurses' assertiveness and 'presumption' might have upon power relations between doctors and nurses. More interestingly, she also rejects the suggestion that nursing expertise should be legitimised through the university, chiefly on the grounds that there was insufficient medical or surgical knowledge in a nurse's or matron's education to justify degree-based study. In her view 'character' and practical ability were the foremost tests of nursing. Moreover, unlike medicine, nursing skills could not be tested by examination:

> It is not the few answers tripping off her tongue about the chemistry of foul air that makes a good nurse but the keeping her patients always fresh air without giving him cold and the thousand and one cares that go to make up a careful nurse.[14]

Sir Henry's proposal that nurses might be registered by the Medical Council or indeed by any authority outside the training institution was quickly dismissed by Florence Nightingale.[15] For her nursing was a 'private' rather than a public matter, requiring local rather than centralised forms of control.

EMPIRICAL EXAMINATION

As we have seen, Florence Nightingale was merely asserting the familiar argument that the character of the nurse was her pre-eminent qualification. A 'bookish' approach to practice and examinations was to be eschewed since it might advantage only the 'forward' and prejudice the 'diffident'.[16] 'Bookish' here implied an over-reliance on the theoretical rather than practical. There may well have been in fact a very pragmatic dimension to the debate, for nursing was not well served by a rich supply of nursing textbooks. One reviewer of nursing texts in 1898 lamented:

> with very few exceptions there are no books compiled for the trained nurse, and she has to fall back on those written for medical men; from these it is very difficult to select what is required.[17]

Florence Nightingale considered that written examinations were insensitive tests of what she considered the important qualities in a nurse. More importantly, under such a system, it could be possible for the 'worst' nurse to obtain the best qualification. Clinical subjects, she claimed, could only ever be tested at the bedside after a matron had prolonged experience of an individual nurse. According to Florence Nightingale, competence consisted in whether the nurse could 'so comport herself as to meet the many emergencies incident to her calling, or whether she has the patience, judgement, firmness, gentleness under all troubles'.[18] Drawing an analogy between nursing and the arts, Miss Nightingale argued that a woman applying for the office of music teacher might be examined on the principles of harmony and certified if shown to know them thoroughly. But only a judge of music could comment on expertise. The same was true of painting: 'no academician was ever elected except on his work, never on his technical knowledge. . . . Nursing is not only an Art but a character and how can this be arrived at by Examination, it cannot.'[19] The quality of a nurse or matron therefore lay in her character, practical ability and treatment. Lectures and making notes on cases were a legitimate but only a small part of the course of treatment and examination. Probationers should record the progress of their ward duties on a weekly basis and the matron keep a similar record.[20] As I have suggested, it was the continuous assessment and supervision of the probationer which testified to her progress.

Florence Nightingale's essentially private views were to find their way into the public debate about registration. For example, in his evidence to the Select Committee of the House of Lords on the Metropolitan Hospitals, William Rathbone, member of the Nightingale Fund Council, cited a letter from Florence Nightingale deprecating the value of examinations as a test of 'good' nursing.[21] Florence Nightingale was adamant that examination by a 'foreign body', such as that proposed by the British Nurses Association, could never guarantee competence.[22] Furthermore, the meaning Miss Nightingale attached to the term 'profession' changed it from a term of approbation to one of disapprobation. She regretted the fashion for using the press to transform every activity into a 'public' one. Nursing to Florence Nightingale was a 'quiet' and 'individual' matter. Patients' subjugation to moral influence could only be justified by their privileged position as the judges and critics of nursing. Moral influence could only ever be displayed by example not by proxy: 'not by belonging to but by being seen to be living up to a "profession" '.[23] Miss Nightingale feared nurses would become nurses by deputy, parasitic upon an intermediary body for the accreditation of their experience and skill. Worse still, nursing might transform itself into a 'book and examination business – a profession not in the high but in the low sense', one where 'we shall be content to let the book and words and the theory do all for us'.[24]

The danger of certification therefore rested in its capacity to act as a disincentive to improving oneself as a woman and a nurse. The only true test of nursing was the work that had been done. Nursing could not be certified like a steam engine, to withstand so much pressure of work.[25] Such an analogy, it was argued, encouraged the growing evil of exalting the mechanical qualities of a nurse at the expense of her 'womanly and best instincts'.[26]

ORGANISING RESISTANCE

Towards the latter part of the nineteenth century those concerned with promoting the registration of nurses began to organise as 'pressure' groups.[27] One of the earliest (but not the first) of these groups was the British Nurses' Association (BNA) established in

1887. This organisation originated as a splinter group from the Hospitals Association. Its main rival was the National Pension Fund for Nurses (NPFN), which owed its origins to Henry Burdett, philanthropist and hospital administrator *par excellence*.[28] The idea of entering the names of nurses along with their qualifications and experience on a common register originated with Burdett.[29] Although the names of probationers at the Nightingale School of Nursing at St Thomas's Hospital had been entered onto a 'register', and although details of training and reports had been recorded, this was intended only for internal use by the hospital and not as a publicly published list for use by prospective employers. Burdett's register, by contrast, was to list the employment history of the nurse and her hospital experience, with the intention of making this information available to potential employers of nurses and to the public where appropriate.[30] Burdett's philanthropic and managerial interests combined in a vision of reform for nursing which linked the welfare of the voluntary hospitals with the provision of an efficient nursing workforce. The Burdett-inspired NPFN was founded in 1887 and was intended to improve conditions of service and establish 'training' criteria as a precondition of qualifying for the Fund's benefits. The NPFN restricted its membership to 'trained' nurses. By defining, then, the 'training' and the maintenance of records of those so qualified, the NPFN could be construed as the first organisation to 'register' nurses.

In 1884, Burdett gave a paper on hospital administration to the National Association for the Promotion of Social Science (NAPSS) in which he declared his views as a committed voluntarist and anti-state interventionist. This meeting was important since it spawned the development of the Hospitals Association, a powerful pressure group representing voluntary hospital interests, which survived as the British Hospitals Association (BHA) until the inauguration of the National Health Service (NHS).[31] The Hospitals Association had a number of subcommittees, one of which was the Sectional Committee on Nursing and Domestic Management. A meeting of this committee was held in March 1886 at Burdett's house, attended by a number of leading matrons, medical and administrative personnel. Amongst those gathered were Miss Wood, matron of Great Ormond Street, Miss Ethel Gordon Manson, then matron of St Bartholomew's Hospital, and Miss Luckes, matron of the London Hospital.[32] Miss Wood opened the proceedings with a paper outlining the ways in which matrons could co-operate for the mutual benefit of nurses and themselves.[33] According to Brian Abel-Smith no contemporary record exists of this meeting, in which he alleges some violent disagreement broke out between Ethel Gordon Manson and Henry Burdett.[34]

FISSION AND SCHISM

Christopher Maggs suggests that far from splitting from the Council, as the 'violent disagreement' suggests, Ethel Manson was elected to the Hospitals Association in May 1886 as representative of the Sectional Committee on Nursing and Domestic Management. Relations between the nursing section and the main Hospitals Association were still cordial at this point, and Miss Manson gave a paper to the Association on 'A Noble Profession: Nursing the Sick in Institutions and Metropolitan Hospitals'. It was at the December meeting in the same year that the Association refused to rescind their decision to promote a registration scheme based on a single year of training. And it was over this issue that relations between Ethel Manson (now Mrs Bedford Fenwick) and Sir Henry Burdett deteriorated. But far from 'storming out' from any meeting as Abel-Smith has alleged, Mrs Bedford Fenwick and her colleagues organised a protest sit-in at the Association's offices. From then on, relations between the Bedford Fenwick and Burdett factions soured, producing the schism which finally led to the establishment of the pro and anti-registrationist camps. The BNA was the break-away group which masterminded the campaign in favour of registration.[35]

At this point support for registration amongst the major hospitals was weak. Mrs Bedford Fenwick and Miss Catherine Woods had been signatories to a questionnaire sent out by the Hospitals Association to inquire into the support for a common register for nurses. It had been sent to thirty-four hospitals in England and Wales. Twenty-four were associated with medical schools, 'ordinary' medical or surgical hospitals, and three were Poor Law Union Infirmaries. No details are given concerning the selection of hospitals. Nineteen hospitals replied, seventeen large ones and two Poor Law Infirmaries. Fewer than half stated they wanted a system of registration for qualified nurses, claiming that they already had a system of registration adapted to their special needs. Entering the names of nurses on a common register was considered as weakening those nurses' loyalty towards institutions. Many hospitals disapproved of an innovation which threatened to dissociate the nurse from her parent school.[36]

AUTONOMY AND AUTHORITY

Lack of support for, and interest in, registration as conceived by the nursing contingent, may have provided an additional stimulus for Mrs Bedford Fenwick and her allies to resign from the Hospitals Association and establish an independent platform for their views. Shortly after the disagreement at the December Hospitals Association meeting, Mrs Bedford Fenwick and Miss Woods set about establishing the BNA in opposition to, and in competition with, the Nursing and Domestic Subcommittee of the Hospitals Association, which was, by this time, in a state of some disarray. The institutions which were particularly aggrieved at the efforts of the BNA were those hospitals that considered themselves pioneer training schools. Spearheading the campaign against the BNA was St Thomas's through the Nightingale Fund Council.[37] St Thomas's antipathy to registration was only surpassed somewhat later by that of the London Hospital. The later retreat of St Thomas's seems to correlate with the withdrawal of Florence Nightingale from nursing affairs. She distanced herself from the public debate on registration, alleging: 'I have kept entirely out of the fray...and earnestly hope to remain out of the fray.'[38] Florence Nightingale refused to sign any public document and was anxious that confidentiality and anonymity be maintained during any consultations she had with Sir Henry Acland and representatives of the Nightingale Fund, such as Henry Bonham Carter and William Rathbone. She intoned, 'When I hear my miserable name mentioned as a final authority it gives me a feeling I cannot describe.'[39]

At the same time, a direct line of descent can nevertheless be traced between the arguments used by anti-registrationists and Florence Nightingale's views. The Central Hospitals Council for London Statement on the State Registration of Nurses, for instance, argued against any system of registration which relied upon testing by examination, and which exalted technical capabilities at the expense of personal qualities. Personal qualities were not examinable, it continued, and it was precisely these rather than technical failings which, anti-registrationists alleged, stimulated complaints from the public.[40] Miss Luckes extolled the virtues of character, mirroring Florence Nightingale's views. She also communicated with Florence Nightingale on training matters:

> But what examination can test those special characteristics of gentleness, quick observation, quiet self control, the innate motherly tenderness, essential [sic] tact which belongs to the real

nurse, and the helpful sympathy with suffering which all true nurses must possess in some degree if they are to be worthy of the name?[41]

The BNA was also intended as a rival organisation to the Burdett-inspired NPFN, launched slightly in advance of the BNA, but with similar objectives. Mrs Bedford Fenwick, although not opposed in principle to the provision of a national pension scheme for nurses, demurred at the participation in nursing affairs by 'non-professionals', by which she meant lay hospital officials such as Burdett.[42] Mrs Bedford Fenwick and her allies objected to the management of the Fund by businessmen, who deprived nurses of the necessary training in business methods.[43] Not only that, but such external jurisdiction was incompatible with the prized professional goal of self-regulation. Part of the nursing vanguard's frustration may well have derived from their resentment of the authority that hospital administrators wielded over matrons in resource control. As such it was a resentment borne of a gendered hierarchy in which 'male' management expertise predominated over 'female' moral authority. But more than that, it was those men who controlled the boards of hospital authorities, and therefore responsibility for the conditions under which nurses worked, who were to be the targets for reform.

Interestingly, freedom from 'managerial' control did not imply independence from medicine, as the original aims of the BNA demonstrate:

1 The formation of registers of nurses and midwives.
2 The formation of convalescent homes and holiday homes for members.
3 The formation of a Benevolent Fund to assist such members as may be in need of temporary pecuniary assistance; the benefits of which will doubtless be extended in due time.
4 The establishment of a medal of merit for nurses to be called the 'Princess Helena Medal'.
5 The foundation of a central home in London, to gather together all nursing interests under one roof, to afford lodgings for country members and other advantages for London nurses.
6 The holding of meetings during each winter session for the reading and discussion of papers on nursing subjects, of an annual conversazione in London and an Annual meeting in some provincial town.[44]

These aims were subtly different from those reported three years later in 1890 to the Select Committee on the Metropolitan Hospitals and suggest that medical control of the organisation had been strengthened:

1 Unite trained nurses together in a purely professional union.
2 Provide for the legal registration of nurses under the control of medical men.
3 Help nurses in times of need or adversity.
4 Improve the knowledge and usefulness of nurses throughout the Empire.[45]

The changing nature of the organisational objectives of the BNA in its early years of 1887 and 1890 suggests that specifying accountability was considered desirable, although the source of such pressure is not disclosed. It had also been the original intention of the Association to promote joint registration of midwives and nurses. This proposal was highly controversial and from the outset met with opposition from members of the Association. Drawing an analogy with medicine, Mrs Bedford Fenwick argued, nurses should be trained in medicine, surgery and obstetric nursing. She insisted that nurses should be trained in all three branches prior to qualification and that midwifery should be a specialist form of nursing undertaken at the 'postgraduate' level.[46] However, the precise history of how registration came to be pursued separately for nurses and midwives has not yet been adequately investigated.[47]

The Select Committee of the House of Lords on Metropolitan Hospitals was the first public forum in which the registration debate was aired. In her evidence to the Select Committee, Mrs Bedford Fenwick expressed her belief in professional self-regulation. She urged that the only way to organise the profession was to give the members a voice in their own progress and education; it was also necessary to establish a controlling body outside the general committees of hospitals in order to regulate that education and the conditions of nurses.[48] The Select Committee investigated nursing conditions in various hospitals. Interestingly, the London Hospital in particular came under fire for its training, employment, housing and welfare arrangements for nurses.[49] A series of letters from ex-nurses was submitted to the Committee testifying to their adverse conditions. It is not clear how these letters came to be solicited but it is unlikely they were submitted spontaneously. Miss Luckes, as Matron, was singled out for particular criticism. Her opposition to state registration was well known and may in part have contributed to the attacks to which the London Hospital was subjected.[50] It is also possible that Mrs Bedford Fenwick was behind the move to involve the aggrieved nurses of the London.

It was never inevitable that the organisations concerned with registration should have divided into two hostile camps. In 1889 a Memorial issued by training schools, including St Thomas's and its allies, asked for postponement of further action on registration until a consensus had been reached on the desirability or otherwise of a public register.[51] However, this apparently conciliatory gesture could be construed as a stalling mechanism to drum up support for the anti-registrationists, since the Memorial also contained the names of institutions that opposed the registration of nurses by bodies such as the BNA. Attempts to contain the conflict within the hospital and nursing world were thwarted as the national press joined the fray. Florence Nightingale, for example, expressed her irritation at the recalcitrance of *The Times*, which had published the Memorial in the first instance, thus signalling its sympathy for the BNA.[52]

HOME FROM HOME

As I have suggested, the idea of a 'common' register was anathema to those hospitals which jealously guarded their antique reputations and relied upon the loyalty, goodwill and commitment of their nursing staff for efficiency. Every nurse, it was argued, should struggle to maintain the prestige of her alma mater, and cultivate that '*esprit de corps* in which it is said, to the discredit of their sex, women are often deficient'.[53] Echoing Florence Nightingale's opinion, Henry Bonham-Carter argued that the training school and hospital should be a 'home' in which moral or spiritual 'helps' would have an elevating and motherly influence on all. It should be a place capable of training good women to withstand temptation and do real work, neither 'romantic' nor menial.[54]

The domestic rhetoric implied a private, 'family-like' relationship of loyalty between nurse and institution, and the prospect that an 'outside' organisation might interfere with it was bitterly resented by the training school authorities. The most intolerable aspect of the proposals was the loss of disciplinary control which the imposition of a common set of rules implied. The BNA's ambitions were also perceived as a significant threat to the economic interests of the training schools. A common register would reduce the control a hospital might exert over the career of the nurses trained by them. The private nurse in particular was considered by Miss Nightingale as at risk of becoming 'an irresponsible nomad'.[55]

REGISTERING DIFFERENCES

It was the representation of nursing as a profession analogous to medicine which divided the Bedford Fenwick faction of the BNA from the Hospitals Association. The implication of state involvement in training matters was perceived as a threat to the economic interests of the prestigious voluntary hospitals, which relied upon their venerable reputations to attract funds and subscriptions. State registration also implied depreciating the value of hospital training certificates and depressing the significance of its testimonials upon the careers of recruits.

The debate on registration revolved around those who wished to reconstruct nursing as a free profession, controlling its own fees and conditions of service, and those who wished to maintain the dominance of hospital management interests in determining the conditions of service. Mrs Bedford Fenwick argued for the emancipation of nurses and nurse training from the control of the hospitals. This was necessary to protect the public and the 'thoroughly' trained nurses from incompetent nurses. As matters stood, the public had no protection against the nurse who had acquired a hospital certificate and subsequently proved to be incompetent. No hospital, it was argued, was responsible for a nurse once she had left its service. By contrast, a general nursing council would be responsible to the general body of nurses and the public for preventing any woman who proved herself unworthy of trust from working at all.[56]

Opponents of the scheme, whose spokesman was Henry Burdett, argued that such a measure was unnecessary, as 'registration' already existed for the adequately trained. Training schools kept a register of their nurses, and issued a certificate to all who had three years' service. A certificate was evidence enough of 'registration'; it was a voucher which could be relied upon.[57] Dr Bedford Fenwick, however, repudiated the notion that matrons could testify reliably for the character of a nurse and match nurses to patients in private cases.[58] The great majority of nurses left their hospitals, he argued, and either undertook private nursing on their own or affiliated themselves to various nursing institutions. Comparatively few remained on the private nursing staff of the hospital where they trained.[59] The value of certificates and testimonials as a guarantor of character and competence was also contested by other commentators. Sir James Crichton-Browne, for example, protested he had seen nurses whom he had dismissed for ignorance and cruelty subsequently engaged at other institutions.[60] In a speech to the BNA in 1887, Sir James, Vice-president of the Association, drew attention to the anomaly whereby plumbers were registered but not nurses:

> Is too much to ask, then, that Nurses, whose duties are no less responsible than those of plumbers... should have an opportunity of recording in a formal way whether they have been properly trained for their work, and that the public should have access to that record?[61]

PUBLIC AND PRIVATE

Mrs Bedford Fenwick and her allies were anxious to break the monopolistic power of the hospital over the employment and career prospects of a nurse, and argued that nursing should be constituted and legally recognised as a distinct profession, with a central controlling body of its own along the same lines as the medical profession.[62] But unlike medicine, where the character of a doctor was regarded as superfluous to his scientific skill, the character of a nurse was regarded as pre-eminent. As Henry Burdett noted, the difficulty was that some nurses might well be excellent institution nurses, but utterly unfitted for private nursing. The matron's job was to fit nurses to the doctors' requirements and the 'character' of the case; a register could not provide such a service. Indeed, he cautioned, 'to take a nurse because she is entered on a register as a nurse, may be to introduce the east wind into your house'.[63]

The nature of a nurse's character was especially important when nurses were sent out to attend to patients in their homes, and were no longer under the surveillance of hospital. The only 'true' guarantor of quality, argued anti-registrationists, was the authority and reputation of the institution which had supervised and observed the conduct of the nurse over a long period of time.[64] Fears of letting nurses 'loose' in households derived from anxieties surrounding their status as unsupervised labour. The stress on self-control and 'character' in nurse training provided an antidote to potential exploitation of the patient's dependency for personal gain. It can also be construed as a response to the embarrassment and fear surrounding intimate ministrations of patients in the secluded environment of private households. Interestingly, fictional accounts of contemporary nursing, in which nurses are portrayed as stealing from or seducing their patients, reveal the gendered nature of the fear induced in men who become dependent upon women to help and assist them at times when they are vulnerable.[65] 'Character' in training, therefore, can be considered a code for ensuring 'decorous conduct', ethical behaviour and emotional self-restraint over sexual matters and embarrassing bodily functions. Guaranteeing a nurse's character provided a form of insurance against the nurse exploiting the proximity of the nurse–patient relationship for selfish ends. From the hospital's point of view, one of the dangers of having women working independently centred on the practical difficulties involved in imposing discipline and sanctions upon employees who flouted rules and regulations. The emphasis on moral purity, modesty in training and certifying character derived from the desire to distance nursing from any other kinds of activity connected with 'private' bodily functions. It is in this sense that nurse training can be considered as part of the 'civilising' process described by Norbert Elias in his work on the sociogenesis of manners.[66] The need for self-control in nurse training seems to have been linked to the rising demand for private domiciliary nursing by an increasingly prosperous middle class. The 'privatisation' of nursing work corresponded closely to the 'privatisation' of bodily functions and the premium set on self-restraint, as the epitome of 'good' manners and gentility, by the middle classes.

The perception of nurse training as the 'internalisation' of self-control was consistent with medical theorising on women's emotional nature. Some medical commentators drew analogies between women and children, claiming that women's skulls were more childlike in structural terms than men's; they were less tilted back on the condyles than men's and their average height was lower.[67] Women were to some extent infantilised in terms of their intellectual, social and political status; they required chaperoning, supervision and patriarchal protection. Education was required, but not of the intellect, rather of the passions. Disciplining the passions and exercising self-control over 'brute' emotions became the touchstone of an essentialist, evolutionary conception of nursing education. The social evolution of nurses through 'civilised' and 'civilising' behaviour ensured their elevation up the evolutionary ladder and correspondingly their distance from the fundamental forces of nature.

MEDICAL MISOGYNY

Medical anti-feminism in the nineteenth century has received considerable attention from researchers.[68] However, little research has
been conducted on the implications of such antipathy for medical
attitudes towards educational improvements for nurses. Doctors were
generally unsympathetic to expanding educational and employment
opportunities for women in the public sphere. 'Scientific' arguments
were advanced to substantiate an antipathy against improving
educational opportunities for women and the working classes.[69]
Members of the BNA, which became the Royal British Nurses'
Association (RBNA) after a royal charter was granted in 1891, were
no exception. A number of medical members published their views on
the benefits and utility of education for women. Education was
considered an important physiological as well as psychological
phenomenon. Psychiatrists and gynaecologists were among the
specialists to offer 'expert' opinion upon education for women in
the latter part of the nineteenth century. A significant number of
medical members of the RBNA were gynaecologists or psychiatrists,
including Mrs Bedford Fenwick's husband and his father, Dr Samuel
Fenwick.

One of the leading commentators on the physiological 'hazards' of
education for women was Sir James Crichton-Browne, self-pro-
claimed 'Doyen of the Medical Psychologists of Great Britain'.[70] In
a paper in the *Journal of Mental Science*, Crichton-Browne asserted
that the brain of the male exceeded that of the female in weight and
that the relatively small size of the female's depended as much on her
intellectual as on her physical inferiority.[71] The participation of
medical men in the debate suggested the issue was politically neutral.
The objectivity of the debate was underwritten by the application of
scientific principles and techniques to the analysis to the data.
Standardised criteria were developed to interpret cranial indices
and correlate these with intellectual attributes.[72] Women's educability
was perceived as being determined by the smaller size of the brain
observed in post-mortem studies, often of the insane. Commentators
seemed untroubled by the apparent inconsistency in applying the
findings from 'abnormal' cases to 'normals'.[73] Femininity was
defined by its biological functions and these had been specially
developed by evolution. Gender determined as well as was determined
by the social order.[74] As one contemporary gynaecologist in 1882
noted:

the word 'Gynaecology'... embraces far more than is expressed in the term 'diseases of women.' In its full etymological meaning it is comprehensive beyond the strict domain of medicine...it is undeniable that to appreciate justly the pathology of women we must observe her in all her social relations, study minutely her moral and intellectual characteristics – that we must, in short, never for a moment lose sight of those physical attributes which indelibly stamp her as a woman, which direct, control, and limit the exercise of her faculties.[75]

The circularity of this argument was regarded not as contradictory to but as proof of its validity, rather than as conflating cause with consequence.

Under the influence of Darwin and evolution theory, medical practitioners and scientists focused their attention upon the physical effects of growth and development.[76] Biological theories of growth had to be reconciled with physical theories of energy production and preservation as Dalton's law of the conservation of physical energy was applied to human physiology. Dalton's zero-sum model translated as meaning energy required for intellectual exertions would deprive other areas of its supply. Any events or activities which made extraordinary metabolic demands were especially costly. The representation of the body as a microcosm of political economy, of which Dalton's law was arguably characteristic, provides an interesting example of the interaction between culture and science. Accordingly, young women were considered particularly vulnerable to enervation and the impairment of their potential fertility if physically or intellectually active and menstruating at the same time.[77] Medical commentators found a willing audience for their views on the negative effects of higher education for women.[78] Children too as growing organisms needed special protection from the over-zealous attentions of educationists.[79]

Interestingly, medical members of the RBNA were at the centre of the debate in which doctors claimed competence in the detection of 'dullness of intellect'. Dr Brudenell Carter commented on the physiological costs of competitive examinations. As early as 1855 he had published a treatise on the implications of education in the promotion of moral and intellectual health.[80] Much of the evidence of 'over-strain' and brain exhaustion was generated by medical practitioners acting as physicians to private schools. Alarmist literature revealed medical preoccupation with 'brain-forcing', malnutrition of the cortical cells and fibres, neurasthenia, congestion of the brain and hydrocephalus. Through participation in these and similar debates, medical men, and psychiatrists in particular, encouraged the 'medicalisation' of education as a means of legitimising their expertise and status in questions of broad public interest.

Crichton-Browne's appointment by A.J. Mundella, Vice-president of the Committee of Council on Education, to report on the school conditions in London seemed to reinforce official confidence in medico-psychological expertise.[81] Crichton-Browne advocated the creation of a 'science' of education through the application of the principles of cerebral physiology. The dangers to women of pursuing 'high culture' were considered a major risk to their fertility and sanity. Dr Langdon Down, senior physician and lecturer in clinical medicine at the London Hospital and RBNA executive member, warned of the dangers of 'over-pressure' in the development of neurotic symptoms.[82]

Concern about the health of women derived from the belief, common among hereditarians, that the burden of responsibility for an embryo's health, and ultimately a nation's racial welfare, rested with women.[83] Accordingly, the two sexes played markedly different roles in heredity. It was believed that maternal rather than paternal characteristics were much more likely to be passed onto the child due to the longer exposure of the foetus to maternal influence *in utero*. While the mother's contribution was primarily that of 'matter', it was the father's energy which animated that 'matter'.[84] Consequently the mother's contribution to constitutional defects of the body or mind were considered potentially greater than those of the male. Maternal influence was enhanced further by the belief that the characteristics which had predominated in the parents at the time of conception would be passed on to the child. Thus women became the guardians of welfare for future generations.[85] The duty of woman, defined medically and subsequently politically, became conceived of in terms of the production of vigorous offspring.[86]

NATURE OF NURSING

Significantly, sick nursing was perceived as an ideal prelude to, and qualification for, marriage and maternity.[87] It is in this sense perhaps that nurses, keen to promote the social and political rights of women, aligned themselves with conservatively minded doctors. In a pamphlet on the status and rights of women, another RBNA member, Dyce

Duckworth, declared his belief that heredity would follow a fruitful and fitful path provided women preserved their womanly qualities.[88] In an address to the Scottish Society of Literature and Art, Duckworth argued that while brain weight, muscular power, length of limb, and capacity for mathematical, classical or philosophical attainments could all be superior in a given woman to those of a given man, training and exposing one sex to influences for which they were not 'fitted' could disrupt 'the natural evolution of perfect womanhood'.[89] Echoing the arguments of many of his contemporaries, he maintained that higher education for women could be taken too far. Over-excitement and strain upon intellectual faculties could make a woman inattentive to her personal attractiveness, unsex her and render her fit only as a companion to philosophers.[90] Higher education, in Duckworth's eyes, implied education for the 'higher' mission of the womanly sex; not just book learning, but the development of womanly graces and qualities.[91] Duckworth invoked Miss Nightingale's assertion that women's work should be done quietly and in private. Not all women were suited to being authoresses, travellers or platform speakers, he asserted. Indeed such women were all too numerous.[92] 'Blue-stockings' with 'cropped heads, ill-fitting dress... and clumsy boots' did little to commend culture to 'weaker sisters', whilst the effect on men was calculated to excite nothing but repulsion.[93]

The opportunities afforded to medical men to influence public opinion were arguably greater than nurses'; it was easier for them to participate in public speaking and to use social connections and publication. The tract *Sex in Education* by Dr Edward Clarke, retired Harvard Medical School Professor, was widely disseminated, went through seventeen reprints and was highly influential in moulding public opinion.[94] Writing textbooks provided another channel of influence, since many contained an implicit form of social theorising. A number of textbooks and pamphlets on nursing were written by medical members of the RBNA, and these were important in policing the cognitive boundaries between the work of nurses and doctors.[95] Satire provided another vehicle for RBNA medical men to comment upon 'reformed' nursing. The doctor-nurse was caricatured in a fictional portrayal of nurse 'typologies' by Dr Frederick Gant.[96] The stress on the nurse as 'Tartuffe', or imposter of doctors, plying remedies and recommending treatments, reveals the seriousness of the perceived registrationist threat to medical men.[97]

TECHNICAL DISAGREEMENTS

As I have suggested, it is in the context of more general arguments about women's educational capacity and intellectual inferiority deriving from evolutionary biology that essentialist notions of nursing education came to the fore. The gloomy prognostications of psychiatric pessimist were countered by advocates of expanded educational opportunities for women stating that there was no incompatibility between scholarly activity and healthy woman-hood.[98] Just as the conservatism of the 'sex in intellect' argument was being challenged by suffragists such as Frances Cobbe, J.S. Mill and (later in the 1890s, following surveys of the first generation of female students) Mrs Henry Sidgwick, so Mrs Bedford Fenwick, herself a suffragist, rejected the essentialist emphasis on personal qualities of the nurse throughout the registration debate.[99] She argued for technical competence, and in doing so she was not denigrating the value of such qualities, but arguing that the accomplished nurse was composed of two parts. The first consisted of the female medical student, and the second the ministering angel.[100] Opponents of nurses' registration rejected any claim for an analogy and, by extension, parity with medicine. They contended that the value of a medical man lay primarily in his 'scientific' skill, knowledge and ability. That he should also be a man of high character and good manners was desirable, but a man defective in those particulars might still make an excellent physician or surgeon. The doctor's function was primarily scientific and his qualifications intellectual. These could be measured with intellectual tests and the result recorded on the professional register.[101]

The question of the relative weight that should be attached to technical and moral qualifications in the nurse was controversial and divisive. For some, technical knowledge was subordinate to personal character in the nurse.[102] Such arguments were not the esoteric concerns of British commentators but flowed across the Atlantic and the Anglo-American axis of nursing reform. Resistance to considering nurse training a form of 'technical' training was depre-cated by Lavinia Dock, an American associate, campaigning journal-ist and suffragist colleague of Mrs Bedford Fenwick.[103] Miss Dock defined technical training as the 'training of hand and brain in harmonious duet', and she was highly critical of the disdain for technical or 'manual' training in nursing.[104] Not only did she consider such views out of step with modern educational thinking, but she argued that technical training was of supreme value in forming character. Miss Dock even went as far as suggesting that technical education could be a corrective to modern 'defects' of character such as those deriving from luxury, idleness, indefinite purpose, aimlessness and useless occupation. So, far from being mutually opposed, Miss Dock considered 'character' and 'technical' training as interdependent.[105]

While some medical men supported registration, others feared its contradictory effects upon nurse–doctor relations. Professor Humphrey, Vice-president of the RBNA, argued that some doctors considered registration would make nurses too presuming. His own experience led him to believe the opposite: trained nurses, in his view, were singularly unpresuming; the greater their knowledge, the less their presumption. For him, ignorance was the greatest cause of presumption, and it was the ignorant who rashly rushed in 'where angels fear to tread'.[106] The possibility that legal sanction for nursing qualifications might lead to the substitution of nursing for medical labour was clearly an anxiety for some.[107] Fear was fuelled by the perception that relations between doctors and nurses had grown in complexity as a consequence of the introduction of 'ladies' into nursing'. Now, more than ever before, the two callings might be drawn from the same class.[108] There is, however, little evidence that the social composition of the nursing workforce was changing radically between the 1880s and 1920s, and on balance, the gains associated with improved training were believed by supporters of registration to outweigh the disadvantages. Such changes would add to rather than subtract from the cultivation of womanly qualities.[109]

ROYAL RIVALRY

The fear that nurses, once registered, might meddle in medicaments and engage in 'amateur doctoring' was not the only one to provoke medical ire. The methods used by the radicals to pursue their campaign were also deprecated. Miss Nightingale, in particular, was aggrieved not only because the campaigning divided the nursing world, but because it 'dragged' nursing, as far as she was concerned, into the gutter. Miss Nightingale accused the rival factions of 'touting' for business and the RBNA of bribing nurses to join and recruit subscribers from amongst their friends and patients.[110]

The question of inter-organisational politics was complicated further by the patronage of the rival organisations by different members of the Royal Family. The Prince and Princess of Wales presided over the NPFN, and Princess Christian over the RBNA. Not only was the nursing world divided but an embarrassing split was threatened in the royal family itself. Some means of conciliation had to be found to re-establish harmony, and Florence Nightingale hoped Sir Henry Acland would be able to build a 'Golden bridge' between the two.[111] The matter was brought to a head when the RBNA applied to the Board of Trade for a licence to act as a registration authority. The principal objection given in evidence against the request was that the RBNA was a self-appointed body and therefore not competent to speak on behalf of the nursing profession or the public.[112] Royal patronage made it difficult for the President of the Board of Trade to refuse a request. Henry Burdett offered to intervene and help find a solution to the delicate problem, ostensibly on the grounds that Princess Christian be 'spared the annoyance and disappointment almost certainly in store for her through the follies of the small clique who really control the BNA'.[113]

A number of options were proposed to justify Princess Christian's discreet retreat. None turned out to be necessary, however, since a resubmitted application on the part of the BNA was successful in securing the granting of a royal charter by the Privy Council to enter onto a 'list' the names of nurses who fulfilled the Association's criteria of three years' training. The subtle change in terminology from 'register' to 'list' added little status to the voluntary register set up by the Association in 1891, but the granting of the Charter was proclaimed as a momentous event for 'professional women'.[114] Interestingly, the stipulation of three years' training automatically excluded nurses from St Thomas's, the London and King's College, where training lasted for one and two years respectively.

CONSTITUTIONAL COMMITMENTS

Significantly, few of the medical registrationists who were office bearers in the now Royal British Nurses' Association seemed to share the views of the radical nursing faction. Sir Henry Acland's attitude may be taken as typical. By 1887 his view about registration seems to have changed from one of approval to disapproval. Miss Nightingale commended Sir Henry on his change of heart: 'I am ... very glad you do not approve of the registration of nurses which the world is going mad about'.[115] Sir Henry's ambivalence is somewhat curious given his

Vice-presidentship of the RBNA. However, this apparent contradiction may reveal the discrepancy between privately held and publicly articulated beliefs. Moreover, membership of a society or group may indicate not so much a whole-hearted subscription to its ideals as the desire to influence and control the direction of policy or business.

It is not possible to amplify upon particular activities of the RBNA, such as the recruitment and voting procedures of its various committees; such details are excluded from available annual reports. Members were most probably recruited, as was the convention for women reformers in education also, for reasons of patronage, power, status and respectability, and not necessarily for their political commitment to registration.[116] Interestingly, the power base of Mrs Bedford Fenwick and her nursing allies was, in actuality, rather small, since they were outnumbered by medical men.[117] No nurses were vice-presidents, and out of twenty-one members of the executive, only seven were nurses. The majority rank-and-file membership may well have been nurses, but the committee composition was weighted heavily in favour of medicine. Medical dominance suggested that political tensions would never be far from the surface, and the early meetings of the Association were rife with controversy.

REGISTRATION IN RETREAT

Shortly after the Royal Charter was granted, the rules for reconstituting the General Council of the Association were changed; more specifically the privilege of permanent offices was removed. Dissension broke out in the ranks of the Association, ostensibly over the manner in which the powers of the new Charter were to be discharged, and in particular whether policy should be controlled by the medical men of the Association or through self government by nurses. The by-laws of the Association were changed during Mrs Bedford Fenwick's absence as superintendent of the English contingent in the Graeco-Turkish War. A new executive was appointed and Mrs Bedford Fenwick was replaced by a nominee of Mr Henry Burdett.[118] Daggers were drawn between Henry Burdett and Mrs Bedford Fenwick.

There were allegations of a series of irregularities, financial as well as constitutional, and influential medical representatives were claimed to be in league with 'the arch anti-registrationist protagonist', diverting the Association from its central objectives.[119] These objections bear the imprimatur of Mrs Bedford Fenwick's rhetoric; but the financial allegations could have been made either by, or against, Dr Bedford Fenwick as Treasurer. The greatest blow to the pro-registrationist lobby was struck in 1896 when, by a narrow majority, the RBNA passed a resolution opposing registration.[120] This breach marked the beginning of the 'internecine treachery' which finally led to the ousting or forced retirement of the Bedford Fenwicks from office.[121]

Mrs Bedford Fenwick was only temporarily diverted from her course. Under the initiative of Miss Isla Stewart, who succeeded Mrs Bedford Fenwick as Matron of St Bartholomew's, the Matrons' Council of Great Britain and Ireland was founded in 1894. Mrs Bedford Fenwick may well have been behind the establishment of the Council as an alternative forum for pursuing registration and as a counterweight to her diminishing control of the RBNA. With registration in retreat, the Matrons' Council became the only organisation devoted to the registration cause until the International Council of Nurses (ICN) was founded in 1899 as an international pressure group for registration. The ICN's first President was Mrs Bedford Fenwick.[122]

A motion proposed by Mrs Bedford Fenwick at a meeting of the Matrons' Council in 1902 was passed to launch the Society for the State Registration of Nurses (SSRN) with Miss Louisa Stevenson LLD as President. The patronage and support of a legal expert was presumably important in offering the Society guidance on parliamentary matters, and in 1904 the society introduced its first Bill into Parliament through Dr Farquarson MP. The very same year the RBNA presented a Bill with similar objectives, having reversed its earlier anti-registration stance. In the same year, following a request from the SSRN, a Select Committee was appointed to consider the 'expediency of providing for the Registration of Nurses'.[123] Many of the arguments originally articulated in the Select Committee of the House of Lords on the Metropolitan Hospitals, and in anti-registrationist tracts, were reiterated. Anti-intellectualism combined with the 'separate spheres' ideology reinforced fears that nurses were developing ideas above their station.[124] The Hon. Sydney Holland, Lord Knutsford, Chairman of the London Hospital and co-author with Miss Luckes of *State Registration of Nurses*, referred to nursing as 'childishly simple'.[125] Dr Norman Moore, senior physician at St Bartholomew's, considered book learning of little value to the nurse.[126] The pro-registrationist challenge had repercussions not only for the particulars of relations between doctors and nurses but for the gender order of health care more generally.

CONCLUSION

I have argued that the 'dangerous' analogy between nursing and medical registration provided the centrifugal force separating the protagonists from the antagonists of registration for nurses. The many points of contact between the nursing and medical registration 'movements' make it difficult to resist the conclusion that nurses attempted to emulate doctors in their bid for registration. Indeed, the symmetries between the principal architects of medical and nurses' registration, Thomas Wakely senior (medical campaigner and founding editor of the *Lancet*) and Mrs Bedford Fenwick are striking, in terms not only of the reforms they promoted but of their temperaments, characters and careers. Both Wakely and Mrs Bedford Fenwick were aggressive, passionate and committed reformers. As editors of the journals they owned, they were uncompromisingly frank in their denunciations of their opponents.[127] Their intemperate language and satirical attacks, however, also carried the potential risk of alienating sympathisers, thus undermining their cause. The *Lancet* was as important an organ for medical reform as was the *British Journal of Nursing* for nursing. Both sought to combine dissemination of clinical information with political commentary and both used their journals as vehicles for exposing abuses. In Wakely's case, these consisted in highlighting the alleged clinical incompetence of elite practitioners and nepotism in hospital appointments.[128] Wakely's published exposes of alleged incompetence by 'reputable' and high-standing members of the medical elite led him into the courts defending charges of libel.[129] In Mrs Bedford Fenwick's case, the main target for her critique was hospital managements' exploitation of nursing labour.

Both Thomas Wakely and Mrs Bedford Fenwick identified the lack of any uniform standards of education as a major obstacle to rationalising the existing diversity of practice; both advocated consolidating a common portal of entry with a common foundation curriculum followed by specialisation in education.[130] 'Quacks' in nursing and medicine alike provided useful ammunition in mobilising support for legal regulation. In both cases appeals to 'science' and 'technique' were used to establish social and epistemological distance between legitimate and 'illegitimate' practitioners.

Wakely's fight for a comprehensive extension of medical training, following a universal course of study granted by a centrally constituted authority, was designed to break the monopoly power of the medical corporations and theoretically free practitioners to move from one branch of practice and location to another.[131] Similarly, Mrs Bedford Fenwick sought to break the captive labour markets established by the London teaching hospitals cartel and establish employer-independent credentials which would enable nurses to migrate more freely throughout the labour market. In doing so, she was advancing the radical proposition that women could organise and pursue their careers independently of men, in spaces where women would be removed from sponsorship, supervision and superintendence. The nursing co-operative was to provide the conventual model that allowed nurses to live and work together as a group, and conferred the economic and social self-sufficiency characteristic of the much-maligned 'new woman'. Wakely was, as far as can be discerned, no advocate of medical co-operatives, but such was the sympathy between the two parties that the *Lancet* provided a campaigning platform from which pro-registrationists could attack the antis.[132]

One point which separated the two protagonists, however, was their political attitudes towards the role of the state in health care and that of radical journalism as a vehicle for change.[133] Wakely maintained that the state should take a more active role in, and assume responsibility for, all aspects of health. There is nothing to indicate that Mrs Bedford Fenwick foresaw the state's role as anything more than that of providing state registration. Significantly, although she published the deliberations of the Poor Law Matrons' Association in her journal, she seems to have overlooked the Poor Law sector as a possible precedent for registration.[134] Instead, through her contact and friendship with American suffragist reformers such as Lavinia Dock, Mrs Bedford Fenwick evolved a view of nursing as a high-status occupation for women whose organisation and economic relations with patients would be comparable to those of medicine.[135] Rather than contextualising nursing within the political economy of health care in general, she concentrated her attention upon the supply of well-educated women for the private nursing market. Moreover Mrs Bedford Fenwick courted politicians from all parties to support her version of the nursing 'cause'. Wakely's political sympathies, on the other hand, lay with the radical politics of William Cobbett. Wakely was elected to Parliament in 1835.[136]

Although a suffragist, Mrs Bedford Fenwick did not stand for election to Parliament.

Similarly, both ultimately failed to achieve their original anti-monopolistic legislative objectives. Opposition to the 1858 Medical Bill, from the medical corporations and Royal Colleges in particular, ensured measures were less liberal and comprehensive than intended.[137] The *Lancet* was sanguine in acknowledging that one Act of Parliament could hardly be expected to remove all grievances, yet, at the same time, criticised the Act as deficient and ill-equipped to meet the difficulties which beset medical qualification and the right to practice. It conceded, however, that it was, after a thirty-year struggle, 'a step in the right direction and the commencement of a series of important changes'.[138] Similar statements were ultimately to apply to nursing. Yet although the professionalisers of nursing had helped to shift the emphasis in nursing education away from the domestic academy model of training propagated by Florence Nightingale and her supporters, they substituted the contradictory gendered strategy of a model of professional educational organisation borrowed upon medicine. How could a female-dominated profession succeed in advancing an agenda of self-regulation by emulating the professional tactics of the group whose dominance depends upon subordination of the group seeking independence? The anomalies inherent in the pursuit of this particular form of autonomy continue to plague reformers of nursing till the present. The next chapter considers the denouement of the registration debate and its transition from a 'professional' issue to an issue on the public policy agenda.

Chapter 4

The Nurses' Registration Act

INTRODUCTION

In organising for registration British nurses were not influenced exclusively by their medical predecessors. Nurses in America and the dominions had also been active in seeking legal legitimation of their status.[1] Co-operation between the protagonists of nursing reform in Britain and the USA was motivated by a shared political vision of the structure and organisation of professional nursing; suffragist sympathies and registrationist politics condensed into a heady brew of emancipatory politics expressed most forcibly in the early ideals of the International Council of Nurses (ICN). Bonds forged between nurse leaders across the Atlantic provided a source of social and intellectual support, reminiscent of an 'invisible college'. Invisible colleges (the term is more current in the history and sociology of science) comprise informal networks of contacts through which information is sifted and exchanged. They act as gate-keepers of information and 'state-of-the-art' technology.[2] The Americans and British crossed the Atlantic to visit each other and were members of the same organisations. This chapter considers the interactions between British and American registrationists. It examines the extent to which the registration question in England and Wales was shaped by contact with American nurses, and by pressures in the administration of health care more generally. It argues that ultimately, however, the achievement of registration in Britain can best be understood in the context of the Ministry of Health's plans for reconstructing the health services.

INTERNATIONAL INFLUENCES

Mrs Bedford Fenwick and her sympathisers moved from a position of organising collaboratively with other groups, such as hospital managers and doctors, to organising alone. In this respect British nurses differed from their American counterparts. Celia Davies has argued that democratic management was a marked feature of the organisations initiated in the USA, but it was not a declared intention of those in Britain masterminded by Mrs Bedford Fenwick.[3] Indeed the idea that nurses should organise themselves into alumnae associations and superintendents' organisations was attributed to Mrs Bedford Fenwick by Isabel Robb, Principal of Bellevue School of Nursing, New York, in her introductory speech at the World Fair in Chicago in 1893.[4] Both Miss Robb and Mrs Bedford Fenwick were founding members of the Matrons' Council of Great Britain and Ireland; indeed Mrs Bedford Fenwick's break with the Royal British Nurses' Association (RBNA) may have encouraged closer links between American and British Nurses. These connections were formalised through the participation of both parties in the ICN, founded by Mrs Bedford Fenwick in 1899. The internationalising impulse in nursing towards the end of the nineteenth century was very much in tune with that in other fields of activity such as medicine, science, botany, agriculture and technology.[5] Such activity was often associated with the establishment of international societies, conferences and congresses. For example, the International Dental Federation was formed in 1900, and the International Society of Surgeons in 1902.[6] These provided the means for trades and professional organisations to exchange ideas and ideologies as a means of expanding intellectual and professional 'capital', and as hothouses for the cultivation of influence and professional networks.

Not surprisingly such organisations, including the ICN, drew upon a common vocabulary in order to articulate their ideals and mission. Although the ICN drew its organisational inspiration from the International Council of Women (ICW), its prototype, model and early rhetoric resonated with other movements which had internationalism at their heart. For example, drawing upon the language of the international labour movement, Mrs Bedford Fenwick suggested that 'if the poet's dream of the brotherhood of man is ever to be fulfilled then surely a sisterhood of nurses is an international idea, and one in which the nurses of the women of all nations, therefore, could be asked and expected to join'.[7] Mrs Bedford Fenwick's closest

American ally in terms of her commitment to feminism was Lavinia Dock.[8] Here the political similarity apparently ended. Miss Dock was a socialist, whereas Abel-Smith refers to Mrs Bedford Fenwick as a 'very blue Tory'.[9] In terms of her social credentials and career pattern, Mrs Bedford Fenwick was closer to Miss Hampton, later Mrs Isabel Hampton Robb, who also married a doctor and worked for registration in the United States of America. Miss Robb helped to found the American Superintendents' Society and Nurses' Alumnae Association. Mrs Bedford Fenwick was reticent about her political allegiances, although it is possible that she belonged to that group of conservative suffragists who objected to the illogical exclusion of the educated, well-to-do lady from the franchise enjoyed by her 'ignorant and propertyless gardener'.[10] Conservative support for women's suffrage, including that of its four party leaders between 1867 and 1914, was justified on the basis of its reinforcement of the existing property-based electorate.[11]

But the argument for a stronger political parallel between Mrs Bedford Fenwick and Miss Dock emerges from some recent evidence regarding Mrs Bedford Fenwick's participation in suffrage politics. Mrs Bedford Fenwick was a well-known suffragist and suffragette and subscribed to the Women's Social and Political Union (WSPU), the militant organisation, headed by Mrs Pankhurst in 1903, endeavoured to promote women's interests within the labour movement from 1908 to 1914.[12] The *British Journal of Nursing* had petitioned for 'Nurse Pitfield' to be released from prison following a militant suffragette demonstration in London, and allegedly led a fund-raising campaign to achieve this.[13] Miss Dock, on one of her many trips to England, came with the intention of volunteering her services to Mrs Pankhurst in February 1914. Unfortunately there is no note of this in ICN records.[14] Miss Dock's pro-feminist politics extended to her advocacy of, and participation in, the settlement movement in New York, where middle- and working-class women worked and lived together. The theory surrounding such social relations was that women who might otherwise be the object of charity would be 'improved' by exposure to the example of their 'social betters'.[15]

By contrast, Mrs Bedford Fenwick's notion of 'community' was one where women of equivalent status lived together and worked to earn their independent means and careers, for example in a nursing co-operative, 'institute' or association. This translated in nursing terms into her support for nursing-led co-operatives managed by and for nurses themselves, catering mainly for the private nursing market.

The achievement of registration in different states of America and different British dominions was used as a precedent by Mrs Bedford Fenwick in arguing for the benefits that registration would confer on nurses and patients alike. The implication of these comparisons was that Britain was falling behind the rest of the world, including those countries over which it had sovereignty, in the provision of 'progressive' welfare measures. One early historian of nursing referred to the export of British-trained nurses as part of Britain's 'civilising' mission to the world. In stimulating support for improvements in nurse training, the author suggested that failure to sustain a steady supply of leaders could depress Britain's status as an imperial power.[16] Locating nursing within the wider context of Britain's imperial relations, while doubtless exaggerating the importance of nursing, was nevertheless tactically useful in playing on the fear that Britain's colonial fortunes might be plummeting.

Opportunities to exchange ideas about registration were mediated through the participation of nurse leaders in the ICN, nursing journalism and testimonies before official and semi-official committees on nursing matters. Miss Dock, for example, gave oral and written evidence to the Select Committee on Registration of Nurses in 1905. She asserted the importance of registration in improving uniformity of standards for nursing education.[17] This proposal was first articulated publicly in America by Isabel Hampton Robb, then Principal of Bellevue Hospital Training School, New York, at the International Congress of Charities, Correction and Philanthropy at Chicago in 1893.[18] Mrs Bedford Fenwick also attended this conference.[19] International meetings were one of the most important channels through which American ideas on registration and organisation were disseminated. Like many women's international organisations formed before World War I, the ICN was a communication and support network for national nurse leaders who subscribed to a common set of values. It was also a pressure group whose political ethos revolved around a shared commitment to improving the economic and social status of nurses. This commitment translated into regulatory activity of state registration of nursing and the provision of nationally determined standards of nursing education. Together these two variables defined what it meant to be a trained nurse. Definition of standards of training, indeed the structure of the nursing profession, nationally and internationally, was remarkably uncontentious. This was mainly because those standards reflected the priorities and aspirations of the Anglo-North American nursing elite who tended to dominate ICN affairs at this point in time.

Great Britain and the USA portrayed themselves as the organisational models for others to follow. At the Cologne conference in 1909, Miss Dock invited nurses to: 'follow our example and unite amongst themselves'.[20] The USA in particular was represented as an example of dependence transformed into independence:

> To our English colleagues we of the United States owe more than we can re-pay and if in our swift American fashion we have broken from their leading strings and made paths for ourselves, we none the less acknowledge our indebtedness with gratitude, and display our accomplishments with the same pride, mingled with a little doubt, with which sons and daughters display theirs to the friends at home.[21]

Nevertheless, as Miss Dock was to argue, the USA could provide a model of support for what could be achieved in reform by less favourably and strategically placed sister countries. The purpose of international meetings, she was careful to point out, was not to have a 'glorious jaunt', nor to return home self-satisfied, complacently criticising that which is different in other countries from our own, but to encourage nurses from other countries who were fighting the same battles 'but do so under a much heavier handicap than we have in our country'.[22] Patriotism mingled with chauvinism in Miss Dock's proud declaration of the pre-eminence of the USA in international nursing affairs:

> Those who fail to realise that we Americans go as a reinforcing army to strengthen the position of our allies in their campaign for a higher civilisation, fail entirely to grasp the elementary meaning of the idea of 'internationalism'.[23]

What such statements revealed was an unshakeable confidence in the 'civilising' role of nurses as the vectors of western bourgeois culture and values.[24] Consensus around this and other critical questions of professional standards was built up through the networks of communication that ICN leaders had established in the course of working for reform. Bonds forged between nurse leaders across the Atlantic provided a source of social and intellectual support, reminiscent of an 'invisible college'. The concept of the invisible college originated with Robert Boyle and was first applied to the 'inventors' of the Royal Society, who were bound together by humanitarian aspirations and projects. Later the term was used to describe a network of socialist-minded Cambridge scientists in the 1930s.[25] Nurse leaders communicated with each other and their constituencies both informally and formally through journals and journalism. Mrs Bedford Fenwick owned and edited the *British Journal of Nursing*, formerly the *Nursing Record and Hospital World*, in which she wrote an international column, one on American nursing called 'Our American Letter', and another entitled 'Outside the Gates' in which she discussed issues of interest and relevance to women. Lavinia Dock produced a parallel column in her famous 'Foreign Department' for the *American Journal of Nursing*. The entry of women into Oxford and Cambridge, the meetings of the ICW, the Superintendents of the American and Canadian Hospitals and the American Superintendents' Society, the organisation of American registries such as the Brooklyn Associated Alumnae, and American suffrage – such issues were all made accessible through these publications.[26] Lavinia Dock, Sophie Palmer (editor of the *American Journal of Nursing*), Mrs Hunter Robb and Adelaide Nutting (the first nurse to hold a full professorship at Teacher's College, New York, and one of the triumvirate of American nurse leaders along with Isabel Robb and Lavinia Dock) all wrote in the *Nursing Record and Hospital World*.[27] Miss Dock gave evidence to the Select Committee of the House of Lords on Metropolitan Hospitals and Registration of Nurses. Mrs Bedford Fenwick herself was an Americanophile, referring to the USA in an article on nursing at the World's Fair at Chicago as 'that most marvellously progressive country'.[28] The control of one's own journal was seen as central to the exercising of 'freedom of conscience' and expression.[29] In Paris, 1907, the importance of the nursing press as a campaigning platform and means of shaping the politics of organisation was stressed by Mary Burr, Director of the National Council of Trained Nurses of Great Britain and Ireland: 'organisation minus articulation is impossible'.[30] Through such channels, opinion leaders such as Mrs Bedford Fenwick and Miss Dock could exert significant influence on each other as well as their organisations in the adoption of ideas on reform.[31]

Friendship and social networks were further reinforced through membership of various clubs and societies. For example, in the USA, Miss Dock and Miss Nutting were members of the Cosmopolitan, a New York-based club. Specifically designed for professional women, and established at the turn of the century, it still flourishes today. Such communities have been portrayed as latent feminist organisations, a focus for philanthropy, and 'spaces' in which women could pursue social, political and scholarly interests.[32] The settlement movement, referred to above, was another model of community around which nurse leaders could organise for change. Henry Street was the most celebrated example and was home to Lavinia Dock and public health nursing reformer Lilian Wald amongst others.[33] It was probably in such environments that important decisions regarding political tactics and significant social contacts were made. In the United Kingdom, nursing co-operatives may well have performed a similar function.

I have argued that the ICN was an important vehicle for 'internationalising' nursing, and I have suggested that the communication networks which developed between nurse leaders help to explain the preoccupations and priorities of nurse reformers in their formative years. But the irony is that we know very little of the social activities and connections of the founders of nursing beyond the polarised hagiographies and at times iconoclastic biographies of Florence Nightingale. A handful of biographical studies casts light on the lives of other nursing luminaries, but there remains a dearth of solid and systematic biographical and prosopographical treatments of nursing's founders.[34] If social experiments, ideas and innovations are socially and culturally mediated, then much can be learned from applying techniques of social network analysis and collective biography used in the sociology of science to nursing history. It is not the intention of this book to conduct or report such an analysis, but it seems reasonable to suggest that the class and economic positions of nurse leaders on both sides of the Atlantic, either through marriage or through private means, made it possible for them to devote a major part of their energies and resources to integrating with traditional elites, with whom they could collaborate and organise for reform.[35] Adelaide Nutting promoted a scheme for the preliminary education of nurses. Together three proposals – preliminary education standards, uniform curriculum and state sanction – provided the core of the educational reforms underlying registration in the USA, and ushered in the beginnings of what might be called the 'Americanisation' of British nursing.[36] Mrs Bedford Fenwick's enthusiasm for American nursing was a crucial variable in the cultural exchange equation between the USA and Britain. Nurses in the USA, according to Mrs Bedford Fenwick, had the distinction of being treated as members of a profession, while in Britain nurses were treated as belonging to a trade. 'We shall find amongst American Nurses [sic], as a class, a much better and higher professional feeling than prevails in this country.'[37]

It would be premature, however, to suggest that the flow of ideas operated in one direction only or indeed that both were operating towards some inevitable point of convergence. Three of the most prestigious training schools in the USA had been modelled after the assumed pattern of the Nightingale School in St Thomas's.[38] Little additional comparative work has extended Davies's pioneering analysis of professional power in British and American nursing.[39] Indeed in a more recent study, Davies argues that although the motives and strategies of nurse leaders on both sides of the Atlantic were remarkably similar, important distinctions of social structure separated the two.[40]

CULTIVATING CONNECTIONS

Such social connections reflected in the ways in which American and British nurses aligned themselves with powerful lay influences.[41] Susan Armeny and Karen Buhler-Wilkerson have suggested that nurses in the USA formed political alliances with women philanthropists to gain status as a consequence of such alliances.[42] In explaining the motives of nurses and women philanthropists in pursuing a co-operative and collaborative strategy for reform, Susan Armeny attributes these less to 'social feminism' than to a commitment to older and more conventional notions of sanitarian science. The limitation of Armeny's study, however, is that the argument hinges on the impact of ideological commitments, rather than on an empirical study of how social networks developed, and of the nature of their political significance.

Leading nurses in Britain also sought alliances with women of position and prestige.[43, 44] Princess Christian's sponsorship of the RBNA provided a direct link with the royal family. Lady Helen Munro Ferguson and Lady Margaret Priestley both supported nursing reform and, in the case of the former, published pro-registration commentaries.[45] Patronage was not, however, considered an inevitable 'advantage' by beneficiaries. Lady Margaret Priestley's criticisms of private nursing, although ostensibly made to improve nurse training in general, were perceived by the private nurse constituency as a vicious attack upon the quality of private nurses' service.[46] Miss Catherine Wood, founder of the then British Nurses' Association (BNA) and Matron of Great Ormond Street, accused Lady Margaret Priestley of exaggerating the defects of the private nurse.[47] The effect of social patronage upon the economic conditions of nurses was criticised by Miss Jentie Paterson at the inaugural meeting of the Professional Union of Trained Nurses (PUTN). Patronage, according to Miss Paterson, was no guarantee of a quality service. Indeed she declared it one of the most insidious of evils:

> ladies who elect to give their patronage to cottage hospitals or County Nursing Associations may flood the country with the semi-trained and the villagers are supposed to be grateful for the services of a cheap nurse whom the lady of the Manor would not employ if she or her family were ill.[48]

Negative experiences of patronage, combined with the desire for independent action, may have inhibited the cultivation of an extensive patronage network by some British nurses. As with the movement to improve secondary and higher education for women, links between nurses and the aristocracy tended to be idiosyncratic.[49]

DOMINION AND REGISTRATION

As I have suggested, the achievement of registration in certain states of America was used as a precedent in arguing for similar provisions in Britain, but it was not the only example which was so used. Mrs Bedford Fenwick listed several other countries which had instituted systems of registration in the dominions. These included the Cape of Good Hope in 1891 and Natal in 1899, where nurses were registered under Medical and Pharmacy Acts. Under these Acts, nurses had no direct representation.[50] Under the Nurses' Registration Act 1901, New Zealand became the first state to give representation to nurses. New Zealand was also advanced in its granting of female suffrage. Of the three Acts, Mrs Bedford Fenwick preferred the New Zealand one, since hospitals were grant-aided and government-inspected. Furthermore, examinations had stimulated hospitals into raising standards. Such a system, Mrs Bedford Fenwick claimed, was proving of great benefit to the public, medical men and nurses.[51] Nursing homes were also registered in New Zealand under government auspices and expense through the Public Health Act. Mrs Bedford Fenwick contended that the adoption of such a method at the expense of some local government authority 'was the only satisfactory means of securing the public benefit and safety'.[52]

Given the above, the argument in favour of assigning a predominant influence to American nurses in British nurse registration would appear to be weakened by the high regard and favourable opinion Mrs Bedford Fenwick had for the New Zealand system. In strategies reminiscent of the New Zealand example, three of the Bills for registration proposed by the RBNA between 1904 and 1919 combined nursing home and nurses' registration. Thus nurses' registration became formally and informally linked to state regulation of the private nursing market. Mobilising the evidence of Britain's colonies was intended to embarrass authorities at home into conceding the contradiction whereby Britain's 'dependencies' were more progressive in terms of their support for social policies than Britain itself. Notwithstanding the attraction of the New Zealand model and the role that distance may have played in inhibiting communication, however, the intensity of contact between the architects of American and British nursing registration suggests that it was the Anglo-American axis more than any other that supported lobbying for reform in Britain.[53]

WARRING FACTIONS

The background to the introduction of the various Bills for Nurses' Registration has been discussed elsewhere.[54] Friendly back-benchers introduced private members' Bills for registration on a regular basis between 1905 and 1914, when the private members' procedure for legislation was suspended due to the outbreak of war. Throughout this period the case for registration had been hampered by divisions within the nursing organisations, by strong opposition from the voluntary hospital lobby's lack of significant public support, and, most significantly of all, by a lack of sponsorship from a government department. World War I had a number of important consequences for nurses' registration. The relocation of nursing on the public policy agenda after the war has traditionally been explained by the threat to occupational dilution and unity engendered by an influx from the Voluntary Aid Detachment (VAD), combined with public and political sympathy towards improving the status of women through female suffrage.[55] The 'hauteur' of the VAD was criticised in the columns of the *British Journal of Nursing*. Yet none of the portraits painted flattered either nurses or VADs:

I do not intend to go on with nursing, too much drudgery and too little pay; we educated women must leave that sort of work to the people. We VAD's have seen the type of women the system produces; splendid of course, but with no more moral courage than a mouse. I hope to become a medical woman.[56]

Lack of leadership in the War Office was identified by the above commentator as the reason for nursing being 'trampled in the gutter and splashed on to the hoardings as the most pauperised and negligible of women's work in the War'.[57] Negative portrayals of the snobbery of VADs towards 'professional' nurses was calculated to reinforce prejudice and class antagonisms between the two groups. The flood of volunteers, coupled with the redistribution of nurses between hospital sectors and the return of former nurses to employment, had stretched the capacity of administrators to achieve an appropriate structure for the definition of the trained nurse and matching of skills to 'needs' in the chaotic conditions of wartime. Some means of bringing order and meaning to the multiplicity of qualifications held by the growing numbers of 'nurses' was required.

LEGALISING LOYALTIES

Partly in response to this problem, several individuals prominent in wartime and voluntary hospital services, including the much-maligned War Office, produced a proposal for the establishment of a College of Nursing. The initiative emanated from Sir Cooper Perry (member of the Army Medical Board and Medical Superintendent of Guy's Hospital), Dame Sarah Swift (Chief Matron of the British Red Cross Society and of the Order of St John, formerly Matron of Guy's Hospital), and the Hon. Arthur Stanley (Chairman of the Joint War Committee of the British Red Cross Society and from 1917 Treasurer of St Thomas's Hospital), who estimated that there was strong support for the establishment of a College of Nursing.[58] Initially it was intended that the College, if established, would operate a voluntary system of accreditation with a basic uniformity of curriculum and assessment between training schools. Successful candidates would then be registered with the College. It was intended as a 'voluntary' alternative to the state-backed licensing advocated by the Central Committee, based on the medical Royal College model rather than the General Medical Council. The Central Committee for the State Registration of Nurses had been established in 1908 to unify the various pro-registrationist organisations.[59] The College of Nursing's approach was attractive to the voluntary hospitals, since it left them with considerable discretionary power and flexibility in determining standards of training and discipline. The aims of the College were to promote:

(a) Better education and training of nurses and the advancement of the profession.
(b) Uniformity of curriculum.
(c) Bills in Parliament for any object connected with the interests of the profession.
(d) Recognition of approved nursing schools. This covered hospitals with at least 250 beds staffed by a resident medical or surgical officer which offered at least one course of lectures per year and an examination for qualification.

These constituted the criteria for admission to the College's register.[60] Male and mental nurses were implicitly excluded by these provisions.

RESISTING RAPPROCHEMENT

Having recruited the support of the major training schools opposed to the organisational leadership of Mrs Bedford Fenwick and her allies, efforts were then made by the College proprietors to join forces with the Central Committee. Support for such a move was forthcoming from some medical members of both organisations, Comyns Berkely, Treasurer of the RBNA, and Princess Christian. Mrs Bedford Fenwick objected to what she perceived as the excessive lay control of the College.[61] The RBNA support for amalgamation continued in spite of Mrs Bedford Fenwick's attacks, but as the College grew in strength it became impatient with the dilatoriness of the RBNA and framed its own Bill for Registration. By 1919 the College membership had risen to 13,047 and was becoming a major force in its own right.[62] Divisions within the nursing world seemed inevitable.

Although by 1919 there was a general consensus within the nursing organisations that state registration was desirable, opinion was still divided as to the precise form that it should take.[63] The College of Nursing and Central Committee both introduced their Bills into the House of Lords and the Commons. Commenting on the Minister of Health's report of a conference with the nursing organisations in the House of Commons, Major Nall, pro-registrationist Parliamentarian, concluded that while everybody agreed that the registration of nurses was desirable and necessary, it was clear in the conferences that those concerned were not agreed, or likely to agree, what was implied by registration. The controversy had unfortunately been mixed up with personal and sectional issues which could not be reconciled.[64] Both Bills were carefully constructed to give the impression of equity whilst assigning priority to their respective representatives.[65] Disagreement still surrounded the constitution and powers of the proposed central nursing council.[66] Major differences of opinion concerned the constitution of the registers themselves. Drawing on the medical model of education, the Bedford Fenwick contingent had originally pressed for a single portal of entry for all nurses in which a general foundation programme would be followed by specialisation.[67]

SUPPLEMENTARY DISBENEFITS

The question of specialisation and the supplementary registers had been vexatious throughout the registration debate. Purists, such as Mrs Bedford Fenwick, maintained that their very existence cut at the root of the 'common portal of entry' principle and vitiated entry standards by providing a 'back door' for 'inferior' practitioners. Echoing the medical maligning of 'specialists,' those nurses who qualified for entry on a supplementary register – mental nurses, male nurses, sick children's and fever nurses – were branded as semi-educated. This was the original source of Mrs Bedford Fenwick's disaffection with the midwives, who had pressed for separate registration from nurses.[68] The history of separate accreditation for midwives and its relationship to nurses' registration has received little attention from researchers. The RBNA originally combined proposals for midwifery and nursing registration. This has resulted in the anomaly whereby members of the RBNA were represented on the Midwives' Council but no reciprocal provision could be made for the representation of midwives' organisations on the General Nursing Council (GNC), since none existed when the Midwives' Registration Act was passed in 1902. Mrs Bedford Fenwick preferred a single qualification which combined obstetric with medical and surgical nursing, corresponding to the three pillars of medical education. There was, she claimed:

> no longer any room for the semi-educated specialist. The medical profession . . . is perfectly justified . . . when it objects . . . to legal

status being bestowed upon an 'inferior order of practitioners', for such the three months trained midwives would inevitably become.[69]

According to Mrs Bedford Fenwick a midwifery qualification was to be a 'postgraduate' qualification, in either the undergraduate or postgraduate curriculum of training of every nurse, and a course of obstetric training was to be included in the training of every nurse.[70] Mrs Bedford Fenwick justified her description of midwives as semi-educated on the basis of the three months' training required by statute for certification under the Midwives' Act of 1902. Assigning parity of status to a group with such a short training undermined attempts to standardise and improve uniformity of training. Mrs Bedford Fenwick, arguing by analogy from medical training, insisted that:

> as medical men and women must be qualified in medicine, surgery, and obstetrics, before they are permitted to practice any of the three branches, so nurses should be educated in the duties of nursing medical, surgical and obstetric cases before they are allowed to practise their profession independently for gain.[71]

SUPERINTENDING SPECIALISATION

'Specialists' (which included midwives) were disparaged on account of their susceptibility to medical domination.[72] Mental or male nurses were not originally included in Mrs Bedford Fenwick's plans for professional organisation, although the Select Committee on the Registration of Nurses, 1904–5, had recommended a separate register for asylum nurses. The restrictive meaning attached to 'registered' nurse by Mrs Bedford Fenwick and her followers was challenged by representatives of mental nurses.[73] There is no substantial study of the pressure group politics associated with mental nurse registration. The interaction and conflict between the Royal Medico-Psychological Association (RMPA), the Asylum Nurses' Union, and the organisations pressing for general nurses' registration awaits detailed investigation.

Confrontation occurred particularly in relation to the number of representatives proposed to represent mental and mental handicap nursing interests on the GNC. Dr Thomas Outterson Wood, Senior Physician to the West End Hospital for Nervous Diseases, London, had welcomed the Select Committee's decision as official recognition of the claims of mental nurses for inclusion in any scheme of state registration. He hoped that this would help 'restrain the efforts of those who would restrict the nurse's calling to any single class'. He argued that 'nursing is the birthright of all, and whether it falls to the lot of men or woman to minister to the sick and suffering, it cannot be claimed as the prerogative of any'.[74] Such statements would seem to vindicate Mrs Bedford Fenwick's concern that specialists were vulnerable to medical control. The use of the word 'class' in particular may have been deliberately ambiguous, referring to social and occupational categories as well as attitudes. Thomson objected to the snobbery and 'lofty scorn and opposition shown towards the recognition of our asylum trained nurses, male and female, as being nurses at all'.[75] Mental nurses were rightly sceptical of the extent to which general nurses in the RBNA would be sensitive to their value and 'needs'. Mental nurses were excluded from membership unless already 'general' trained, and only one out of thirty-one places on the executive council was allocated for nurses trained in asylums.[76]

ORDERING GENDER

Debate concerning the supplementary registers raised further questions about gender and class inequalities within the occupation. Anne Summers has drawn attention to the 'caste' system in nursing around which hierarchical relationships between men and women of different social classes were structured within institutions.[77] Male nurses, not trained in mental nursing, were arguably in the weakest position of all. Numerically small and poorly organised, they were subjected to the same strategies of exclusion by which female nurses were subordinated by male doctors. In 1891 there were only 691 male, compared with 53,057 female, nurses (1.3 per cent). By 1901 this figure had risen to 1,092 male, compared with 64,214 female, nurses (1.7 per cent).[78] Separate status for male nurses on a 'supplementary' part of the register originally had been the only concession by the Central Committee to the specialists in terms of occupational closure. Male nurses were trained only in the nursing of male patients; their training excluded nursing not only of women, including maternity and gynaecological work, but of children. This automatically blocked their access to the prestigious teaching hospitals and career opportunities which such an association afforded. The historical 'marginalisation' of men from the power structures of nursing has received little attention from researchers. Yet what is clear is that nurses appear to be no exception to the sociological orthodoxy that a weak group often subordinates a weaker one to improve its status.

The 'invisibility' of male nursing so angered one author that he declared that 'judged by the standards which we apply to women nurses, the skilled male nurse is thought by some to be practically non-existent'.[79] Interestingly this 'invisibility' does not extend to some official records. The term 'nurse' was used to refer to men tending the sick in Census returns between 1851 and 1891, whereas the utilisation of 'nurse' in connection with asylum care only superseded 'attendant' after 1919. Peter Nolan attributes this semantic shift to moves by general nurses and doctors to 'medicalise' mental illness after World War I. The term 'mental nurse' was institutionalised in 1923 with the establishment of the supplementary register of the GNC, and has been retained as the official title since that time.[80]

One of the major criticisms levelled at the College of Nursing Bill by the Central Committee was that it allowed for the formation of an unlimited number of supplementary registers. In a debate discussing the merits and demerits of the College of Nursing Bill, Miss Isabel MacDonald, secretary of the RBNA, castigated the College's position in caustic terms:

> If you are going to establish a supplementary register for fever nurses, perhaps one for children's nurses, it may be for health nurses, then under this Bill you can have, if you like, nurses for the Zoological gardens.[81]

The College Bill could be defended as more egalitarian since it was designed to assimilate all groups of nurses on an equal basis. This attack from the Central Committee was somewhat wrong-footed since by 1919 it too had made concessions to sick children's, male and mental nurses. Nor was the Central Committee as insensitive to the managerial interests of hospitals as its rhetoric suggested. It refused to establish a fever nurses' register on the grounds that it would deprive the infectious hospitals of the most desirable material for training: 'intelligent women would not spend years in training in the nursing of infectious diseases only to be side-tracked eventually.'[82]

SPECIALISING IN ANALOGIES

Whilst the disdain for 'specialists' in nursing corresponded to the much earlier prejudice against 'specialists' in medicine, by the early twentieth century the analogy between the two was strained.[83] By the turn of the century, the term 'specialist' in medical circles was no longer one of abuse. At the beginning of the nineteenth century, specialist practice was conflated with, and condemned as, quackery. A range of practitioners claimed special expertise in the treatment of specific diseases, bodily parts or age groups. In doing so many were accused of 'preying' upon the vulnerabilities of a credulous public to further their own ends.[84] General practitioners feared that specialists would not only expose the deficiencies of their own practice but threaten their economic livelihood by offering a superior service. By the beginning of the twentieth century, however, attitudes towards specialisation had transformed from being negative to positive. Part of this change derived from the perceived benefits of innovations in instrumentation and technology. Social and psychological factors connected with attitudes towards innovation are also likely to have been important.[85] Rosemary Stevens argues that in mid-1870s America, ambitious practitioners entered specialist areas of practice because the work was easier, the hours more regular, and the opportunities for social and financial advancement greater than in general practice.[86] One important incentive to specialisation identified by Granshaw was the exclusion of ambitious practitioners from conventional career pathways. This 'interests' theory, for example, is advanced to explain the development of proctology by Fredrick Salmon, founder of St Mark's Hospital, whose career ambitions were blocked at St Bartholomew's Hospital.[87]

INSTITUTIONALISING SPECIALISATION

Specialist hospitals provided a 'cultural medium' in which scientific knowledge could be translated into social status and prestige. As Granshaw observes, 'specialisation had long been the means by which outsiders in medicine might seek to rise'.[88] The 'bricks and mortar' route to medical entrepreneurship was first exploited by John Cunningham Saunders, founder of Moorfields Eye Hospital.[89] A number of equally ambitious practitioners followed suit.[90] Specialist hospitals and specialists were, however, criticised as superfluous and as forces which fragmented the intellectual and practical basis of medicine. More importantly still, they were seen to syphon off the interesting cases from general hospitals.[91] The tincture of disapproval with which specialists were tainted eventually evaporated under the pressure to professionalise medicine and reform medical education.

Impetus to reform medical education was provided by the

Carnegie Foundation in the USA, which funded a large-scale survey by Abraham Flexner to review medical education in the USA and Europe. The Flexner reports were influential in providing comparative and constructive critiques from which reforms in medical education could be framed in industrialised countries.[92] In the USA, Flexner criticised conditions at most centres except Johns Hopkins Hospital, Harvard and Case Western Reserve Universities.[93] The Johns Hopkins School was taken as the model for developing medical education in other parts of the country. Full-time professorial and laboratory staff were identified by Flexner as the key to upgrading teaching and research facilities. Permanent endowment of faculties was recommended to replace reliance upon income from student fees. The organisation of the Johns Hopkins School of Medicine had been based on the Germanic model of using clinical and laboratory departments in teaching.[94] As standardisation became the keynote of undergraduate medical education, specialisation became the hallmark of the postgraduate level. Sir William Osler, appointed Regius Professor of Medicine at Oxford in 1904 and co-founder of the Johns Hopkins School of Medicine in 1889, had been highly critical of the state of teaching in British medical schools upon his arrival in Oxford. He bemoaned the fact that there was no clinical school in Oxford and no links with cognate university departments staffed by paid officers.[95] Flexner, Osler and E.H. Starling, the distinguished University College physiologist, gave evidence to the Royal Commission on university education in London. Their combined testimonies confirmed the conclusion that professorial units in London hospitals should underpin the 'active invasion of the hospitals by the Universities'.[96] The status of specialist knowledge was legitimised through postgraduate training and qualification and the numerous societies devoted to its development. 'Specialisation' was slowly transformed from being a term of disapprobation to one of approbation; from deviance to orthodoxy in professional advancement. By the beginning of the twentieth century, attitudes towards specialisation were so favourable that it implied someone of superior rather than inferior skill and status.

DISUNITY AND UNIONISATION

The debate in nursing about specialisation took a slightly different tack. It was not specialisation *per se* that Mrs Bedford Fenwick objected to, but direct entry into a specialism without general foundation training. Specialisation was to build upon a common fundamental discipline of general nursing. The 'caste' system in nursing was enshrined in specialist and employment divisions within the occupation. However, Christopher Maggs and others have challenged the view that recruitment to voluntary hospitals in the late nineteenth and early twentieth centuries was as socially exclusive as the nursing leadership suggested.[97] The social class differences separating rank-and-file nurses in the different employment sectors were arguably much less than leaders were willing to concede. In the effort to 'gentrify' the occupation, leaders projected their own social origins and aspirations on to the occupation as a whole. The character and strength of the different industrial organisations through which nurses expressed their identity has been surveyed by Mick Carpenter and Christopher Hart.[98] Unions and associations recruited initially from specific employment sectors. It was only in the upper echelons of the general and Poor Law hospitals that common membership between organisations could be found. Poor Law matrons, for example, were represented on the Matrons' Council of Great Britain and Ireland, and later, after it was founded in 1919, in the Association of Hospital Matrons (AHM); and Mrs Bedford Fenwick published reports of the Poor Law Matrons' Association meetings in the *British Journal of Nursing*. Cross-membership did not appear to extend to rank-and-file organisations which catered for specialised employment sectors rather than grades of workers. Some were deliberately socially exclusive. Poor Law and asylum-trained nurses were excluded from membership of the RBNA on the grounds that they had not trained in a 'general' hospital. Mrs Bedford Fenwick was concerned that opening the register of trained nurses to men as well as women would, 'considering the present class of persons known as Male Attendants . . . hardly be likely to raise the status of the association'.[99] Fear of losing control of the Association to members more militant than herself may further explain Mrs Bedford Fenwick's exclusive criteria.

Nurses organised into unions as well as associations for professional ends. The end of World War I witnessed a wave of industrial assertiveness which induced some general nurses to unionise. Women workers had become increasingly assertive in their demands for improved pay and conditions. Female membership of unions had risen from 183,000 in 1910 to 1,086,000 by the end of 1918.[100] The Asylum Workers Association had been formed as an alternative to the RBNA by doctors prominent in the RMPA, but it eschewed any connection with trade unionism. Ten years later it was eclipsed in membership strength by the National Asylum Workers Union (NAWU), and it was finally superseded by the latter in 1919. The first paid secretary of the union was George Gibson, who later became leader of the Confederation of Health Service Workers.[101] By 1920, membership of the NAWU stood at 16,000, of which 7,000 were women.[102] The Poor Law Workers Trade Union was established in 1918 and its officer counterpart, the National Poor Law Officers' Association, became increasingly assertive in the aftermath of the war. The latter's attempts to transform itself into a trade union failed, but it was successfully absorbed within the National and Local Government Officers Organisation. Significantly, the nursing press contained extensive comment on the question of unionisation in nursing but was divided in its support for such moves.[103] Mrs Bedford Fenwick provided a forum for the newly formed PUTN to publicise its meetings and activities in the *British Journal of Nursing*. Little is known of the history of this organisation, but it was constituted as a union of nurses working in co-operatives and in the non-institutional sector.[104] An outspoken and founding member of the PUTN was Maude MacCallum, also a prominent member of one of the strongest and most successful nursing co-operatives in London. She was later appointed member of the first provisional nursing council and was a loyal supporter of Mrs Bedford Fenwick.

Miss Isabel MacDonald, secretary to the RBNA and long-standing ally of Mrs Bedford Fenwick, was also a vocal member of the union and at its opening meeting identified several dangers which threatened the livelihood and welfare of the nurse. One of the most potent 'dangers' was the hospital with private staffs who trained nurses and then 'grasped . . . the income arising from their labours'. Their 'tentacles' were spreading to absorb not only private nurses but their independence too.[105] Fears that hospitals were expanding their private staffs, even forming co-operatives of their own, ran high. Hospitals had considerable competitive advantage over the nurses' co-operatives: they could charge less by offsetting fees against emoluments and draw upon the social networks of former medical graduates. Theoretically doctors could send for all their nurses to the hospital where they trained.[106] The hospital could in theory become a monopoly supplier of labour in the institutional and non-institutional spheres in a given locality. This was perceived as the major threat to the operation of a 'free' nursing market. Mrs Bedford Fenwick was prepared to condone trade union activity by nurses provided it was directed towards emancipatory ends.[107]

The Lloyd George coalition administration had been disturbed by the threat of industrial disorder, particularly in the cities of the north. Clashes between police and strikers in Glasgow were referred to by Lloyd George in alarmist terms as 'Bolshevik risings'.[108] Adams argues that Lloyd George, although himself no revolutionary, was prepared to use revolutionary rhetoric for dramatic effect. His approach to industrial relations was conciliatory only where it was necessary to contain social upheaval.[109] Capitalising upon the government's sensitivity to unionisation, Mrs Bedford Fenwick claimed the passing of a Registration Bill would have a pacifying effect upon nursing unrest and predicted 'organisation throughout the nursing world will follow'.[110] The use of the term 'organisation' was ambiguous, suggesting 'disorder' as well as 'order' were equal possibilities depending on the outcome of Registration. Anxious to contain the spread of industrial unrest, the government had set up arbitration machinery and later, following the Whitley report of 1917, urged employers to establish national bargaining machinery.[111] The state was seeking to establish itself as a model employer for others to emulate. Dr Christopher Addison, First Minister of Health, was sympathetic about what he termed the 'discreditable' payments made to nurses, 'much less than the wages of an ordinary cook or kitchen maid'. He considered it essential that nursing become a properly paid profession.[112]

ADMINISTERING INTERVENTION

Government intervention in nurses' registration can be understood in the context of plans for reconstructing the health services and the need to incorporate the nursing services within those plans.[113] The Ministry of Health had been created to rationalise the overlapping confusion of health functions undertaken by a multiplicity of unco-ordinated government departments, including the Local Government Board, the National Insurance Commission, the Privy Council and the Board of Education.[114] Hitherto, twenty-one government departments had been undertaking what Dr Addison referred to as the 'odds and ends of health work'.[115] The Machinery of Government Committee, which reported in 1918, had been established to correct the overlapping confusion of functions and 'Lilliputian administration' which characterised different areas of government policy.[116] The coalition government's post-war social reconstruction plans were designed to inspire a 'land fit for heroes' as well as containing the labour unrest associated with a disrupted economy. Extension of public-funded health services presupposed a mobile workforce with standardised credentials and rates of remuneration. Registration was described by Dr Addison as an 'essential element in any real improvement of existing medical services, particularly for the industrial population. It is a reform which is ten years overdue.'[117] Registration provided the means of promoting industrial stability simultaneously with regulating the conduct of nurse training and discipline.

The nursing organisations, however, were still irreconcilable in their definitions of registration as enshrined in the rival Bills put forward to Parliament. Dr Addison suggested both parties drop their present Bills and allow the government to introduce its own Bill as early as possible. Rosemary White has argued that the Local Government Board, of which Dr Addison was President prior to the absorption of its functions within the Ministry of Health in 1919, was put off the idea of registration by its experience of midwifery registration, when voluntary interests were alleged to have been promoted at the expense of Poor Law in the approval of institutions for training.[118] Little direct evidence that the Midwives' Act exerted any impact upon Dr Addison's attitude towards nurses registration is contained either in Ministry of Health files or in the Addison Papers in the Bodleian Library. While evidence from the Departmental Committee on the Workings of the Midwives' Act (1909) suggests that the action of the Central Midwives Board (CMB) had reduced the supply of midwives from some Poor Law hospitals, this was limited mainly to the earlier part of the Board's career.[119]

COMPROMISING POSITIONS

Dr Addison was openly sympathetic to nurses' registration and on conditions in the nursing services.[120] A series of conferences between Ministry of Health officials and nursing associations were held prior to the drafting and introduction of a government Bill on Nurses' Registration. The organisations concerned were the Central Committee for the State Registration of Nurses, the AHM and the College of Nursing. There was considerable cross-membership between the executive council of the AHM and representatives from the College of Nursing, which potentially increased the chances of certain individuals being appointed to the first Provisional Council by the Minister of Health. The new AHM supported the College of Nursing Bill.[121]

The Association was established in 1918 as a rival College of Nursing-backed organisation to the Bedford Fenwick-led Matrons' Council for Great Britain and Ireland. Very little is known about the activities of the Matrons' Council except from published reports of meetings in the nursing press and short accounts in the early history of nursing textbooks.[122] The aims of the Council, founded in 1894, were 'a uniform system of education, examination, certification, and State Registration for nurses in British hospitals'.[123]

The objects of the AHM were:

1 To enable members to take counsel together on matters affecting their profession.
2 To consider and if necessary take action upon legislative proposals calculated to affect the interests of the nursing profession.
3 To maintain the honour and further the interests of the nursing profession.

Membership of the Association was open to trained nurses who held or had held the position of matron or superintendent of hospitals and institutions concerning the training of nurses and the care of the sick.[124] The establishment of an additional organisation so close to the passing of the legislation can be seen as an attempt by College Council members to capture as much representational power as possible on the new council by creating an additional channel for representation. Cross-membership in the governing bodies of the College of Nursing and the AHM would theoretically favour candidates with dual appointments. Positions on the Council could in such a way be more easily concentrated in the hands of the College and Association elite. Amongst the supporters of the AHM were matrons of the leading London and provincial training schools. The President of the Association was Miss Lloyd Still, matron of St Thomas's hospital. Miss Rachel Cox-Davies, matron of the Royal Free Hospital, was Honorary Secretary of the Association. Both Miss Cox-Davies and Miss Lloyd Still were founder members of the College of Nursing Council but denied any motivation to set up a rival to any existing nursing organisation. Unity and strength were their chief objectives.[125]

COMPREHENDING POWERS

The Minister resolved to avoid burdening the registration authority with duties that did not properly belong to it, or promoting the interests of any sectional institution. The Bill would attempt to deal with 'public interests in concert with the parties' wishes'.[126] In presenting the proposed measure to his Cabinet colleagues, Dr Addison reassured them that the council's functions would be limited. The Bill would be 'confined within the smallest possible compass', setting up a suitably composed council charged with working out detailed regulations. These would be subject to the approval of the Ministry of Health, 'avoiding the discussion of highly technical details of nursing work, and training, and the conflicting personalia of the nursing world, in the unsuitable arena of the House of Commons'.[127] Cabinet agreed to sanction the introduction of a Bill provided agreement was obtained from the parties principally concerned. Consultation was also required with the Secretary of State for Scotland, the Chief Medical Officer to the Ministry of Health and the Secretary of State for Ireland.[128] The Central Committee's Bill had originally sought to have one central United Kingdom registration system, but nationalism ensured separate arrangements were made for England and Wales, Scotland and Ireland, with reciprocity between each.

Mrs Bedford Fenwick and her supporters had hoped that the legislation would empower the council to exert some control over conditions of service and that this would eliminate 'sweated labour' from nursing. Dr Addison explained during his separate meetings with the nursing organisations that the council would not deal with questions such as conditions of service and hours of labour. These would be the policy of the Ministry of Health to safeguard.[129] The means by which safeguards would be put into operation was not specified, but plans for rationalising the health services may well have been what officials had in mind.

Sir Robert Morant, Permanent Secretary to the Ministry of Health, explained that a government Bill would only succeed if there was substantial agreement. Both sections of opinion would have to be satisfied with something less than they had hoped for. The parties were swiftly disabused of any notion that the government would allow appointees to the Council to exercise a high degree of autonomy in the conduct of their affairs. Whilst the matrons regretted the failure of the College of Nursing's Bill they conceded that they would be prepared to accept a Bill on the general lines indicated by Sir Robert Morant.[130] On the question of nominations to the Council, Dr Addison insisted the Council should be as representative of the profession as possible. He disagreed strongly with any suggestion that ministerial nominations implied persons would be subservient. He was determined not to allow his choice to be fettered and gave a formal assurance that neither the Central Committee nor the College would be given 'such numerical representation as to enable them to dominate'.[131] The cleavages of opinion which had separated the rival factions were temporarily subordinated to the short-term goal of securing the best compromise which political necessity permitted.

RESERVATIONS AND RESOURCES

The final point which had to be settled was the financing of the Council. The Central Committee, the Treasury and College of Nursing advocated that the Council should be self-supporting.[132] Others believed that it should be partly financed by some 'rich' outside body such as the College of Nursing Limited; or that fees exacted by the Council from nurses should be high enough to ensure an adequate income for fulfilling the various functions conferred on the Council. The weakness of the latter scheme was that it required a higher fee than the government could allow, while the former was deemed inadmissible within a national scheme. The Ministry decided it would be prepared to supplement the Council's initial income from fees, with a grant to meet any deficit arising from the setting of a lower fee. It was envisaged that this would be quite a small sum confined to pre-negotiated conditions with the Ministry and subject to Treasury sanction.[133]

The cost of establishing and running a nurses' register was difficult to estimate due to the difficulty of forecasting the number of nurses who might register.[134] Ministry officials projected that, given the hypothetical numbers of nurses eligible to register under various conditions, the cost of establishing and running a register was likely to be £16,000. Assuming an income of £25,000, the records stated that this would yield a small income for the Council of £1,250 per annum.[135] If the Council attempted to be self-supporting, a permanent fee of five guineas would have to be extracted from nurses wishing to register according to the variables identified by officials. This would then obviate the need for any Treasury subvention. The point on which there was even less certainty was the cost of examinations, which would depend upon the number and nature of papers to be set and the frequency with which exams were to be held. Dr Bedford Fenwick's earlier estimates of Council costs were dismissed by

Lawrence Brock, the Assistant Secretary to the Ministry of Health, as 'grossly extravagant'. Dr Bedford Fenwick's budgetary and policy proposals were criticised as overambitious and requiring a much more elaborate examination than seemed necessary. The allowance for the appointment of six permanent inspectors was decried as particularly profligate.[136]

RE-ENACTING REGISTRATION

The radicals, led by Mrs Bedford Fenwick, were initially jubilant and rejoiced in the registration victory.[137] In a letter to Dr Addison, Mrs Bedford Fenwick thanked him for 'the splendid Christmas gift you have so marvellously bestowed upon the profession of nursing'.[138] Hopes for professional self-regulation, elimination of competitors and majority representation for the radical contingent evaporated as the full implications of the legislation were realised. The Council was not to be self-governing or professionally exclusive and accountable to the 'profession'. It contained representatives of the Privy Council and Board of Education, and all members were responsible in the first instance to the Minister of Health. Nor was a single portal of entry instituted. It was the College rather than the Central Committee's Bill which finally predominated, reinforcing the hierarchy of specialisms.

A register was to be established but its status was voluntary, and no legal monopoly of practice was afforded to the registered nurses against their unregistered competitors. The immediate effect of the Act on improving the status of the trained nurse was debatable. The Act failed to meet the high expectations of the radicals and in this sense was similar to the Medical Registration Act of 1858.[139] However, rank-and-file interests were to be represented on the new nursing Council. George Webster, former chairman of the radical London-based British Medical Association (BMA) noted: 'it has to be much regretted that the general practitioners were not likely to be represented on the medical council by members of their own body'.[140] The legislation fell short of the ambitions cherished for it. Furthermore it failed to command the resources necessary to fulfil these. The scope and limits of the Council's powers were trimmed and tailored to a minimalist view of the educational functions it could perform. Clear lines of accountability were written into proposals; the expenditure of the Council was subject to Treasury scrutiny and ministerial audit through the submission of an annual financial report.[141] This 'niggardly' view was represented as the price necessary to recruit Cabinet commitment for a government Bill.

CONCLUSION

The battle for nurses' and medical registration disguised a deeper struggle for control of the private nursing market and the establishment of independent careers for nurses against the monopolistic tendencies of certain elite institutions.[142] The private nurse was in many respects analogous to the mid-nineteenth-century general practitioner. Both perceived they required protection from prestigious institutions which controlled important areas of the medical and nursing markets. Thomas Wakely attacked the medical corporations as Mrs Bedford Fenwick criticised the teaching hospitals for their imperialistic attitudes and actions in the nursing and medical markets. However, in her endeavour to protect and promote the interests of the private, freelance nurse, Mrs Bedford Fenwick ignored the needs of the poor for nursing care. Her 'hemianopia' left her sensitive only to the supply of nurses for the paying public. Mrs Bedford Fenwick's was a gender- and class-specific strategy in which the 'new' nurse was cast in the image of the 'new' woman, with all the contradictions that entailed. The radicals' partisanship was expressed in their rejection of existing measures used to regulate the 'quality' of nursing labour in the state sector.

The Scottish Poor Law Nursing Service had possessed a 'register' of nurses since 1885.[143] The Lunacy Commission in London kept a 'blacklist' of nurses dismissed for any serious fault from a lunatic asylum under the jurisdiction of the Commissioners.[144] In theory, reformers could have adapted the available public rather than a private model of organisation. Instead they opted for a professional model based on the organisation of medicine. Such a narrow definition of 'public' interest may have strengthened government resolve to restrict the powers of the GNC. As with the Medical Act of 1858, there was surprisingly little expression of dissatisfaction from the 'consumers' of health care that existing medical or nursing care was deficient. Nor was there much evidence from the public that they suffered significantly from the ministrations of the 'unqualified'. Evidence of unsatisfactory practice relied heavily, if not exclusively, upon evaluations by suppliers of nursing services.

I have further argued that international connections and suffragist sympathies provided important support for legislative reform within

British nursing. Yet the achievement of registration cannot be understood without reference to the government's plans for post-World War I social reconstruction. The government's promise of extended provision of state welfare measures was part of a strategy intended to head off industrial unrest. The registration of nurses was a corollary to such measures. It was fortuitous that governmental and occupational objectives coincided, but both were working to different agendas. The nature of these agendas and the fragility of the consensus forged by registration are discussed in the chapter which follows.

Chapter 5

Crisis and conflict in the Caretaker Council (1919–23)

INTRODUCTION

The Nurses' Registration Act brought only a temporary peace to the warring factions which vied for supremacy during the debate. The Act received a mixed reception in the nursing press. Some anticipated a 'golden future' and 'honourable status' for nursing and welcomed the victory against apathy and antagonism.[1] Others were sceptical of the prospect of radical reform and compared the passing of the Act to 'applying sticking plaster to a gumboil'.[2] As a step towards the establishment of an elected nursing council, a Caretaker Council was established. The Caretaker Council provided a fresh battleground for old and new contests to be fought. Differences which had divided registrationists before the passing of the Act re-emerged in the Council's early work. Its composition by unreconciled parties provided a recipe for strife and disaster. The conflicts revolved around rival interpretations of what the powers of the Council should be and how it should be constituted.

These and other unresolved tensions put the consensus forged between the registration factions under severe strain. So divisive were the issues which separated the radicals, led by Mrs Bedford Fenwick, and the moderates, represented by the College of Nursing, that the future of registration itself was jeopardised. Clashes between radicals and moderates forced the government to intervene, ushering in the first of a series of defeats for the radical view. Mrs Bedford Fenwick survived deselection from the Caretaker Council's Registration Committee, but only to exert limited continuity of authority through other channels. This chapter discusses the forces which ultimately brought about the defeat of Mrs Bedford Fenwick and the incipient extinction of her professionalising view of nurse training and recruitment. Furthermore, it considers the implications of the early political dynamics between state officials and a nascent body of 'professional' women as a case study in professional/bureaucratic conflict.[3]

NOMINALIST CONTROVERSY

The appointment of the Caretaker Council proved a delicate political balancing act for officials. The two main officials responsible for implementing the Act were Sir Robert Morant and Laurence Brock.[4] The Council was to be composed of twenty-five members, nine 'lay', including medical appointees, and sixteen nurses. Two appointees of the Privy Council were to be supplemented by two from the Board of Education. Five representatives were to have 'knowledge' of training schools and sixteen were to be involved in the provision of nursing services to the sick.[5] Of the lay members, two were to be appointed by the Privy Council to represent the public and two by the Board of Education to provide more general educational experience. The five remaining members provided the Minister with the only opportunity of appointing medical men in general or specialist practice.

Nominations were first invited from interested parties. Sir Robert Morant insisted everyone on the Council should be justified as a useful person in his or her own right, 'not merely to placate'.[6] Dr Addison had indicated that he intended to secure, as far as possible, a fair geographical distribution so that the Council would not be London-dominated. He had given a pledge in Committee that he would appoint two representatives of general hospitals for children. This in fact was the only parliamentary pledge, but he was also keen to ensure that the rank and file should have some representation and that the Council should not consist entirely of matrons.

Geographically, however, nominations clustered around the London area. Although the list included representation from Manchester, Liverpool and Cheshire, only slightly more than half the nominees originated from the provinces. A total of sixteen matrons were nominated for consideration, some several times over by different organisations, thereby enhancing their chances of appointment. Interestingly, Mrs Bedford Fenwick was supported by the largest number of organisations: the Royal British Nurses' Association (RBNA), Society for the State Registration of Trained Nurses (SSRN), the Matrons' Council, the National Union of Trained Nurses and the Association of Hospital Matrons (AHM).[7] Although the AHM was ostensibly a rival to the Matrons' Council, Mrs Bedford

Fenwick may have been nominated by her ally, Miss Barton, Matron of the Chelsea Infirmary and Poor Law representative on the AHM executive, who was also appointed to the Caretaker Council.

Anxious to balance hospital with public health interests, Sir Robert Morant interviewed several candidates with this in mind. Few were forthcoming with the necessary experience or personal qualities necessary except a Miss Swiss, a health visitor, who was appointed. She was allied with the new Professional Union of Trained Nurses (PUTN) and thought more likely to side with Mrs Bedford Fenwick. District nurses received eight nominations, mainly from the AHM. Miss Peterkin, superintendent of the Queen's Jubilee Nurses, was an executive council member of the AHM.[8] The alignment of district nurses with hospital matrons points to the poor organisation of district nurses at the grass-roots level and the concentration of the nursing elite in hospital-dominated organisations. As may have been anticipated, nominations for matrons from the large London teaching hospitals predominated, only two of whom had experience of public health work.[9] Selecting matrons seemed unavoidable, since talented women tended to become matrons and insufficient numbers of the rank and file had come or been put forward for selection.[10]

The second largest number of nominations (fifteen) came from nurses in private practice selected in roughly equal proportions by the AHM, PUTN, Matron's Council and RBNA.[11] This reveals the political strength of this section of the occupation. The Poor Law sector, which employed the majority of institutional nurses, however, offered only two names from the National Poor Law Officers Association. This suggests that trade union support for the Council was weak. Significantly, the majority of Poor Law nominations originated from the College of Nursing, AHM and Matrons' Council.[12] Only one of the nurse members of the provisional council had a Poor Law training and only three matrons worked in Poor Law hospitals. Officials conceded that a larger claim to representation by the Poor Law was justified, but their estimations of the numbers on which to base representation were vague.[13] Part of the problem related to the fact that the Ministry did not publish statistics on the numbers of nurses employed in the Poor Law sector. The only routinely collected statistics were those for the numbers of nurses registered with the General Nursing Council (GNC), published in Ministry of Health annual reports.[14] Conceivably, the Minister of Health may have anticipated safeguarding Poor Law interests through his sanctioning power over the Council's rulings. Alternatively, given the more active union organisation in the public sector, the pressures upon government to concede to demands originating from that sector may also have been more difficult to resist.[15]

Thus, notwithstanding official pronouncements on the meritocratic basis of appointments, political considerations were very much to the fore in officials' selection of candidates. Miss Smith, for example, Welsh superintendent of the Jubilee Nurses, was selected on the basis of her dual representation of Wales and non-institutional nursing. Miss MacCallum, secretary of the PUTN, although 'unpopular' with some sections of the occupation, was included in case her union members set the dangerous precedent of refusing to register.[16] Prominent among officials' concerns was whether members were likely to vote with the College or Central Committee group and whether they could combine multiple representational interests.[17] Political and personal rivalries were also involved. Miss Cox-Davies, Miss Lloyd Still, and Miss Sparshott were strong protagonists of the College and 'greatly disliked' by the Bedford Fenwick contingent. Mrs Bedford Fenwick, Miss MacDonald and Miss MacCallum represented the opposing group. Appointees of the Board of Education, namely Miss Steele and Miss Batty Tuke (Principal of Bedford College for Women), along with Hon. Mrs Eustace Hills, Lady Hobhouse, Mr J.C. Priestley (chair of the Council) and Rev. Cronshaw (chairman of the Radcliffe Infirmary), were all thought likely to act with the College.[18] Five candidates from mental hospitals were put forward, two male and three female, and five from general hospitals for children. Six 'sundry' persons were also proposed on the basis of their supposed 'expertise'; one on the strength of her marriage to a government inspector of factories![19] Of the five Ministry of Health appointees, fifteen nominations were received, including the erstwhile anti-registrationists Lord Knutsford and Lord Sandhurst. They were excluded, but medical men were selected who could add representational strength to weaker elements. Consequently Dr Bedford Pierce from the Royal Medico-Psychological Association (RMPA) supplemented the mental side.[20] Although the political sympathies of all the specialists were not known, taking those which were, it looked as though some balance had been achieved in combining College and Central Committee loyalties. Having achieved this distribution, the Minister claimed to have fulfilled his pledge about appointing a representative Council. With 'probably equal disgust on both sides', officials considered they had hit 'the right mean'.[21]

The distribution of members on the first Council roughly reflected the membership of the various nursing organisations, but trade union and Poor Law representation were artificially low.[22] By 1925, the College of Nursing claimed 23,500 members.[23] Mr Herbert Paterson, Medical Honorary Secretary of the RBNA, quoted a membership of 5,000.[24] Miss MacCallum, secretary to the PUTN, reported its membership as 1,000.[25] The Registered Nurses' Parliamentary Council, formerly the SSRN, claimed 4,000 members.[26] General hospital matrons predominated over all other interests on the Council, domiciliary, public health, rank-and-file and specialist.[27] It is not possible to identify which nurses had also been trained in fever nursing from either the Council Minutes or the 'official' history of the Council.[28]

CHAIRING CHOICES

A chairman had to be appointed, and although the Minister had no such power in the Act, Morant maintained that both College and Central Committee representatives expected the Minister do this.[29] The Privy Council was asked to nominate a lawyer of standing to preside over the judicial subcommittee of the Council. Mr Joseph Priestley KC, son of the late Sir William and Lady Margaret Priestley, was recommended by Sir Almeric Fitzroy, Secretary to Privy Council, as a man of 'agreeable manner and tactful'.[30] Mr Priestley was considered appropriate since he was associated with neither the College nor the Central Committee and could therefore be regarded as impartial. The alternative to a ministerial nomination was to leave the Council to select its own chairman. But this was considered impractical since the two sides were so evenly balanced that neither was thought likely to sacrifice a vote.

Brock, sensitive to the task that any chairman would face in handling the committee, implied that it was an unenviable one: 'the three College protagonists will glare at the three Bedford Fenwick protagonists'.[31] While regretting that selecting 'standard bearers' was unavoidable, since those who were sufficiently well informed tended to be those who could not be omitted, Brock anticipated antagonism from the outset. Even where the two groups would not necessarily differ on principle, the mere sight of one another seemed sufficient to arouse 'reciprocal hatred and combat for the sake of combat'.[32] In the event, however, it was hoped that historical animosities would be subordinated to Council business.

Controversy plagued the Council, even extending to the appointment of the first registrar. A series of objections were raised to the
nomination of Miss Marion Riddell. As a former employee of the War
Office, it was argued she might be tempted to exercise the same
'autocratic methods...which had aroused much resentment amongst
large numbers of British and Colonial Nurses during the war'.[33]
Moreover, as she was Secretary to the College of Nursing Council,
Miss Riddell's appointment, it was claimed, would represent a
disincentive to registration for nurses opposed to the College of
Nursing.[34] It was on this basis that the Minister was asked to receive a
deputation from the PUTN. Priestley suggested the Minister receive
the Union's representatives if only to point out the impracticality of
inviting ministerial intervention every time a minority decision was
over-ruled. Morant advised against receiving a deputation to avoid
implying that the Minister regarded the Union's opposition worthy of
consideration. Morant suspected Mrs Bedford Fenwick as the *agent
provocateur* behind the protest, on the basis of its epistolary style.[35]
Miss Riddell was duly appointed as the best candidate.

PRECARIOUS FOUNDATIONS

But the appointment of the Caretaker GNC revealed the true extent
of the radical registrationists' defeat. The College of Nursing, with lay
support, had a comfortable majority. The RBNA had only five votes it
could rely on. The founding members of the GNC faced a formidable
challenge. They were required to devise a set of rules which would
define admission to the register and elections for future Councils.
They were to administer the process of registration and establish rules
for the conduct of business by various standing committees. One of
their key tasks was to ensure sufficient numbers of nurses were
registered to elect the first Council. As with the Midwives' Act, *bona
fide* practitioners were eligible for admission to the register. They were
required to produce evidence of good character, experience of practice
for three years, and adequate knowledge and experience of nursing
the sick. In addition, the Council was expected to rationalise training
in a heterogeneous health care system and harmonise rulings between
the three national Councils; Scotland, Ireland, and England and
Wales each had its own Councils and different legal and administrative systems, and they jealously guarded their autonomy.

Imposing some form of common identity upon the various
branches of nursing was a major political undertaking. Part of the

heterogeneity of training derived from the diversity within the health care system itself. The Council was concerned with rationalising training provision in some 1,500 training 'schools'. This was a task far in excess of that which had previously confronted the General Medical Council's (GMC) supervision of medical education in only twenty-four centres.[36] In many other respects, however, the challenges were similar.

The GMC had no legal power to compel licensing bodies to accept the minimum standards laid down by the Council. The lack of a common entrance examination to medical schools meant that universities sifted applications through individual examinations which they themselves conducted. Although the Council had attempted to make uniform standards a reality, idiosyncrasy still prevailed.[37] It was not simply the scale of provision which differentiated medical from nursing education, but the place of students in the economy of health care.

Hospitals depended upon probationer nurses much more than on medical students. However, medical schools were not immune from problems of resources. These were expressed in terms of a conflict between the proprietary interests of hospitals and scientific ideals. Attempts to consolidate pre-clinical scientific teaching in well-resourced institutions were thought likely to disadvantage institutions where resources were poor. Abraham Flexner, in his survey of British medical education, recommended St George's, Westminster and Charing Cross Hospitals for closure due to the poor quality of their scientific teaching and laboratory facilities. This was attributed directly to the poverty of the institutions.[38] Any proposal by the nursing Council to change the contribution of probationer labour to hospital economics was likely to be strongly resisted by administrators and policy-makers.

QUALIFIED STATEMENTS

The Caretaker Council held its first meeting on Tuesday, 11 May 1920, when the rules for admitting existing nurses were drawn up. The minimum age for entry on to the register was set at 21, and candidates had to supply evidence of good character from three responsible persons to cover the three years preceding application. To qualify as an 'existing nurse', candidates were to have had one year's training in a general hospital or Poor Law Infirmary before 1 November 1919, in addition to two years' subsequent practice. The registration fee was set at one guinea, with an annual retention fee of 2s 6d.[39] A series of standing committees – finance, education and examination, disciplinary and penal, registration and mental nursing – were then appointed.

The rules for admitting nurses to the general and supplementary registers proved anomalous; in some instances the standard for entry on to the sick children's register was higher than that governing general nursing alone.[40] Heated debate revolved around the recording of qualifications already held by nurses. Indeed this proved so divisive that a crisis erupted which threatened the viability of registration itself. At the centre of the controversy was Mrs Bedford Fenwick, who insisted upon a medical analogy in her assertion that all qualifications held by nurses should be recorded on the register. This was interpreted by ministry officials as an attempt to convert the register into a kind of *Who's Who*.[41] Mrs Bedford Fenwick insisted that nurses would have a genuine grievance if their hard-earned certificates were not recorded.[42] Several members, who disagreed with Mrs Bedford Fenwick's resolution, suggested it should be excluded from the Registration Committee's report to the Ministry. Miss Cox-Davies contended that the word 'certificated' should be reserved until future nurses were admitted to the Register by state examinations.[43] Mrs Bedford Fenwick used the occasion to accuse members of misrepresenting Council business.[44] But she herself did not escape criticism, and was, in fact, subjected to similar accusations; her publication of Council business in her journal being described as a 'travesty of the facts'. Particular exception was taken to the publication of Council business in advance of important decisions being made. This was perceived by Mrs Bedford Fenwick's opponents as an attempt to incite nurses into pressurising Council into policies and decisions favoured by Mrs Bedford Fenwick herself.[45] The precise method used to record early Council minutes is unclear. No secretary seems to have been employed for the task. As chairman of the Registration Committee, Mrs Bedford Fenwick was in an ideal position to influence reported Council business.

Quarrels regarding propriety of procedure spilled over into questions of individual competence. Mr Priestley's qualifications as chairman of the Council were even challenged in Parliament.[46] Addison defended his choice of chairman and strongly repudiated any suggestion of discontent within the Council as 'foolish gossip'.[47] Brock identified the immediate source of the questions as either Miss MacCallum of the PUTN or Mr Christian of the Asylum Workers

Union. He was convinced, however, that neither would take action independently of Mrs Bedford Fenwick. Brock considered that the action was a deliberate attempt by Mrs Bedford Fenwick to discredit Priestley, who had not proved as amenable to her influence as she had expected.[48] Priestley took the accusations levelled against him very much to heart. He refused to continue as chairman on the grounds that he did not enjoy the full confidence of the Council, and Sir Almeric Fitzroy agreed, albeit reluctantly, that Mr Priestley's resignation was in order.

CRISIS OF CONFIDENCE

Brock assured Priestley he had the full support and confidence of the Minister, but Miss Cox-Davies intimated that if Priestley left this would induce several other members to resign in sympathy.[49] Moreover, the departure of College members was likely to stimulate the exodus of neutral members. The College would then have the excuse, which Ministry officials believed some had always wanted, to boycott the register. The future of registration was imperilled further by inefficiency in processing applications for registration. As matters stood, the administrative system obliged nurses to send their original certificates for verification. Many were reluctant to part with their original papers, afraid they might be mislaid. This had prevented many nurses from coming forward to register. As a practical solution to this problem, it had been proposed that copies of certificates could be sent in by individual nurses via the Roll of the College of Nursing, whose membership qualification was more stringent than that proposed by the Council.

In the four months from the opening of the register some 3,235 applications were received, but only 984 were completed. Applications came into the office at the rate of 800 a month, but less than one third were passed by the Council. The Council was under great pressure to process these applications quickly, since it was due to leave office on 23 December the following year and had to ensure a sufficiently large and representative number of nurses were registered to elect a new Council. Out of an estimated 50,000 nurses, only 1,550 were on the register five months after it had opened. The Minister criticised the over-meticulous methods used by the chairman of the registration committee, Mrs Bedford Fenwick, in scrutinising certificates. He was quick to point out that if the status quo continued 'many of the nurses would be dead and buried before they got on to the register'.[50] Ministry officials regarded Priestley as an excellent, impartial and hard-working chairman but unfortunately 'not a fighter'.[51] Priestley was asked to reconsider his decision. If he persisted, it was likely that half the Council would resign in sympathy. Thereafter it could prove difficult, if not impossible, to induce people of any standing to accept appointment to the Council, thereby reducing it in effect, to what officials referred to as a 'rabble of nonentities and camp-followers of Mrs Bedford Fenwick'.[52]

Priestley, however, was resolved to resign. As predicted, his departure provoked the resignations of the majority of the Council.[53] Officials were frustrated that fifteen members tendered their resignations ostensibly in protest against the 'uncontrolled ill-temper of one particular member'.[54] Sir Jenner Verrall and Miss Dowbiggin expressed their intention to resign unless Priestley could be persuaded to return. Only four members, in addition to Mrs Bedford Fenwick, chose to remain.[55] But even within this coterie, support for Mrs Bedford Fenwick was not unanimous. Miss MacDonald felt she could not resign in view of her long association with the RBNA, but was prepared to undertake not to attend any meetings or to give Mrs Bedford Fenwick any active support.[56] Presumably she thought that Mrs Bedford Fenwick had gone too far. In effect all Council business was brought to a standstill, since there was no possibility of a quorum for meetings. Brock played down the severity of the crisis and asked the editor of *Nursing Times* to make any statement concerning the resignations as anodyne as possible. Sir Alfred Mond, now Minister of Health, made only a brief comment to the nursing press.[57] The intervention was too late. A *Nursing Times* editorial alluded to the event as a 'tragedy', regretting that the nursing profession, which it declared should be a 'gentle sisterhood, seemed fated to be the ground for bitterness and quarrels'.[58] Mrs Bedford Fenwick extracted maximum political capital from the fiasco, condemning resigning members' action as 'irresponsible striking behaviour.'[59] Mr Robert Richardson, Labour MP for Houghton-Le-Spring, in a similar rhetorical style, condemned the matrons for having driven off the committee 'the only friend that working nurses had'.[60]

Charges levelled against Mrs Bedford Fenwick by Council members included:

1   Free and open discussion was prevented on the Council and subcommittees.

2 Publication of the Children's Hospital syllabus occurred prior to it being officially given to the press.
3 Claims to the effect that the country would be 'stumped', and that opposition stimulated from outside to support her views would be mobilised, threatened to wreck the work of the Council.
4 The conduct of the registration process was unduly delayed and staff hampered.
5 Views contrary to Mrs Bedford Fenwick's were suppressed in the minutes of the registration subcommittee.
6 When appealed to in the Council she refused to modify the minutes, stating that the views opposed to her own were not worthy of being recorded.
7 The Council by a large majority decided upon the deletion of the paragraphs to which objection had been taken. In spite of this, these paragraphs were published in the next issue of her journal.
8 The work on the Council was a painful and distressing duty, chiefly because of the domineering and unconciliatory attitude of a certain member, which prevented proper deliberation and discussion, and which was felt injurious to the nursing profession.[61]

The resignation of Council members left Mrs Bedford Fenwick more isolated than she could have anticipated. Shaken at the resignation of a number of members whom she normally counted her supporters, she nevertheless claimed to be unaware of the extent to which her behaviour had alienated her former colleagues.[62] The whole future of registration was now in jeopardy. Officials feared that the departure of the College of Nursing members would induce the majority of College nurses not to register. College membership was estimated at 19,000 and considered by Ministers 'the pick of the profession'. If the College boycotted the register it would hardly be worth printing.[63] Once again, the Ministry was left to act as conciliator between the two rival factions. Had Priestley been willing to reconsider his resignation, the matter could have been settled, but this he was only prepared to do if Mrs Bedford Fenwick tendered hers.

The Minister agreed to mediate between resigning members and Mrs Bedford Fenwick to work out a solution to the catastrophe. The resigning members submitted the minimum terms under which they and Priestley would consider withdrawing their resignations. These were:

1 Mrs Bedford Fenwick's resignation from the Chairmanship of the registration committee, a post considered inappropriate to the owner and editor of a nursing paper.
2 A formal undertaking from Mrs Bedford Fenwick not to publish in her paper any documents not given to the nursing press generally on any matters under consideration by the Council, and to desist from all attempts to incite nurses to pressurise the Council into adopting any particular policy.
3 A formal undertaking not to visit the offices of the Council except for the purpose of attending committee meetings. Mrs Bedford Fenwick was reported as insisting upon scrutinising each application for registration personally, interfering with the staff to a point which caused the breakdown of the administrative machinery.

Evidence of animosity between Mrs Bedford Fenwick, the resident Council staff and other Council members, however, is not apparent from their early correspondence with each other. Conversely, the tone of such correspondence suggests good, rather than poor relations existed between various parties. In a letter to Priestley, Miss Riddell refers to Mrs Bedford Fenwick's almost daily attendance at the Council headquarters. Far from her being criticised, Miss Riddell represented Mrs Bedford Fenwick as a strong ally, sympathetic to the demands of the registration work. By the same token, Mrs Bedford Fenwick's resolution to check and verify applications met with little opposition when originally proposed to Council.[64] Nevertheless, notwithstanding the dubious validity of the accusations against Mrs Bedford Fenwick, Ministry officials held out little hope for reinstating members on any terms. There was, however, no legal means of removing Mrs Bedford Fenwick, and even if there were, it was feared she might be driven, perversely, to launch an anti-registration campaign. Dissolving the Council was not considered as an option since there was still no electorate and the rules for elections had not yet been framed.[65]

Three options were suggested for ministerial action. The first recommended that the Minister tell Mrs Bedford Fenwick the present Council members would not serve with her, and there was no prospect of inducing other qualified and representative persons to take their place. In such circumstances he would have no alternative but to ask her to resign. If she refused, the Minister would indicate that he would not take steps to fill the vacancies which had arisen and, in the absence of a quorum, the Council would become defunct. If Mrs Bedford

Fenwick refused to resign, she might either apply for an order of mandamus to compel the Minister to make some fresh appointments, or raise the question in Parliament at the beginning of the next session. In the case of the order of mandamus, it was thought the Court would probably refuse to grant the application in the face of a strong affidavit from the Minister. Alternatively, if the question were raised in Parliament the Minister could state the facts without fear of any proceedings for libel. Such a debate, was likely to render Mrs Bedford Fenwick's position untenable.[66] The second, more risky possibility, suggested by Priestley, was to dissolve the Council and appoint a new one, even without an electorate. It was not clear, however, whether the Minister could assume powers of this kind, since this was a situation for which the Act had made no provision.[67] The third option, suggested by Morant and most favoured by the resigning Council members, was to amend the rules relating to the election of committees and to arrange for the re-election of all committees at the beginning of the following year. This would enable the majority of members to prevent Mrs Bedford Fenwick's election to any committee. As a member of Council only, then, it was felt that 'opportunities for mischief would be greatly reduced'.[68] Arrangements could then be made to admit to the state register *en bloc* nurses on the register of the College of Nursing. The Council could then press on with the preparation of rules for future elections. As soon as 20,000 nurses were on the Register, the present Council could be dissolved and an election held under conditions which would give Mrs Bedford Fenwick little chance of being elected.[69]

The Minister, accompanied by Sir Arthur Robinson and Brock, received a deputation of the majority of members who had resigned from the Council in December 1921.[70] With some irritation, the Minister remarked how curious it was for the majority of a Council to resign in protest against a minority. Somehow it seemed quite ludicrous for the majority to resign due to their inability to control 'one elderly lady of uncertain temper'.[71] Acknowledging that Mrs Bedford Fenwick's posturing and bearing could doubtless give offence, he claimed that she herself seemed unaware of any offence given.[72] Unfortunately the constitution of the Council gave him no power to call on a member to resign. However, Section 2(2)(e) of the Nurses' Registration Act probably gave the Council the power to submit a rule for approval making it possible to call on a member to resign. If the Council failed to take this course of action, he would then be placed in the ridiculous position of going to the House of

Commons and asking for the repeal of an Act 'because the people who had asked for it were incapable of carrying out its provisions'.[73] There was, it seemed, no easy solution to the problem since Mrs Bedford Fenwick, as the individual most responsible for the passing of the Act, could equally wreck its success.[74] Meanwhile, Sir Arthur Robinson sought the advice of Sir Cooper Perry, member of the College of Nursing Council and Dean of Guy's Hospital Medical School, to identify a prospective chairman. Thus, with the help of a mutual friend, the Minister hoped to come to some understanding with Mrs Bedford Fenwick.

The 'friend' referred to was Sir Wilmot Herringham, consultant physician at St Bartholomew's Hospital. Sir Wilmot and Mrs Bedford Fenwick had been brought up in the same Morayshire village. But the association appears to have ended with kinship of birth and work-place. Relations between the two seem always to have been strained.[75] In the event Mrs Bedford Fenwick refused to resign, but Sir Wilmot agreed to take on the chairmanship of the Council.[76] This was endorsed by the College contingent, whose support was crucial to the success of state registration. With the College in control, Sir Cooper Perry gave assurances that he and Sir Arthur Stanley, Chairman of the College of Nursing Council, would do all they could to secure the adhesion of the College of Nursing membership to make up a respectable electorate.[77]

A number of suggestions were offered by the Minister to enhance the efficiency of registration itself. A system of block registration was recommended. Thus qualified nurses would be automatically admitted from recognised organisations. With such a scheme it would be theoretically possible in twelve months to create an electorate and for an elected Council to assume administration of the Act. A Council elected by only a small minority of the qualified nurses in the country was regarded as potentially disastrous.[78] Miss Cox-Davies agreed that existing registration methods were hopeless but that block registration had been the original intention of the College of Nursing, in the hope that, had their Bill become law, all nurses on the College register would automatically become state registered without incurring a further fee. The College would then simply hand over its funds to the GNC.[79] The question of a double fee for state and College registration had been a major source of contention within the College Council.

But designing the mechanics of registration was considered an issue for the Council to settle. Deferring action for fear of reprisals in the *British Journal of Nursing* was untenable. While Mrs Bedford

Fenwick could always comment upon decisions taken by the Council, the Minister would ask her to stop publishing proceedings. Sir Arthur Robinson pointed out that a small amendment to rule 44(2) would enable the Council to reappoint all committees at the beginning of the year, and that this could provide a mechanism for securing a more 'satisfactory' composition for the registration committee.[80]

Interestingly, amendments to the rules used for the new registration procedure were questioned in Parliament. Mr Kenny, a Labour MP, alleged that the new rule practically instituted a 'dictatorship' and delegated the business of the Council to a paid official, the registrar.[81] This opened the door to 'irregularities and evasions of the Act'. He requested that these rules be reconsidered. Sir Alfred Mond retorted that the functions of the Council were to settle questions of policy, adjudicate on doubtful cases and regulate practice. The precedent existed to delegate responsibility for the examination of all clear cases, and this was the practice of similar bodies. He strongly deprecated the suggestion that such a rule was conducive to evasions of the Act.[82]

RECONCILING NATIONALISM

Amending rules for registration, however, had repercussions for reciprocity with the other Councils and admission standards for existing nurses, and it seems that various parties sympathetic to Mrs Bedford Fenwick's views were not slow in pointing these effects out.[83] The original Act stated that there was to be reciprocity of rules governing the conditions of admission to the register of nurses registered in Scotland and Ireland. The objective of the Act had been to secure uniform standards of qualification in all parts of the United Kingdom, and in doing so, the GNC for England and Wales was to consult with similar Councils in Scotland and Ireland. A parliamentary question from Major Barnett, an open supporter of Mrs Bedford Fenwick, alleged that the rules for admission to the English register had been framed without reference to the other Councils. Nationalistic tensions were increased when it was suggested that it was unusual for a state body to accept entrants at second hand. Any register accepting such entrants, it was argued, was potentially weakening its position in the eyes of the profession and the public, and reciprocity in such cases could theoretically be considered void. A nurse, for instance, failing to register in Scotland might conceivably come to England and, under the looser provision, register there. She could then claim registration in Scotland under the reciprocity rule. Such a rule, it was maintained, should be considered *ultra vires*.[84]

The debate over reciprocity not only increased nationalistic tensions between the different Councils but raised further questions around the criteria for absorbing existing nurses onto the register. After heated debate, an amendment was tabled by Dr Chapple to the criteria originally set out by the Council in the House of Commons on 14 June 1923.[85] The criteria for assimilating existing nurses had originally been drawn up to exclude those from the Voluntary Aid Detachment (VADs). Candidates were to have been engaged in practice three years before November 1919 and to have completed a year's training. Dr Chapple's amendment challenged the latter point. His amendment substituted medically vetted competence in medical and surgical nursing and suitability to sit an examination, if necessary, set by the Council.[86] The Chapple amendment was regarded as a dilution of standards and a retrograde step by critics, but revealed the limited extent to which the Council could resist outside pressure and exercise independent action.[87] The amendment was perceived by some as the final insult to the status of the register and training. One nurse complained that trained women felt 'let down so badly by the Registration Act . . . there would be little incentive to register'.[88] The editor of *Nursing Mirror* echoed the sentiment, writing that she would probably withdraw her name from a register which had 'ceased to be of the slightest value to a properly trained nurse'.[89] Some complained of deception on the part of the Council, and of the amendment as the defeat of registration.[90]

CONCLUSION

Unresolved tensions between the moderate and radical sections of nursing opinion resurfaced in the Caretaker Council. Tempests and tirades vitiated the early Council business, reducing the number of nurses on the register by July, the month for the first elections, to only 12,000.[91] By then only dubious cases were being passed to the Registration Committee for consideration. Mrs Bedford Fenwick failed to be elected to the Council in July 1923. Opportunities for any direct influence upon the body she had done so much to create receded, but did not disappear entirely. Through her contribution to the early Council debates on training, Mrs Bedford Fenwick ensured a legacy for her vision of professional status for nurses.

The history of the Caretaker Council reveals the need there was for the Council to look to Ministry officials for leadership in the interpretation of its duties. The Council experienced a crisis of its legitimacy. Not only did the crisis reveal nurses' inexperience in policy-making, but the antipathy towards Mrs Bedford Fenwick's leadership weakened College of Nursing support for state registration still further. Indeed it raises the question of whether the College of Nursing was ever greatly committed to state registration. Mrs Bedford Fenwick's uncompromising attitude may well have provided the College cadre with the ideal escape from any statutory responsibilities. The College maintained a strong interest in substituting its own register for a state-backed system, even after the passing of the Act. By August 1920 the College of Nursing register claimed to have the names of 19,000 trained nurses and was regarded as the largest and most reliable list of qualified women by Ministry officials.[92] Consistent with this spirit the *Nursing Times*, as late as August 1920, warned that it was a serious mistake to assume that state registration would render unofficial registers useless.[93] But with the College of Nursing's co-operation secured and the radicals dispatched, the Ministry could assume moderation in the Council's proceedings would prevail. Conventional professional/bureaucratic conflict was not in evidence during the early days of the Council's existence; friction came from within more than from without, and there is little evidence of adversarial politics separating Ministry officials from nurse leaders. This was set to change. The relation of the Council's nurse education policy to wider government objectives in health policy and the consequences this had for professional/bureaucratic relations are discussed in the chapter which follows.

Chapter 6

The education policy of the General Nursing Council (1919–32)

INTRODUCTION

Although Mrs Bedford Fenwick lost her place on the Council in 1923, her vision of nursing education was not immediately extinguished. A number of standing committees were established after the passing of the Registration Act, including one connected with education and examinations.[1] As a member of that subcommittee, Mrs Bedford Fenwick found a channel for her ideas on the aims, content and structure of nursing education. Her unyielding views on the highest possible standards being applied to nurse training brought her into direct confrontation with a large section of the committee's members. The question of educational standards proved so controversial that a Select Committee was required to impose a settlement.

High hopes were cherished for the education and examinations committee as a vehicle for realising the Council's ambitions. These were dashed and diluted by a number of changes in the wider political economy of health care. This chapter explores the impact of the changes in the political economy of health care upon nurse education policy formulated by the Council. I consider the objectives and content of the Council's education policy, as well as the pressures shaping its determination. I argue that nurse education expressed in microcosm some of the tensions involved in adjusting the supply of female labour to the changing demands for welfare in the inter-war period. The discussion focuses primarily upon the general register, but other registers are considered as appropriate.

One of the first tasks of the newly convened Education and Examinations Committee was to devise a draft syllabus for use in the general hospitals and an affiliation scheme aimed at grouping hospitals to provide a balanced range of clinical facilities. The affiliation scheme and syllabus were interdependent and raised the question of resources and responsibility for training. Ideally standards were to be improved without compromising poorly resourced institutions. But this issue extended far beyond the epistemological details of curricular design; it drew attention to the piecemeal and unco-ordinated growth of health care more generally. Nurse training raised a number of crucial questions about responsibility for the funding and organisation of public and voluntary hospital agencies.

The first problem confronting the Council was the dearth of information about current training facilities. This undermined its capacity to plan for training provision on a rational basis. In medical education, a comprehensive survey had identified the distribution and characteristics of training resources, but no such data were available for nurse training.[2] One of the first tasks undertaken by the Council, therefore, was to conduct a survey of training facilities. This was perceived as an important preliminary to drawing up plans for the co-ordination of training functions and facilities. Information was requested on nurse–patient ratios, varieties of clinical department, numbers of beds, types of case, frequency of examinations, numbers of lectures given, details of administration, teaching staff and use of independent examiners.[3] This was the first survey of training facilities for nurses in England and Wales. It gave no details of the response rate and its findings were limited to the Poor Law Sector. The data included accommodation for patients and types of training schools. There were 640 Unions, with 94,000 beds for the sick. Facilities for training were divided into ninety major and twenty-five minor schools recognised by the Ministry of Health. Major schools maintained a resident medical officer and had 250–1,400 beds. Minor schools had no resident medical officer and had 110–280 beds. A certificate of training from a recognised school qualified a superintendent nurse for the office of matron. Roughly 1,400 probationers completed their training annually, including a small number of male nurse probationers. These numbers were expected to increase with the reduction in the working week from fifty-six to forty-eight hours.[4] Recognised schools required three years' training, and some offered massage and midwifery in the fourth year.

Notwithstanding a common authority to oversee training, there was no uniform pattern to training or examination. Training tended to rely upon the personnel and staff, the amount of teaching material available on the wards, and the extent of the guardians' interest in the matter. Whilst a few Boards were renowned for providing every facility for training, including sister tutors, preliminary schools and extra experience, most did not. Theoretical training consisted of a six- or seven-month course of lectures and demonstrations for two years during the winter, followed by an examination by the doctors and the matron at the end of the year. The third year was generally spent on revision.[5]

The Education and Examinations Committee was hampered in its efforts to devise policy sensitive to the conditions in institutions by the poor quality of data available. Consequently it was forced to rely upon the experience of its members when formulating rules for the conduct of examinations, training experience, and criteria for admission of candidates to the register.[6] A draft syllabus was drawn up by Miss Lloyd Still, chairwoman of the Education and Examinations Committee.[7] Like many of her contemporaries, Miss Lloyd Still was educated at home, largely by her father. She complained in later years she was 'not really educated', but her biographer, Lucy Seymour, claimed her enthusiasm as a reader compensated for any lack of formal instruction. Miss Lloyd Still took considerable interest in post-qualification training and in 1913 had made preliminary inquiries at King's College, London, in order to establish a one-year course for qualified nurses. A scheme and syllabus were drawn up and discussed with King's College and the Nightingale Fund Council. The war intervened, but in 1924 these proposals evolved into the Diploma in Nursing of the University of London, first awarded in 1926. Miss Lloyd Still became one of the first Advisory Committee members and an examiner for the university in hospital administration.[8]

Miss Lloyd Still's contribution to nursing education was not reflected in her published writings. Her influence needs to be deciphered from discussions in policy documents. She seems to have viewed nursing as a practical craft rather than an academic endeavour. As late as 1937 she warned the International Council of Nurses (ICN) against the dangers of making 'a study. . . instead of an informed and skilled practice of nursing'. Science and art were necessary but should be applied.[9] She was similarly pragmatic with respect to the pace of reform: 'Do not let us be in a great hurry to make reforms. Take Time. Go slowly.'[10]

No explicit details are provided in the Council minutes as to how the content of the syllabus for the general register was determined. The syllabus was conceivably based on what was already taught at St Thomas's. Miss Lloyd Still claimed that only subjects already taught in hospitals were included, although they were drawn up in a different way; they represented a synthesis of what already existed.[11] Critics were not reassured. Some perceived the syllabus as the product of a large teaching hospital. Even members of the Examination and Education Committee considered it too comprehensive for the smaller hospitals to cope with. The appointment to the Council of representatives from the Board of Education had intended to bring general educational expertise within the reach of the Council. However, no consultation seems to have taken place with representatives of the Board of Education to ensure that general educational principles were adhered to in the programme.

The question of whether the syllabus for teaching and examination was to be a compulsory or advisory measure was also controversial. The status of the syllabus was critical in determining the standard of entry for future nurses on to the register. Mrs Bedford Fenwick insisted that only a compulsory syllabus, which would 'command the respect of intelligent women and qualify them to follow their duties efficiently', should be recommended; the 'national vice' of expediency, she argued, should be avoided at all costs.[12] Concern was also expressed by individual members of the Committee about the stringency of examination and its effect upon recruitment. Anxiety revolved around the need for the examination to be of sufficient standard to protect the public, but without excluding the average institutions of nursing. Miss Lloyd Still attributed complaints to a lack of understanding.[13] Miss Worsley stated that the Liverpool hospitals were much against the statutory syllabus. Mrs Bedford Fenwick reminded the committee that practices in some of the training schools exceeded the standard laid down by the Council. A uniform standard would not be possible without statutory powers, and she hoped the Council would support the Education Committee in enforcing the standard laid down in the syllabus.[14] The Council was undecided on whether the syllabus at this stage should be compulsory or advisory, one of training or examination.

PRESSURE FROM WITHOUT

To test opinion and defuse criticism, it was decided that the syllabus should be circulated to all heads of training schools for comment. Several letters of complaint had been received from the County Medical and Poor Law Officers. A deputation was received from representatives from Poor Law training schools. These related to four main points: the overloaded nature of the first year, the need for post-registration training for ward sisters, the strain the syllabus would impose on hospitals with less generous facilities, and the narrow outlook of nurses after hospital training.[15] As it stood the draft syllabus required remodelling to ensure the theoretical instruction and elementary science subjects could be treated in outline only. Second, examination rather than training standards should be represented by a syllabus. Third, certain subjects, such as the metric system, could be omitted until established in the elementary school curriculum. Finally, examiners should include matrons and medical officers from Poor Law infirmaries only.[16] A number of deletions were requested from the curriculum, including that of drainage systems. Miss Lloyd Still defended the introduction of drainage systems in the interests of simplifying the first year: 'the keeping clean of lavatories, the ventilation of rooms, was in quite a simple form . . . gave the nurse something to think about'.[17] Elementary science was considered useful, especially if the nurse were later to take up district work; gynaecology was a subject which, Miss Lloyd Still considered, every nurse should know, especially for private work. Such questions were of national significance and not merely of parochial concern.[18] Mrs Bedford Fenwick replied that a resolution had provided for a proportionate division of responsibilities between doctors and nurses and that Poor Law Officers and matrons would also be given consideration.[19] Mrs Williams of the Swansea Board of Guardians asked the Council whether it intended to recommend preparatory schools in different districts. Mrs Bedford Fenwick confirmed the Council's acceptance of the principle of preliminary schools but added that such provision would depend upon economics.[20] Mr Frater, Councillor and Chairman of Tynmouth Union Board of Guardians, stated that training schools welcomed the high standard of training and would endeavour to fall in line with the excellent syllabus the Council had drawn up.[21]

The County Medical Officers of Health for England and Wales lobbied on behalf of public health and district nurses. They argued that nurses should be involved in educating the public by 'bringing the scientific information we have on such matters as food, exercise, the effect of fresh air, spread of infection within the reach of the public'.[22] Medical practitioners were neither trained nor available for this kind of work. Moreover, the nurse's work was concerned with the management of the patients' personal and environmental hygiene. A thorough course of hygiene based on physiology and anatomy was considered far better for a nurse than the 'smattering of medicine and surgery which she is at present taught'.[23] Current hospital training programmes were criticised as being oriented towards work requiring 'much less thought and initiative than that of a district nurse'.[24]

Defending the syllabus, the Council stressed that some attempt had been made to accommodate public health and sanitation in the curriculum. Including such material represented a deliberate attempt by the Council to 'widen...outlook and to counteract the limited vision sometimes acquired in sick wards'.[25] Public health and welfare work was mentioned in the syllabus partly as an inducement to recruitment for such work.[26] Nurse training was seen as fulfilling wider social objectives; it could help the nurse 'realise her duty towards (patients) as a responsible citizen'.[27] However, the precise effect that these preliminary comments had upon the shape of the final syllabus is difficult to estimate.

Wider reaction to the syllabus was to be gauged publicly by an informal conference of hospital matrons and sister-tutors in April 1921. This 'Great Conference' was a unique consultation exercise in the Council's history. In her introductory address to the meeting, the chairwoman outlined the statutory duties of the Council. She explained that its business was to set a uniform standard of education in nurse training schools, and to formulate rules and regulations for the examinations which future nurses would have to take prior to being registered. One of the chief tasks of the Council was to co-ordinate the essentially competing systems of training which prevailed and to devise a means of forging these into a national system. Hitherto each hospital had been a law unto itself, catering for its individual needs only. Parochialism had promoted widely varying standards of training and resources. Localism was to give way to the national interest. The chairwoman continued by claiming that the syllabus of training was intended to unify training schools by providing some definite material upon which to organise facilities. Training should aim to produce a clinical assistant without excessive theoretical training, or 'an efficient machine at the expense of the vitalising spirit...[to] develop the mind as well as the heart and hand'.[28] Vestiges of liberal educational and individualistic principles are evident from this concern with the probationers' development. Probationers were to be encouraged to increase their knowledge of scientific, social and practical subjects, and to broaden their perspective beyond that fostered by the narrow confines of an institution. Curative and preventive work was to be undertaken, and particular emphasis was placed on that which concentrated on the nation's child and maternal health, its racial inheritance and economic and social state.[29] This comprehensive training was intended to enable the nurse to develop along any one of the allied branches of practice at the end of training.[30] It was hoped that a flexible system of training would be developed to accommodate all schools irrespective of the prior education of recruits; a rise in standards was to be achieved without imposing excessive strain.[31] This was the most explicit and comprehensive statement of education policy produced by the Council.

A barrage of criticism was aimed at the syllabus. The first year in particular was regarded as over-weighty. Many regarded the terminology as intimidating and the entire content as overcrowded. Miss Cummins, Matron of the Liverpool Royal Infirmary, complained that the language used throughout the syllabus was too complex: 'it was impossible for the rank and file to see into the minds of those who had composed it'.[32] Miss Lloyd Still urged that words and terms could be translated by the teacher into 'kindergarten language . . . and . . . understood by the most illiterate nurse'.[33] This rejoinder exemplifies the Council's key dilemma: how to raise standards in a population whose scholastic achievement was low.[34]

Miss Musson, Matron of the General Hospital, Birmingham, declared atmospheric pressure, drainage systems, antenatal care and child welfare were out of place in the first year.[35] Smaller training schools were considered particularly disadvantaged in reaching the standards, due to the difficulty in attracting probationers of even a moderate level of education.[36] Similar fears were articulated by other matrons: the candidates with whom they had to deal were girls with elementary education, 'of the reticent class,' who began earning their living at about 14 years of age. As a consequence the smaller hospitals tended to attract the 'failures' of other occupations.[37] The volume of elementary science included in the syllabus was perceived as of no practical value to the nurse; it took up time better spent on the wards.[38]

Objections were not confined to small hospitals. Miss Cummins hoped the Council would not lose sight of the fact that it was moral and not only theoretical qualifications which made up the nurse.[39] Miss McIntosh from St Bartholomew's endorsed the view that the syllabus might be overcrowded: 'it took the shy probationer three years to find her feet'. Probationers would get a very superficial idea of the range of nursing work and might be confused in assimilating the proposed volume of material. Indeed, it was feared that first-year probationers might break down under the strain of work and study.[40]

The ambitious scope and objectives of the syllabus threatened many representatives at the 'Great Conference'. The plan for co-ordinating schools was one in which it was hoped all of them could participate, irrespective of the educational level of nurses. An elastic system had been evolved to allow a steady rise in standards without imposing undue strain on less advantaged institutions.[41] It was hoped the Council would introduce a uniform standard of training on comprehensive lines to ensure a one-portal examination for admission to the state register of trained nurses. The syllabus was intended to provide a guide to a minimum level of attainment expected of probationers.

As a preliminary to imposing common standards upon hospitals differing in size, wealth and patient mix, the Council proposed a number of schemes for the grouping of hospital training schools. These would allow probationers to obtain a more diverse and comprehensive training experience and would also enable consortia of hospitals to share a more extensive range of teaching staff. Mrs Bedford Fenwick applauded the scheme, which utilised 'all available material' in hospitals for training.[42] Conjoint schemes for reciprocal training between registers were proposed as the means by which hospitals could affiliate into a comprehensive network. This presented the Council with one of its most difficult challenges: the evolution of a scheme in which the many small hospitals could be assimilated without compromising standards. The resulting measure was a complicated formula involving permutations of bed numbers, residency of medical officer and specialism. Complete training schools were those which had satisfied the Council that medical, surgical, gynaecological and children's diseases services were provided. At least one resident medical officer was to be kept and the period of training was to be not less than three years. The ratio of medical to surgical beds was not to exceed 2:1 or be less than 1:2. Affiliated hospitals were not considered sufficiently large to give a complete training, but they could be affiliated to a complete training school. In such institutions four years training was compulsory, with two years being spent in the affiliated hospital. The preliminary state examination was to be taken at the end of the second year.[43]

Implicit within the scheme was a hierarchy of institutions ranging from the large general teaching hospitals to the small specialist ones.

Specialist hospitals were potentially disadvantaged by proposals which required them to extend the training period from three to four years. In language reminiscent of a conventual model of organisation, small 'satellite' specialist institutions would be grouped around a 'mother' hospital.[44] The longer period of training required for conjoint training schemes was perceived as an indication that Council considered such institutions inferior. Payment of Poor Law nurses training in voluntary hospitals was also raised as a potential problem. Although the guardians were identified as the appropriate paymasters, there was no guarantee that they would agree. The Council, however, attempted to circumvent the resource problem by devolving 'grouping' arrangements upon hospitals themselves.[45] Smaller hospitals, though, were again particularly loath to sacrifice their identity in a group configuration; in particular they were highly critical of the scheme which used number of beds as an index of quality in assessing the training merits of institutions.[46]

The Council faced a formidable task in formulating an educational policy for a heterogeneous occupation whose complexity was compounded by the diversity of the health care system. It was estimated in 1919 that there were about 1,500 training schools. This made the Council's task very different from that of the General Medical Council (GMC) in 1858, which had been required to oversee medical education in only 24 centres.[47] The Council was therefore required to rationalise the provision of training and bring some order to the existing chaos of nurse education. In short, it had to rebuild educational resources from its very foundations. All this was to be achieved at a time when major changes were being planned in health service administration.

Government intervention in nurses' registration can be considered complementary to the establishment of the Ministry of Health and the centralisation of administrative arrangements for health policy more generally. Shortly after his appointment as the first Minister of Health, Dr Christopher Addison appointed Lord Dawson of Penn as chairman of the newly formed Consultative Council on Medical and Allied Services.[48] One of the first tasks for this Council was to make recommendations on a scheme for the systematised provision of medical and allied services.[49] Existing health services involved considerable administrative complexity and division of responsibility. A chasm existed in the hospital system between the public and voluntary hospitals. The Cave Commission on Voluntary Hospitals was established to investigate the question in detail, and with remarkable speed produced its first report in 1921.[50] Indeed it reported so quickly that it gave the impression of having prejudged the issue.[51] Although it drew attention to the limited co-ordination, overlap and disparity of resources within the hospital sector, its recommendations were concerned merely with shoring up the existing system rather than effecting fundamental change.

Robert Morant, first Permanent Secretary in the Ministry of Health, viewed the financial position of the voluntary hospitals with deep pessimism. This was a view shared by some leading proponents of the voluntary system. A deputation of representatives from the voluntary hospitals for London met with Dr Addison in April 1920 to discuss their plight.[52] Government subsidy and co-ordination with Poor Law facilities were suggested as a means of easing hardships. Addison mentioned that supervision would be a condition of government subsidy and that this could most readily be channelled through major local authorities. He added that he was anxious to preserve the voluntary effort and in the short term was prepared to make arrangements to help the hospitals over their current financial crisis. This was intended only as a stop-gap on the way to establishing an improved and more permanent scheme for the provision of services for the community as a whole.[53]

EDUCATION FOR HEALTH

Morant favoured municipalisation as the solution to the precarious financial position of the voluntary hospitals.[54] Such thinking echoed the Fabian socialism of the Webbs.[55] Charles Webster has emphasised the importance of the Webbs–Morant connection in the dissemination of socialist ideas on health service reform. Morant was friendly with Beatrice and Sydney Webb, who were given to patronising and promoting the careers of promising public servants.[56] Morant was also well known to Lord Dawson, responsible for the *Interim Report on Medical and Allied Services*. Indeed Morant was on the best of terms with Dawson.[57] Dawson's scheme for a stratified and integrated system of primary, secondary and tertiary health centres borrowed the terminology and organisational principles of education. Before being employed in the Ministry of Health, Morant had been Secretary at the Board of Education, where he had been the chief architect of the 1902 Education Act. The symmetries between the recommendations of the Dawson report and the Education Act of 1902 suggest that Morant worked on health issues by analogy with education. In a handwritten note to Addison, Morant revealed the parallels between the two areas:

> Elaborate a little the Health Services e.g. Arrange for every place of suitable size to have its primary health centre (just as naturally as its elementary school) . . . and for every area of a larger size to have as its secondary Health Centre (just as naturally as its secondary school) with its higher health services . . . eight contiguous counties to have its tertiary centre (just as naturally as its university).[58]

The Education Act of 1918 was intended to promote a constructive partnership between the central and local authorities. Moreover, it was designed to organise education on a progressive, systematic and comprehensive plan.[59] Similar assumptions underpinned Ministry of Health plans for the extension of health services. An analogical pattern of thinking was applied by Morant to nursing education. College of Nursing Council minutes for 1919 reveal that before the government's legislation on registration was prepared Morant had already indicated that nurse training schools should be recognised by the Board of Education. Training schools were expected to fulfil certain conditions concerning length of training and curriculum, to submit to inspection and to demonstrate an adequate staff of teachers. Such schools were expected to receive assistance from the grant for technical education based upon returns from schools of probationers in training. Schools duly recognised in this way would be recommended to group themselves to form an examination board. Board of Education assessors would then be appointed to take part in qualifying examinations, and nurses who passed such examinations would be placed on the register.[60]

The possibility of grants being made available to hospitals for nurse training and administered by the Board of Education was seriously considered by officials before and after the General Nursing Council (GNC) was created.[61] What is less clear is the extent to which such arrangements were expected to operate in concert with, or independently of, the Council. The prospect of grants being available for nurse training was one of the reasons behind the Ministry of Health's decision to include Board of Education nominees on the Nurses' Registration Council.[62] Morant maintained that Board of Education views on training would carry more weight if associated with the leverage of a grant. He hoped too that Board of Education views would be formulated in close consultation with the Ministry of Health.[63] Superficially it also seemed logical that the training of nurses should be dealt with by the same central department which dealt with the training of health visitors and midwives. Such a strategy was calculated to strengthen government control over decision-making within the Council. The Treasury, though, was resistant to any proposal that grants for nurse training should be provided. It was argued that the administration of grants for the training of health visitors should be undertaken by the Ministry of Health and not by the Board of Education. Morant, however, claimed that he had managed to convince the Treasury that their view was erroneous and succeeded in widening the scope of the measure to include midwives and nurses.[64]

The question of grants for nurse training lay dormant until the GNC had produced its training proposals. It received renewed impetus from the publication of the Cave Commission report, which recommended grants should be made for the training of nurses. Support for this measure came from the British Hospitals Association (BHA), which argued that nurses trained in hospitals were a national resource, who were regularly absorbed by the general nursing service of the country. The costs of training, hitherto borne by private bodies, should therefore be subsidised by the state. Grants should be administered by bodies in charge of funds for technical education.[65]

Brock shared Morant's views that facilities for technical training were primarily a matter for the Board. He was sceptical of the reasoning offered by the Committee to support their request for state aid. He considered it a camouflage device to obtain state assistance without prejudicing private generosity. Brock was unconvinced that the training of nurses involved a net cost to hospitals. The probationer provided the hospital with cheap labour, certainly during the latter part of training. The consequent saving of salaries resulting from the employment of probationers more than compensated for the cost of any instruction. It was not necessarily the case, however, that future regulations would enable such a situation to persist. Hospitals might be compelled to increase considerably their spending on training.[66] Janet Campbell, Senior Medical Officer for Maternal and Child Welfare in the Ministry of Health, conceded that ultimately the training of nurses would have to be organised systematically, but warned the time was not propitious for approaching the Treasury. Besides, Morant's view was not universally accepted in either Ministry of Health or Board of Education circles.[67] As part of the 'hospital machinery', nurses were learners as well as workers. The finance of training was therefore inextricably linked to the financing of the hospital itself. It was therefore claimed that it was difficult to specify how far any grants given would be expended on the purpose for which they were given.[68] Estimating the potential cost of grants was also problematic. On the basis of figures received from the College of Nursing, Brock calculated that a £25 per capita grant to hospitals would cost approximately £269,000 per annum.[69] On the basis of its current probationer complement, the London Hospital would be entitled to a grant of £10,000 per year. By the end of 1921 officials within the Board of Education were pessimistic about securing Treasury support for such proposals.[70]

Addison and Morant held similar views on the future financing and administration of nurse education.[71] The departure of Morant and Addison from the Ministry of Health removed the major sources of pressure for government-sponsored reform of nurse education. Morant's sudden death from pleurisy in March 1921, and Addison's demotion from the Ministry of Health to become Minister without Portfolio, left the GNC in an isolated position in pressing for further change. Addison's expensive housing project, proposed as part of his reconstruction programme as Minister of Health, brought him into conflict with Lloyd George, who was anxious to curb expenditure. Addison was replaced by Sir Alfred Mond, also a radical Liberal, but who substituted slum clearance for a new building programme.[72] Although Brock acted as a vehicle for Morant's views, he lacked Morant's visionary and crusading commitment. More important still, he was forced to operate in an economic climate hostile to increasing state expenditure. How far the GNC's decisions on inspection and grouping of hospitals were indebted to Morant's model of technical school education is open to question. Superficial similarities may obscure deeper differences and more independent strands of thought. Morant's formulation of plans for reshaping nurse education in advance of the establishment of the Council suggests he perceived only a limited role for it in controlling its policy. The word 'technical' was left loose by Morant, possibly deliberately so. Was it intended to imply a broadly based secondary school education or practical instruction for adults? Secondary school leavers were usually destined for the upper echelons of the labour force, whereas adults undergoing technical instruction were more often drawn from the semi- and unskilled levels.[73] Defining such a distinction would have revealed much about Morant's views on the social status of nurses.

Although the GNC's educational proposals were ultimately a pale reflection of Morant's vision of technical education, they were nevertheless in tune with his thinking on health service integration. The Council's strategy had been designed to unify the nursing services, mirroring unification of the health services. The syllabus had been issued with the object of welding together the various branches of nursing and giving training schools a new orientation towards health as a whole: 'it is a question of a new relationship, focus, and outlook, and is a big step in a national scheme of unification'.[74] Scotland had produced a report on the planning needs of hospital and nursing services after World War I, but no comparable document was prepared for the nursing services in England.[75] The Dawson report recommended a separate inquiry into nursing services, but its findings fell on the stony ground of economic retrenchment.[76] The impetus and rationale for harmonising governmental and Council policy were consequently lost. Although originally the GNC was perceived as an important ally in implementing government policy on social reconstruction, government influence receded as its policies gave way to the Geddes Axe.[77] However, governmental priorities were only one of a number of pressures influencing the Council's decision-making. Those emerging from within the Education and Examinations Committee will now be discussed.

DEINSTITUTIONALISING TRAINING

If the Council's policy had a modern ring, it was not because of any contact with and contribution from Board of Education experts. The Council's policy implied a student-centred and broadly based approach to learning, but there is no evidence that Board of Education appointees were involved in framing proposals at any stage. The Council's proposals were intended to foster the nurse's powers of development whilst increasing her capacity through a more extensive knowledge of scientific, social and practical subjects. A major priority was 'to train her mind to a wider outlook than usually obtained within the four walls of an institution, bringing into line with the curative measures the no less important branches of preventive work'. If the dominance of the institutional ethos in training was to be corrected, a comprehensive training was required to equip the nurse for any branch of nursing she might wish to undertake on the completion of training.[78] Furthermore the nation's health was to be promoted through its mothers, infant and child life, racial inheritance, economics and social state.[79]

THEORY AND PRACTICE

The correlation of theory and practice was a further major concern of the Council policy-makers. Introductory lectures on cell structure, the skeleton, joints, muscles and skin were intended to stimulate greater interest in clothing, personal hygiene, care of feet and hands and methods of cleaning. Instruction on instruments and wound dressing would be preceded by discussion of infecting agents, tissue reactions, disinfection and sterilisation methods, the composition and impurities of air, atmospheric pressure and heat.[80] Treatment of the alimentary tract for gavage and lavage presupposed a knowledge of the anatomy and physiology of the gut and 'food values'. Knowledge of the therapeutic action of drugs was a prerequisite for competent drug administration.[81] Venereal diseases and their transmission were considered a particular priority on account of their 'devastating effect on the race and the publicity given to these questions'.[82]

A nurses' chart, containing an inventory of tasks for the nurse to work through under supervision, was intended to give structure and system to clinical experience. This too provoked a number of objections: the ward sister was being 'robbed' of her prerogative as teacher and the guidelines produced for teaching were rigid and inflexible.[83] The syllabus for the second and third years provided headings as signposts to what specialists in the various fields might teach: bacteriology, materia medica, hospital economy, diseases of children, the eye, ear, nose and throat, and orthopaedics. These subjects were to be dealt with in outline only, being more suitable for 'postgraduate' courses.[84]

DOCTORING EXAMINATIONS

Although the nurse was to understand the bearing each subject had upon her work, it was also stressed 'how little of [medicine] . . . she herself touches or can know'.[85] This assertion contradicts the more liberal aims of the curriculum and reveals the enduring preoccupation with epistemological demarcation between medicine and nursing. In particular the Council was concerned 'that a nurse should be an inferior kind of medical practitioner'.[86] Dr Goodall, the medical spokesman for the Council, declared that doctors would probably play a smaller part in teaching elementary subjects than hitherto. Anatomy, physiology, chemistry and physics would, however, continue to be taught by medical men. He conceded that the role of medical men in nurse teaching had been abused in some instances: often it had been relegated to the junior members of the profession. Although this could be justified in relation to scientific subjects, pathology required more experienced practitioners. Teaching by medical men had also been overly theoretical, addressing subject matter more appropriate to the work of a matron or sister-tutor. Examinations in nursing subjects were no longer to be conducted by medical men but by trained nurses. Extolling the curriculum, Miss Barton, President of the Poor Law Matron's Association, expressed appreciation at what she considered a most 'stimulating syllabus'. She was convinced the standard of education would improve the calibre of recruits. Nurses, she argued, should be taught how to think and how to learn.[87] Miss Bodley, matron of Selly Oak Hospital, Birmingham, agreed and suggested that a preliminary course of training and examination could 'screen' out unsuitable candidates. There was general consensus that increasing the standard of education would have a positive effect upon recruitment provided the reputation of the hospital was enhanced at the same time.[88]

A meeting of the Education and Examinations Committee held after the 'Great Conference' discussed how best to accommodate the anxieties of the smaller hospitals within present arrangements. Many members were sympathetic to the difficulties of matrons and acknowledged that support for the syllabus originated from the larger hospitals.[89] Changes to the content and terminology used in the syllabus were recommended. Mrs Bedford Fenwick ridiculed such amendments as 'childish'.[90] Nurses had been denied justice in the organisation of their training and the syllabus was designed to remedy this deficit. However, incorporating criticisms was bound to under-mine the integrity of the syllabus; prejudice against the use of precise terminology represented the major obstacle to nursing reform.[91] Dr Goodall maintained that nurses were taught too much as if they were medical students. The texts he had read on nursing had all been written by medical men and gave the impression that the nurse was an inferior kind of medical practitioner.[92] Mrs Bedford Fenwick noted that junior medical men were put in the position of teaching nurses things they did not know themselves. She hoped nurses would refuse to be taught by untrained people, such as doctors![93] Miss Worsley denounced the curriculum as 'invertebrate and wobbling', but it was Mrs Bedford Fenwick who was most vocal in articulating construc-tive alternatives.

The question of encouraging the establishment of central preliminary schools to reduce the strain on smaller schools during the first year was welcomed by most as a useful strategy. It was strongly supported by Miss Tuke, Principal of Bedford College and representative of the Board of Education.[94] A resolution that a scheme of central preliminary nursing schools be recommended as part of the prescribed training for admission to the register for future nurses was submitted to the Council.[95] It was felt that a thorough preliminary training involving the pooling of resources might help reduce wastage and attract better candidates. Mrs Bedford Fenwick was convinced that the 'class' of nurse recruited twenty years ago had been lost and that the standard of 'culture' in nursing needed to be raised: 'at present nurses are classed as domestic servants'.[96] It was not clear by whom nurses were classified, whether by officials or in the eyes of the public. Miss Villiers confirmed the poor educational attainment of nurses in fever hospitals, her own area of expertise, many of whom she claimed could not even write a report on their patients.[97] This raised the question of minimum standards of entry into the occupation. No firm conclusions were reached, but this was soon to become a major issue which preoccupied the Council.[98]

COMPROMISING CONCESSIONS

Notwithstanding Council's efforts to take into account the varying resources of schools, ultimately it did not appear to have had a marked effect upon policy decisions. Indeed, Council was dismissive of criticisms and disinclined to make any real concessions.[99] The Council's consultations served more as a public relations exercise than as an occasion for promoting changes. Shortly after the conference, the Council wrote to Boards of Guardians inquiring whether they would be willing to adopt the syllabus as a precondition of being 'approved' for training. The Poor Law Unions were incensed at the Council's approach and communicated their anxiety to the Minister of Health. A subsequent move by Council to devise regulations on the status of the syllabus alarmed officials.

If the syllabus were intended to provide guidelines for nurse-training institutions, it need not be incorporated into the regulations and would not require ministerial approval. The question revolved around the meaning of 'prescribed'. Brock drew a distinction between the legal and policy implications of the term. Ministry legal advisers maintained that 'prescribed' meant prescribed by rule. This did not necessarily mean that, in policy terms, Council should issue rules laying down the detail of training. However, in all recent statutes the word 'prescribed' had carried a power to make rules. Requiring the Council to prescribe training was intended to give the Minister, and hence the legislature, the power of approving and modifying the proposals of the Council without tampering with the details of administration. Parliament had deliberately refrained from giving an entirely free hand to a body composed mainly of experts, 'who inevitably tend to look at the matter from a professional point of view'.[100]

Brock recommended a latitudinarian approach be taken in the definition of educational standards. Rules need not include details of a syllabus, but could well indicate the compulsory subjects in which candidates would be examined. Although the Council had issued the syllabus on its own authority, this did not necessarily compel its application. Attention was also drawn by Brock to the Council's lack of power to prescribe conditions pertaining to the approval of institutions. 'In neither case', the Council was reminded, 'are the Council given uncontrolled discretion.'[101] The standard for admitting nurses by examinations should follow those already applying to existing nurses. The Act did not empower the Council to make their approval conditional upon the adoption of the syllabus unless it was incorporated in the rules. It would in all likelihood be impossible for any institution to give the prescribed training without at the same time adopting the syllabus.[102] The test by which the rules can be judged, Brock added, was not whether the standard was ideal but whether it was a workable compromise between the ideal, 'which you and I would like to see realised', and what was practicable to demand of existing nurse-training institutions.[103]

Ministry officials adopted a strong line in setting out the Council's position. They were notably irritated at having to intervene in Council combat once more. The Council was instructed to emphasise that in future dealings with the Guardians, the syllabus was provisional and contingent upon the Minister's sanction to rules not yet submitted. The Minister recommended a simple rule providing for the total period of training for each part of the register, indicating that the instruction each nurse received in subjects for examination would be acceptable.[104] As an alternative route to achieving compulsory standardisation, the Council turned its attention to producing a syllabus of examination for scheduling to the rules.

POOR LAW PENALTIES

The Poor Law Unions complained that the Council had made little attempt to simplify the syllabus as they had requested.[105] Implementing such a policy would, they claimed, create a 'disastrous shortage' of applicants for training.[106] The Association urged the Minister to ask the Council to combine one syllabus for examination and adopt a gradualist stance towards improvement. Yielding to pressure from the Poor Law Association, Ministry and criticisms in the nursing press, the Council recommended that the training syllabus should occupy an advisory status only. In subsequent correspondence with the Ministry of Health, it was recommended that the only compulsory measure in training should be the examination syllabus. The ultimate test of the efficiency of an organisation would therefore be the performance of candidates in the prescribed examination. Thus the Council could gradually raise standards of training with the 'minimum of friction and without appearing to exercise their statutory powers in an arbitrary manner'.[107] An advisory syllabus had the advantage of elasticity in terms of its content and structure, but did not preclude Council from substituting a compulsory syllabus at a later stage.[108]

The nurse's chart, which listed the practical objectives of experience at each stage of training, was perceived by the Ministry as an attempt to introduce compulsion surreptitiously into the syllabus. Brock's annoyance with the apparent recalcitrance of the Council was provoked by Sir Willmot Herringham's request to have the matter considered speedily.[109] Herringham was anxious to point out that the chart was simply a method for recording the detailed practical work upon which the examination of theory and practice of nursing was to be based. It was not intended to have any examinable status but was simply to be deposited in the matron's office at the conclusion of each ward experience.[110]

The status of the training and examination syllabus remained controversial until resolved by a Select Committee in 1925. The Committee's terms of reference considered the scheme of election to the Council, specifically the reservation of seats for matrons, as well as rules respecting the prescribed training for nurses.[111] Mrs Bedford Fenwick and her supporters fought a determined rearguard action in defence of a vision of a rigorous training modelled on that of medicine and indifferent to the needs of training schools.[112] The early years of the GNC were marked by the institutionalisation of a regime which assigned priority to the development of a much wider dispersion of skills and local arrangements in the rationalisation of training provision. Arguments in favour of standards and safety, similar to those that had previously been advocated in favour of registration, were applied to the case for a compulsory syllabus. Permissive measures were dismissed as inadequate for improving standards. Without a compulsory syllabus, training was likely to remain haphazard and dependent upon the interests of the matron.[113]

A number of witnesses insisted a compulsory syllabus was essential to defining the standard of proficiency and encouraging more than a smattering of knowledge. Miss MacCallum argued for a uniform curriculum. The training of some nurses had omitted such crucial elements as the 'giving of hypodermics or the treatment of a case of haemorrhage'. Both of these were essential in private work. Nurses, she insisted, should be trained for the care of the sick, not for the convenience of the hospital.[114] Miss Kent, President of the Registered Nurses Parliamentary Council, drew an analogy with higher education. She argued that an advisory syllabus would be counter to the practice of every university, not only in England but abroad.[115] Brock warned that any attempt to drive up the standard too high would provoke resistance. He was careful not to specify the source of such reaction but tactfully implied a kinship between radical and ministerial aspirations: 'It is not that we do not want to get into the millennium, the danger is that we get into the millennium in one go.'[116]

The Select Committee disappointed radicals' aspirations. It concluded that 'training' did not necessarily involve anything more than existing rules. The Council was advised to take steps to ensure a minimum standard of training was available to all probationers and that inspection and advice, rather than a cast-iron syllabus, should constitute the measures of efficiency.[117]

The scheme of election to the Council, and therefore the criteria for selecting policy-makers, were also considered by the Select Committee. In particular it was debated whether the reservation for six out of the eleven seats allocated to matrons as general nurses should be perpetuated. Places had originally been reserved for matrons on the grounds of securing educational experience from 'experts'. Most witnesses advocated free elections on the grounds of precedent; Scotland and Ireland both had free elections, with results which differed little from those in England. Miss MacCallum was sceptical that a free election would alter the distribution of matrons. Nurses could not compete with matrons: they had neither the time nor the money to do so. Mrs Bedford Fenwick drew attention to the advantages of the richer nursing organisations in putting forward their candidates for election: matrons had significant advantages over nurses in any election due to their reputations.[118] Miss MacCallum considered the matrons' and nurses' interests mutually exclusive: 'ordinary nurses are barely allowed to call their souls their own'.[119] Although not referring directly to elections for the GNC, of which there had been only one and even then mismanaged, prevailing methods of selecting candidates were regarded by Miss Mac-Callum as at best undemocratic, if not blatantly corrupt. She declared: 'I myself have seen in a nurses' sitting room a list signed by the matron . . . containing the names of people to vote for.'[120] Brock was concerned for the opposite reason – that free elections could provide for the all too efficient selection of the most numerous category of nurses, those in the Poor Law sector.[121] Underlying many objections to free elections was the anxiety that nurses could not be 'trusted' to elect those with requisite experience. Such arguments were recognised by some witnesses as echoing earlier objections to extending the franchise to women.[122] The Committee concluded that little would be 'lost' by democracy and, irrespective of the election method used, it was unlikely to disturb the dominance of the nursing elite. In future, elections to the eleven seats for the general register were to be open to any nurse registered on the general part of the register.[123]

The failure to secure a mandatory syllabus was the final insult to the Bedford Fenwick vision of a unified profession with statutory standards of education. The Council had made some attempt to impose a unified foundation on the special branches of the occupation. All nurses, irrespective of specialism, would be expected to sit a common preliminary examination. This was intended as a minimum national standard which would increase mobility and accelerate training for other parts of the register. In reality, however, it tended to devalue the supplementary registers, since it implied that 'general' training should precede all other forms of nursing.

GENERALISTS AND SPECIALISTS

While some groups of nurses had welcomed being absorbed into the Council's registration system, others, notably male mental nurses, were not enthusiastic. Mental nurses had had their own nationally recognised credential since 1891 under the auspices of the Royal

Medico-Psychological Association (RMPA). Under the Nurses' Registration Act, the RMPA had expected to obtain delegated powers of examination to continue its established system of training and examination.[124] The Council were reluctant to volunteer powers to a medically controlled body and were determined to substitute their own Registered Mental Nurse examination and certificate. Union hostility to 'general hospital snobs' who represented a potential source of cheaper female labour, combined with the support of medical superintendents, ensured the primacy of the RMPA certificate throughout the inter-war period.[125] Although there is little direct evidence to suggest women were excluded from joining asylum unions, negative attitudes towards female nurses, and the existence of exclusionary practices in other male-dominated unions, may have prejudiced female recruitment.[126] The tendency of employers to demand multiple qualifications for promotion in the supplementary areas underlined the greater prestige of a general qualification. This strategy was reinforced by the economic imperative, which obliged nurses to work for probationer rates of pay for longer.[127]

The enormous variation in the sizes of different institutions, their geographical distribution and clinical facilities, raised the question of grouping hospitals to provide efficient facilities for general training. Conjoint and reciprocal schemes were devised to allow students to obtain more diverse experience and to support more elaborate educational staff and resources.[128] Such a scheme presupposed some means of monitoring training provision. The Council had no powers to inspect institutions. Poor Law hospitals were under the jurisdiction of the Ministry of Health, which already employed an inspectorate, many of whom were nurses. Council members criticised the Ministry's inspection procedure as perfunctory and sporadic. The Council considered its own system of self-completed questionnaire and random visits as inadequate.

Miss Dowbiggin described the conflict which occurred between the Guardians and matrons with respect to training and discipline.[129] Discipline was considered an important aspect of training and the Guardians insisted on maintaining control over the conduct and selection of staff. This implied dual responsibility in the supervision of training. A meeting was held between the Examinations and Education Committee and representatives of the Guardians to clarify responsibilities for training.[130] Joint consultation between Guardians, the Clerk and matrons was agreed upon to deal with matters of conduct and examinations.[131] Conditions for approval of general and

Poor Law hospitals were a chronic source of tension between the Council and the Ministry of Health. The Council was anxious that all hospitals should be treated alike in relation to the provision of training facilities, irrespective of the authority which controlled them. In particular, the Council sought to ensure that the provision for teaching in the hospitals under the Ministry of Health's authority was as satisfactory as those under the voluntary hospitals' and public health authorities' jurisdiction.[132] Successive attempts by the Council to gain powers of direct inspection for all training schools, using a full-time inspectorate, were rejected by Ministry officials throughout the inter-war period.

Shortly after the Council had been established, a verbal agreement had been made between Ministry officials and Sir William Herringham for Poor Law Hospitals to be approved automatically by the Council for training on the basis of procedures already operated by the Ministry's own inspectorate. This was regarded at the time as only a temporary measure occasioned by the lack of documentary evidence available on all hospitals. With the impetus of a favourable recommendation from the Select Committee behind it, the GNC pressed to have its criteria for approval of training institutions accepted universally.[133] The Ministry was against any change in existing inspection procedure in spite of support for the Council's terms by the BHA, Board of Control and Association of Poor Law Unions.[134]

The Ministry was petitioned on a number of occasions between 1925 and 1930 to allow the Council inspection rights in Poor Law institutions, but action was deferred. Latterly the Council were deflected on the pretext of allowing local authorities the opportunity to adjust to the Local Government Act of 1929. The Ministry doubted the Council's legal right to inspect approved training schools, and the more innocuous term 'visitation' was recommended. Following the Local Government Act, an increase in the number of inspections was invoked as contradicting the policy of minimising central control over local services. The scrutiny of local expenditure, and the search for economies by the associations of local authorities at the request of the Chancellor of the Exchequer, suggested that it was an unfavourable moment to put forward a proposal for increasing the number of inspections in hospitals.[135] The Ministry retaliated that dual inspection was wasteful at a time of pressure on public expenditure.

By the mid-1930s, resources could not be invoked as the major obstacle to inspection. The Council had accumulated a surplus of

£80,000 in liquid assets, which it proposed to use to appoint full-time inspectors. Ministry officials auditing the Council's accounts had commented unfavourably upon the large balances accumulated by it. Although no expense would be incurred by bodies other than the Council, the Ministry refused to sanction the use of the Council's assets for this purpose and suggested instead that it should reduce its registration fees. In 1933, following a deputation of the Council to the Ministry concerned with the training of probationer nurses in public assistance hospitals, a scheme of reciprocal accreditation for institutions based on joint consultation was evolved.[136] This collaboration did not reflect any weakening of the Council's resolve to gain direct inspection rights. However, the Ministry was not prepared to leave the approval of training schools in the hands of a professional body whose criteria for approval it considered rigid, arbitrary and capable of jeopardising the provision of services.

The final strategy for setting standards to which the Council had recourse was to withdraw accreditation from hospitals, or to deny it to them. The Registration Act had provided for an appeal mechanism against the Council's decision to deny approval by the Ministry. While this was perhaps initially intended as a means of exerting some positive control over planning operations, in the bleak economic environment of the 1920s it operated as a brake on the Council's powers. Loss of accreditation could impose further financial strains on an already compromised institution. The Ministry was anxious to protect the operation of local services and unwilling to have these jeopardised by the actions of a body not directly concerned with service responsibilities. On the two occasions where approval for training was not given owing to the low number of occupied beds, strong reaction was provoked by back-bench MPs, and the Council's decisions were over-ruled by the Ministry.[137]

As the government's plans for introducing a more unified and comprehensive health service became the casualties of economic retrenchment, the Council remained in an isolated position in attempting to co-ordinate health services. The 'millennium' of social reconstruction evaporated, with deflationary measures and cuts in public expenditure occasioned by the Geddes Axe. Divisions between voluntary and public-funded hospitals persisted throughout the inter-war period in spite of the insolvency of the voluntary hospitals. As mentioned above, the departure of Addison in April 1921 and the premature death of Morant from pleurisy in March 1920 removed the prime sources of pressure for reconstruction of the health services.[138]

Dawson lamented lugubriously, 'thereafter . . . the Ministry passed on stony ground'.[139]

CONCLUSION

The Council was only ever able to exert limited influence upon the quality of training provided in individual hospitals. Its early vision of a broadly based educational strategy was whittled down to the resource capacity of the average institution. The GNC's attempt to introduce national standards of nurse training, to promote unity and mobility within the various branches of nursing, was seriously undermined by wider administrative and economic factors. The financial plight and vested interests of the voluntary hospital system provided the major obstacle to the GNC's proposals to undertake a radical reorganisation of nursing training.

The inter-war period saw the comprehensive defeat of the elitist Bedford Fenwick vision of professional nursing education. The GNC was forced to accept a significantly diluted version of its educational proposals and only a minor regulatory role in upgrading the standards of nurse education. In principle, the Council's plans to co-ordinate hospital and community health services around nurse training schools can be considered a form of 'hierarchical regionalism'.[140] Daniel Fox argues that hierarchies of services were organised in geographic regions based on medical schools in the inter-war period, and that these provided the template for regionalisation under the National Health Service (NHS). Webster criticises this thesis on the grounds that Fox fails to produce evidence of the geographical and administrative boundaries implied by his term.[141] Furthermore, the operation of 'hierarchical regionalism' assumed a degree of co-operation between the different health service agencies which Webster argues did not exist.[142] The GNC's records do not reveal how conglomerates of hospitals were organised for teaching purposes. Examination pass rates did not distinguish between the various routes to the register, and consequently the success of affiliation schemes is difficult to evaluate. Although the Council seem to have taken account of impending changes in health service administration when drawing up their training proposals, there is little evidence of lobbying or any attempt to influence planning decisions or put forward a nursing alternative by the Council or nursing organisations.

In the face of such powerful and entrenched vested interests, it is hardly surprising that the Council failed to make an impression on the existing pattern of hospital and health service provision. On the occasions when the Council tried to implement a more idealistic version of policy, it was rapidly brought to heel by the Ministry of Health or Parliament. The first strategy adopted by the Council to improve the status of the occupation used education as the means for attracting high-calibre recruits. Failure to secure sufficient numbers of recruits forced the Council to reconsider its policy and seek alternative methods of exerting 'quality' control over its educational and gate-keeping functions. The Council therefore substituted a strategy of selection to reduce 'wastage' and enhance its educational results. Drawing its inspiration from educational psychology, the Council moved away from a medical model of curricular organisation to one involving closer identification with secondary education. Education continued to be perceived as the key strategy for remedying labour market problems in nursing.

Chapter 7

Commission and committee in nurse education policy (1930–9)

INTRODUCTION

Throughout the 1930s the General Nursing Council (GNC) was forced to respond to the intensifying demographic pressures which threatened to reduce the supply of nursing labour. Through its work as a validation body for training institutions, it was confronted with the effect of its decisions upon the workforce. As the gate-keeper of entry into the occupation, it had to contend with the interdependence of the service and educational implications of its work. Early in its history the Council assumed conditions of service as part of its routine responsibilities. One of the first issues debated by it was its stance on the Hours of Employment Bill. This was quickly dropped from the Council's agenda, however, when the Ministry of Health pointed out it did not strictly fall within its remit.[1] The length of the working week was a continual subject of debate and national negotiation throughout the inter-war period. Industrial strife and the political mobilisation of labour, both directly and indirectly, provided strong pressures for the reform of nurse training and conditions of service. Throughout the 1920s and 1930s the Labour Party and Trades Union Congress (TUC) produced blueprints for action which were adopted by policymakers before and after World War II. Questions of labour supply and regulation continued to plague the Council until they culminated in the first of several semi-official investigations into nursing conditions and training.[2] This chapter considers the impact of the political pressures which impinged upon the nursing labour market in the late 1920s and 1930s. In particular, it addresses the effects of industrial organisation upon the reform of nursing education.

INDUSTRIAL INFLUENCES

A number of tensions began to brew in the industrial sector as the social aspirations of the post-World War I era evaporated and gave way to economic orthodoxy. In particular, pledges to enforce a forty-eight-hour working week failed to materialise legally. Paradoxically, the only concrete effect of the tortuous negotiations between government, the TUC and employers was an extension of the miners' working week under the Coal Mines Act of 1926.[3] During the nineteenth and early twentieth centuries, hospitals had been exempted from most of the legislation passed to regulate the conditions and hours of industrial workers, including the Workmen's Compensation, Hours of Employment and Unemployment Insurance Acts. Great resistance was expressed by nurse leaders imbued with professional sensitivities to including nursing within any legislative measures promoted by the Ministry of Labour. However, the possibility of including nurses in the Hours of Employment Bill, designed to reduce the working week to forty-eight hours, was debated by the College of Nursing Council between 1919 and 1920. In other words, the exclusion of nurses from the legislation was not a foregone conclusion.

The Hours of Employment Bill underwent several permutations. The College was sympathetic to nurses being included in the second Bill of 1920, which was to bring nurses' statutory working week into line with other workers', but the College did not agree with overtime payments or time taken in lieu. It was claimed that the adoption of such a principle was not applicable to a 'profession founded upon a spirit of service to the community'.[4] A report of the Salaries and Superannuation Committee of the College demonstrated that hours worked by nurses varied from seventy-one hours for day and eighty-four hours for night duty to fifty-two and a half hours' day and fifty-nine and a half hours' night duty.[5] Inclusion of nurses in the Unemployment Bill implied that nurses employed in voluntary institutions could be treated as domestic servants. In any case, the committee regarded unemployment among nurses as small and at a level that could be met by special funds from the College. Furthermore, a referendum of College members revealed opposition to the inclusion of nurses in the Act.[6]

Incorporating nurses within either the unemployment or hours of employment legislation detracted from their claims to professionalism.[7] The inclusion of nurses in the Unemployment Insurance Act was rejected by the College on the grounds that in spite of this some individual hospitals, notably St Thomas's, persevered in classifying their nurses as domestic servants for contractual purposes.[8] The College recoiled at being included in any legislation sponsored by the Ministry of Labour.[9] The recommendation of a maximum forty-eight-hour week for nurses was, however, consistent with the College's earlier proposal from the Report of the Salaries Committee in 1919. The Parliamentary Committee of the College had initially recommended inclusion in the provisions of the Bill. However, the College Council was less convinced of the costs and benefits to be derived from inclusion in employment legislation. The position of nurses was further confused by the policies of the various institutions responsible for employing nurses. The British Hospitals Association (BHA), for example, offered to press all hospitals within its jurisdiction to establish a fifty-six-hour working week.

A resolution passed by the West Ham Board of Guardians in April 1924 urged all Board employees to be trade union members and that this be a condition of appointment.[10] The College protested against such a 'coercive' policy on the grounds that it would limit the number of candidates for posts of responsibility.[11] The College's attitude reflected its wider opposition to what it perceived as the rigidity of trade union organisation. But it was keen to maintain a membership profile in the Poor Law Sector, arguing that 'hard and fast rules could not be applied to those engaged in nursing without detriment to patients'.[12] The College was later forced in 1925 to open membership to probationer nurses on account of trade union competition. Certain Boards of Guardians made membership of a trade union a precondition of employment for all nurses, including those in training.[13] In the early 1920s the only group of nurses to be included in Whitley Council negotiations were those employed by the Ministry of Pensions. The result of the College's policy on pay and working conditions meant that salaries were left to the vagaries of market forces or whatever benefit or degree of industrial organisation could be secured from hostile employers.[14]

Towards the latter half of the 1920s, concern began to grow that the supply of nurses was insufficient to meet the demand for nursing labour. The Labour Party arranged a special conference in 1927 on nursing and kindred occupations.[15] The conference was conducted in two sessions, the morning session by the Right Hon. F.O. Roberts MP, ex-Minister of Pensions and Chairman of the Executive Committee of the Labour Party. The afternoon session was chaired by Beatrice Webb. A welcome address was given by Mr Ramsay MacDonald, who claimed that the nursing profession was in the throes of 'revolutionary change... intellectual and social ferment into which the minds of men and women are plunged at certain times, when as it were, the pot is coming to the boil'.[16] The issue apparently 'coming to the boil' was the demand by nurses for dignity and status as well as material improvements. The Labour leader declared himself 'a tremendous believer in status. We want to emphasise that status is just as important for the Nursing Profession as pay itself.'[17] According to MacDonald, the Labour Party was as interested in the nursing and medical professions as it was in coal mining or factory work. Nurses were as essential to the full conspectus of the Labour Party and central to the planning of any readjustments in the social services.[18]

Findings from a questionnaire survey of institutions and associations employing nurses confirmed that nurses were worse off with regard to remuneration, hours and general conditions of service than other groups of similar workers. However, the identity of comparable workers was not defined.[19] A forty-eight-hour week was recommended, with an eight-hour day, inclusive of lecture hours. Unionisation was advocated as the best means of dealing with conditions and exercising equality in bargaining power.[20] Whitley Council negotiation facilities were suggested for nurses employed by the state.[21]

The Labour Party used its report as the basis for a policy statement on nursing, recommendations from which were echoed in later reports produced by other bodies. Nursing education was criticised, in particular, for using probationers as cheap labour. A parallel was drawn with medical education, under which training schools were no longer to be subservient to the needs of the hospital. They should be organised and financed separately. Probationers were to be treated as students and domestic labour was to be delegated to ward maids. Preliminary schools of training were to be established and organised centrally to spread resources to less well-equipped areas. Training schools were to receive grants from educational authorities and maintenance scholarships were to be awarded to approved students. The GNC was to demand a prescribed syllabus and all students were to pass through a three-year programme of general training prior to specialisation.[22]

These issues, however, lay dormant until the Labour MP Fenner Brockway, chronicler of contemporary social problems, resuscitated the issue of hours of employment for nurses in 1930. An inveterate campaigner, he turned his attention to nursing as an extension of his commitment to workers' rights. Although he does not refer specifically to his involvement in nursing in his autobiography, a family photograph contains an inset of one of his daughters, Joan, in a nurse's uniform. It is not, however, clear precisely when his daughter entered training and what impact this may have had upon her father's interest in nursing affairs.[23] In any case, Brockway introduced a private member's Bill in 1930 to establish a maximum working week of forty-four hours for nurses when the average was fifty-six hours.[24] It was against this background of pressure to regulate the working hours of nurses that the *Lancet*, the campaigning medical journal, established a commission on nursing. Brockway's initiative provoked resentment from the now Royal College of Nursing (RCN) Council, which demurred at the introduction of a Bill without prior consultation. Firm in its anti-industrial stance, the College took considerable pains to oppose the Hours and Wages Bill.[25] It invited the secretaries and members of its various branches to write to their MPs. It wrote to the Minister of Health, women MPs and *The Times*, and published its views in the *Nursing Times*, then an organ of the College. The College Council was gratified to receive letters from a number of MPs assuring them that the Bill would be opposed.[26] The Council invited Mr Brockway to a meeting of its Parliamentary Committee to give an account of the reasons why the Bill was introduced, but took no further action on the matter beyond that meeting.[27]

In November 1930 the College's education committee seized the initiative and, in view of the difficulties involved in attracting sufficient suitable candidates, recommended a conference to be held on the recruitment and training of nurses.[28] The conference was to be convened with representatives of the medical and teaching professions, hospital governors and the nursing profession. Coincidentally the *Lancet* notified the College of its intention to arrange a commission of inquiry into recruitment and conditions of service in the profession. The editor of the *Lancet* acknowledged the College's proposal, but hoped that nevertheless the College would be prepared to co-operate with the journal in its investigations. Upstaged by the *Lancet*, the College seems to have decided to drop its original plan for a concurrent conference and offered instead to give evidence before the Commission. It proposed to go ahead with its own conference after the Lancet Commission had reported. A 'flagship' project such as a major review of nursing education could well have helped the

College's application for a royal charter, which was being considered at the same time. Opponents of the granting of the charter denigrated the achievements of the College, arguing: 'what had it done to earn such a signal honour?... Very little money had been spent on education.'[29] Nevertheless, the College was to play a significant role in the collection and collation of evidence for the Lancet Commission and was therefore in a strong position to influence its findings.[30] The Salaries and Superannuation Committee of the College was one of the first to be asked to prepare and submit evidence.

THE LANCET COMMISSION

A letter in the *Lancet*, predicting an impending crisis of nurse recruitment, particularly in smaller hospitals and sanatoria, seems to have provided the stimulus to the establishment of the Lancet Commission.[31] The author, Dr Esther Carling, was superintendent of Berkshire and Buckinghamshire Joint Sanatorium. Some sanatoria were forced to employ ex-patients as staff in the attempt to solve staffing difficulties.[32] Recruitment problems in sanatoria were notoriously acute. Indeed, as one of the most depressed areas of nursing work, tuberculosis (TB) nursing was a barometer of the climatic changes in the nursing labour market. Fear of infection combined with social and geographical isolation compounded the recruitment difficulties in this part of the profession. The Prophit Survey published after World War II found that nurses working in general hospitals with TB wards had a risk of infection four times that of women in the general population.[33] The *Lancet* had published a report of the incidence of TB in Canadian and Norwegian nurses in 1930 in which it was concluded that nurses were 'specially liable to contract TB'.[34] Along with Dr Jane Walker, also medical superintendent of a sanatorium, member of the Socialist Medical Association (SMA) and author of a textbook on TB nursing, Dr Carling campaigned throughout the inter-war period to have TB nursing approved for state registration by the GNC.[35] Petitioning was not successful and the Council demonstrated little sensitivity to the problems of sanatoria. The absence of a TB register exacerbated the depressed status of TB nursing, compounding the problems of recruitment and diminishing the prestige of staff posts.[36] The situation was only eased when TB rates declined. The exception was Scotland, where sanatoria experience became a compulsory part of 'general' nurse training after the National Health Service (NHS) was instituted.

Dr Carling identified one of the main 'causative' factors of the shortage as the unattractive conditions in nursing compared with other occupations: 'opportunities to recruit well-educated' girls were being 'lost' to other occupations. Hospitals as a consequence had resorted to employing temporary nurses and 'elevating' ward maids to nurses. The modernisation of education, attitudes and conditions was required in order to bring conditions in nursing into line with those of other fields of employment.

Dr Carling's definition of 'crisis' was not accepted without dispute. Some argued that nursing was only one of a number of occupations requiring 'rationalisation'.[37] Gladys Carter, Canadian nurse and graduate in economics, criticised nursing education as confused in its objectives. Did doctors want a highly trained expert and assistant in the prevention and cure of sickness, or someone who had spent the larger part of her training 'scrambling' through the work of the hospital? Nurses, she claimed, often completed training without sufficient knowledge to support medical practice. Educated women were unlikely to enter a profession which was evidently so dissatisfying.[38] Miss Carter was one of the first to call for the application of work study techniques to nursing work as a means of establishing practice on a scientific basis.

It is not clear what finally prompted the *Lancet* to take action and fund the inquiry, although the journal's historical involvement in reformist activity may well have been important.[39] The Commission was arguably launched as a private initiative on the model of its great public health investigations of the nineteenth century.[40] TB had moreover featured prominently in the journal's columns, and the status, prestige and recruitment problems of sanatoria in particular were certainly given unprecedented attention by the Commission's report.[41] The GNC's determination to pursue a 'single portal of entry' policy had led to the rejection of claims by representatives of TB nurses for registration. TB nurses could undergo specialised training, initiated in 1920 by the Society of Medical Superintendents of Tuberculosis Institutions. The Society conducted courses until 1927, when its training functions were taken over by the Tuberculosis Association. The Tuberculosis Nursing certificate was recognised as a statutory qualification for TB visitors employed by local government under the Local Government Act of 1929.[42] It was possibly partly the changes anticipated in the organisation of health services following the Local Government Act that influenced the course of the *Lancet* initiative.

COMMISSIONING METHODS

The Commission's terms of reference were to:

> inquire into the reasons for the shortage of candidates trained and untrained, for nursing the sick in general and special hospitals throughout the country and to offer recommendations for making the service more attractive to women suitable for this necessary work.[43]

Details of the criteria guiding appointments are not available, but metropolitan, voluntary hospital and academic interests were strongly represented.[44] Dr Dorothy Brock, President of the Association of Headmistresses, and Miss Edith Thompson, council member of Bedford College, represented the elite element in girls' education.[45] The first meeting of the Commission was held on 8 December 1930, and the Commission took two years to report. In addition to taking oral and written evidence from individuals and interested bodies, it also conducted its own investigations by questionnaire survey regarding conditions of service and recruitment to nursing. The paucity of statistical data on the characteristics of the nursing workforce and educational background of nurses forced the Commission to rely heavily upon the RCN as a source of evidence and information.[46] There was no centralised agency for the collection of statistics. The Ministry of Health, for example, did not collect figures routinely on the numbers of nurses employed under its own jurisdiction. The only regular nursing returns were the numbers of cumulative and new registrations with the GNC published in the Ministry of Health Annual Reports. The RCN had undertaken two surveys of the salaries and conditions of service in various branches of the occupation in 1919 and 1931.[47] Data were not sufficiently detailed to enable the Commission to draw independent conclusions. Responses to the Commission's questionnaire were collated and analysed by Professor Austin Bradford Hill, founding father of medical statistics in the UK. These were published in three stages: first and second interim reports followed by a final report in early 1932.[48]

The method used to select hospitals for the questionnaire sample was to identify all voluntary or municipal hospitals in counties whose names began with C, S, K or M, these being the initial letters of the names of the officers of the Commission. This was rather a far cry from the randomisation procedure that Bradford Hill would make his own in the design of randomised controlled trials. Questionnaires were also sent to hospitals in other counties in special circumstances – for example, a random sample of sanatoria were selected from a variety of counties. A total of 1,251 hospitals was sampled. Shortages of all grades of staff were reported by all types of hospital. These were most marked in hospitals not approved as training schools, and least acute in the London voluntary hospitals.[49] The shortage was found to be one of quality as well as quantity. Although 57 per cent of London voluntary and 63 per cent of provincial municipal hospitals stated that they required an entry educational standard of secondary school education, this was only enforced where practicable.[50] Nearly one third of all hospitals were willing to accept probationers of the seventh elementary standard. One tenth made no stipulation. Amongst these were a number who stated they must be content 'as long as the candidates can read, write and spell'.[51] To counteract the effects of 'wastage', every year hospitals had to re-recruit half their establishment of probationers in order to replenish their complement of trainees. The greatest part of this loss occurred in the first year and was attributed to 'inefficiency', examination failure, 'unsuitability', ill-health or dislike of the work.[52]

Of the probationers who sat for state examinations, only between one sixth and a quarter qualified annually. Voluntary hospitals secured a higher number of passes than the municipal or children's hospitals. Even the most prestigious schools experienced difficulties. The Nightingale training school had lost a seventh of the total probationer strength, 24 out of 167, the previous year.[53] The major difficulty for probationers lay in combining theoretical with ward work. To overcome some of the difficulties, education authorities were invited to co-operate with hospitals to provide schools for the preliminary training in the GNC's syllabus.[54]

While each body laid a slightly different emphasis upon the evidence it submitted, there was considerable consensus regarding the diagnosis and treatment of problems between organisations. The RCN attributed the 'surmised' shortage of candidates to the increasing demand for nurses, not to the failure of supply. The more favourable competitive position of other professions, particularly those offering higher salaries and greater liberty, was crucial. As important, however, was the 'hostile and un-reliable' correspondence in the press, which conveyed an erroneous impression of nursing work. Both the Association of Hospital Matrons (AHM) and the RCN Council stressed the importance of educating public opinion about the improving conditions in the occupation.[55]

As far as pre-nursing education was concerned, the College recommended selected subjects should be taken by senior students intending to enter the profession. It advocated matriculation as the basis of entry, with the establishment of a central preliminary training schools' examination at the end of the first year, run in conjunction with education authorities. These were to organise and offer maintenance grants from the Board of Education. When the student entered the hospital she would therefore be able to concentrate on practical nursing duties and receive organised bedside teaching.[56]

The memorandum submitted by the Salaries and Superannuation Committee of the College identified lengthy training, stiff examinations, off-duty time taken up with lectures, and even 'the dole' as contributing factors to recruitment difficulties. Elevating nursing to a university degree, with scholarships for schools to encourage study in anatomy, physiology, hygiene, cooking and elementary chemistry before entry into hospital, was also advocated.[57] Any solution would have to comprehend educational, economic and social factors.[58] According to one witness, the problem was partly one of physique: 'the standard height and health of nurses had been allowed to drop. . . . Girls of good physique are seen more often as sales girls in shops and warehouses, whereas too often one finds little women as nurses in hospitals for adults.'[59]

The College assumed that nursing was losing ground to other middle-class professions; it was teaching and social work rather than nursing which were seen as 'suitable' forms of employment. Consequently the popularity of nursing needed to be restored. No statistical evidence was provided to justify this assertion, and recent research suggests it is doubtful whether nursing ever did attract substantial numbers from the middle classes.[60] The association between nursing and the middle-class educational market for girls was reinforced by the career literature sponsored by the RCN and published in the educational press.[61]

REPORTED REACTION

The reforms advocated by the Commission were designed to adapt rather than radically reconstruct existing facilities. Many of the shortcomings identified by the Commission were not new. It consolidated and gave formal expression to earlier criticisms.[62] The financial insolvency of the voluntary hospitals ensured that the findings were confined to non-monetary measures. Recommendations that schools of nursing should be linked to universities reflected the social aspirations of organisations exerting the greatest influence over the Commission's deliberations. Furthermore, it was recommended that two grades of nurse should receive official recognition.[63] Most attention, however, was devoted to bridging the so-called 'gap' between leaving school and entering the occupation. A trial of scholarship and maintenance schemes was advocated to enable girls of 16 years or even younger to remain at school. Scholarships were to be supplemented with periodic visits to hospitals to stimulate and sustain interest in hospital work. Some such schemes were already operated by Worcester and West Riding Education Committees. The London County Council's Trade Scholarships scheme was suggested as a model which might be extended to other areas.[64] 'Bridging' courses were intended to cover the theoretical part of the syllabus for the preliminary state examination. Thus the elements of anatomy, physiology and hygiene would all be taught before probationers began ward work. Transforming the teaching of such subjects required only slight modification of existing courses provided for under the Regulations for Further Education.[65]

The plan to 'split' the theoretical and practical teaching of the preliminary examination was rejected by some members of the RCN subcommittee on the Commission.[66] Allowing candidates to sit for the preliminary state examination whilst still at school was welcomed as a useful strategy to relieve the pressure on hospitals overburdened with the teaching of preliminary subjects. The groundwork which occupied so much of the time of the sister-tutor could then be devoted to the teaching of nursing subjects.[67] The GNC was not convinced: the preliminary examination was not an 'entrance' exam, but preliminary to the final examination. It was the sole entry route into the occupation. The integrity and regulation of the single portal were regarded as sacrosanct.[68] It was hoped that considerable benefit would be derived from concentrating upon improving the general education of girls between 16 and 18, rather than teaching specialist subjects at school.[69]

The press response was sympathetic to the criticisms of conditions in hospitals. *The Times* echoed the *Lancet*'s diagnosis that many occupations now offered better salaries, prospects, freedom and social amenities than nursing. Nurses were frequently overworked, underpaid and compelled to undertake work which ought to be done by other people. Nursing would nevertheless always be a calling apart, a service based on vocation rather than the hope of reward. It was regarded as inevitable that it would 'always be hedged round with restrictions and governed by rigid regulations'.[70] Although it was regarded as advisable to try to 'fill the gap' between school and hospital training, there was also the argument that encouraging girls to participate in co-operative schemes between education and hospital authorities could confuse a 'mere romantic enthusiasm [with] a true vocation'.[71] The corollary of this position was that nursing ought to draw its recruits from the more highly educated members of the community and that entry should be narrowed rather than widened. Such a solution was bound to compound rather than repair existing difficulties. The prominence given to the criticisms of petty discipline and the need for 'modernisation of educational policies and attitudes' were endorsed in the press.[72] The role of discipline in training provoked contradictory responses from commentators. If the 'right' type of probationer could be attracted, severe discipline would be unnecessary. Yet such discipline was regarded as an intrinsic part of the care of the sick.[73]

The response in the nursing press to the report emphasised the conflict of ideals between senior nurses who regarded long hours of routine work as an important part of training, on the one hand, and those who recognised that hospital training failed to cater for the intelligent girl, on the other. The educational methods employed in hospitals were condemned as depressing rather than stimulating curiosity. The restrictions on the social life of the probationer and the inconsistency between the responsibilities placed upon her on and off duty were also identified as negative influences.[74] The report was applauded by the *Nursing Times* as infusing a new spirit into the nursing profession without disturbing present methods.[75] The *British Journal of Nursing* deplored the splitting of the preliminary examination and proposed division in examination responsibilities between the secondary schools and hospitals.[76] Hospitals should rather place the education of the nurse on a sound economic footing.

Opinion was divided amongst sister-tutors as to the best means of streamlining the overcrowded syllabus. Using an architectural analogy, Margaret Hitch, tutor to St Bartholomew's, argued:

> We are trying to construct a building within the space of three years upon little or no foundation, and I am reminded of those New York

architects who have now discovered that no reliance can be placed in the stability of a sky-scraper of fifty floors which occupies only half an acre of land![77]

Medical reaction was sympathetic but added nothing new to existing interpretations of the report.[78] The National Council of Women of Great Britain endorsed splitting the preliminary examination at its October conference.[79] The one issue on which there was universal agreement was the recommendation that probationers' salaries should be raised to attract more recruits.

REGISTRATION REFORM

The recommendation of the Commission to institute a simpler form of registration, with one register and supplementary diplomas, was perceived as desirable, but only when the hospital system was more unified.[80] Until the systems of hospital administration articulated more smoothly with each other, it was difficult to promote educational measures which assumed closer co-operation between agencies. The report favoured maintaining separate registers as a measure to help the mental, fever and children's hospitals enlist probationers by offering them state recognition. The Commission recommended that it might be possible to raise the status of supplementary registers without abolishing them by enabling such nurses to qualify for the general register after short additional courses.

Existing regulations of the Council permitted nurses on the supplementary registers to be admitted to the general part of the register after two years. However, in practice, a registered mental, fever or sick children's nurse usually started afresh as a probationer and worked for three years, at probationer rates of pay, before gaining admission to the general register.[81] The levels of co-operation and of pooling of resources needed to forge collaborative relationships between different hospitals or groups of hospitals were considered 'unlikely to be reached in the near future for reasons quite unconnected with nursing'. The main impediments to co-operation were identified as the autonomy of and competition between voluntary hospitals for the support of the charitable public, and the jealous protection of their reputations as training schools.[82] While in theory specialist hospitals such as the mental and fever hospitals came under local authorities, general hospitals were resistant to shortening courses to promote exchanges and combined forms of training.[83]

COUNCIL CONFORMS

At the meeting of the Education and Examinations Committee of the GNC, held to consider the Lancet Commission's findings, thirteen voted for, compared with eleven against, splitting the preliminary examination.[84] Both the Council and Ministry recognised the problems of filling the gap between probationers leaving school and yet not being old enough to commence training. The Council had to contend with the difficulty that girls who might otherwise be attracted to nursing were being drawn into other occupations before they were eligible for recruitment. Employers of nurses seemed to assume that nurses had to be physically, mentally and emotionally mature to withstand the strain of nursing work. A woman had to be 'well-seasoned all round' to be a successful nurse.[85] Brock cautioned: 'the moral dangers of letting young girls with no knowledge of the world enter hospitals, especially medical schools, at too early an age are too obvious to need emphasising'.[86] Such statements encapsulate assumptions about the role of the 'moral' maturity of the nurse and its potential to counteract the 'temptations' of institutional or urban life. In its evidence to the Lancet Commission, the RCN was reluctant to recommend 'living-out' arrangements for untrained staff. The College's reluctance was occasioned by the fear that the slum nature of the accommodation surrounding many hospitals, and the consequent difficulty of securing suitable accommodation at a reasonable distance from the hospital, might deter parents from sending their daughters to train as nurses.[87]

Nursing was not alone in experiencing difficulties in bridging the gap between school and adult employment. A number of schemes had been devised by a number of authorities to provide part-time education between school leaving and full-time employment, the most notable being that by the London County Council (LCC). Much of the impetus for such schemes stemmed from the need to deal with the problem of juvenile unemployment. Opposition to devolving responsibility for nurse education to lay educational authorities was sustained by hard-liners, such as the Bedford Fenwick lobby, until the late 1930s.[88] The GNC was sluggish in establishing collaborative links with education authorities, but was temporarily relieved of responsibility to act by the upturn in recruitment occasioned by the economic depression of the mid-1930s.

CRISIS TO COMPLACENCY

Although the Lancet Commission proved useful as a consciousness-raising exercise, it produced few tangible improvements in recruitment or conditions. Nevertheless, it helped to consolidate the pressure to divide the preliminary examination and bring nursing education into closer alignment with mainstream education. Opportunities for reform were, however, overtaken by changes in labour market conditions, which allowed employers to lapse into a laissez-faire mode of operation. In 1933, only one year after anxieties surrounding workforce shortages had been articulated, the *Lancet* seemed sanguine: 'the express purpose of attracting candidates for training has during the past year become less urgent, because the influx of suitable young women into the nursing profession has greatly increased'.[89] The deteriorating economic climate had produced an upturn in recruitment 'during which any form of training offering board and lodging and pocket money has advantages'.[90] The temporary improvement in recruitment was considered so significant that the RCN proposed a protectionist employment policy against the admission of foreign probationers to British hospitals.[91]

The instability of labour market conditions provided a convenient excuse for inaction: 'splitting the prelim' was deferred until 1939. Devolving the teaching of elementary scientific subjects had presupposed that resources and the climate of opinion favoured girls being schooled in the biological sciences. The teaching of biology to schoolgirls was notoriously slow to develop and contrasted markedly with the effort directed towards the teaching of domestic science subjects.[92] Collaboration between nursing and general educational authorities was impeded further by intransigent attitudes within the Council itself, which demonstrated a grave reluctance to work closely with experts in general education. Originally the Board's representatives were appointed to provide independent advice to the Council on educational matters. Immune from the original controversies surrounding the establishment of the Council, representatives from the Board of Education were considered a valuable source of neutral advice.[93] Prominent individuals such as Miss Tuke, Head of Bedford College, and latterly Miss Gwatkin, President of the Association of Headmistresses, were difficult to ignore. However, there was no guarantee that educational appointees would, as a matter of course, be elected to the Education and Examinations Committee.

Indeed, the conspicuous absence of Board of Education

appointees to the Education and Examinations Committee was questioned by the Board in 1930. Officials asked the registrar why only one of their representatives had ever been elected on to the Education and Examinations Committee. The Board suspected that the older, 'more reactionary' members of the Council were anxious to concentrate the power of the committee in their own hands.[94]

TESTING TIMES

Alongside proposals to 'split the prelim', the Council had a range of strategies for improving the selection and standard of candidates. One was the application of a general knowledge and intelligence screening test. As early as 1920, Brock had suggested a simple educational test as a condition of selecting hospitals for grant-aiding.[95] Testing techniques were attractive to educational policy-makers in nursing, since they promised a swift and pragmatic solution to the chronic problem of labour and educational wastage. The application of testing techniques to education has been attributed in part to the professionalising ambitions and ideological commitments of educational psychologists.[96] The perceived utility of vocational tests may well have grown as the demand for nursing labour increased throughout the inter-war period. Much of this expansion occurred through the substitution of student nurse for assistant nurse labour.[97] Consequently, selection of the 'fitting' became a major issue for the Council and the Ministry.

The introduction of a simple educational test as a condition of entry into training required amending the Council's rules and seeking the approval of the Minister of Health and Parliament. Miss Musson, the first nurse chairwoman of the GNC, called for a simple test to eliminate the illiterate from training. The ignorance of arithmetic, in particular, demonstrated by certain candidates provoked unremitting criticism from examiners.[98] Medical men marking preliminary papers in anatomy and physiology had consistently drawn attention to the poor standards of performance.[99] The Council had first passed a resolution in 1932 to institute a test examination, and in 1935 a rule was submitted for Ministry approval. The Ministry of Health was sympathetic and indicated that formal approval would be forthcoming. Furthermore, it was suggested that the test might be administered by the Board of Education. However, organisations such as the BHA opposed the test on the grounds that it would depress recruitment, for which, it was believed, the public would hold the BHA and not the GNC accountable.[100] Advocates insisted that the test should be considered a gateway rather than a barrier; it made no pedagogical sense to expend energy training nurses who would never be capable of passing the state exams. The test was designed to select candidates who perhaps had not achieved well at school, but who nevertheless could make efficient nurses.[101] Such arguments, however, could also be counter-productive; they suggested nurses required little intelligence or education to function effectively as nurses. Critics maintained the test was superfluous; most voluntary hospitals already imposed an entry standard. In practice this varied, and a small minority demanded none at all.[102]

Miss Musson drew the analogy with teaching and the Civil Service, both of which required a general educational standard and experienced few recruitment problems. Miss Musson was especially anxious to dispel the notion that it was unnecessary to be educated in order to enter the nursing profession. Low-pass and failure rates ranging from 22 to 48 per cent in 1937–8 in preliminary examinations contributed to anxieties about educational standards.[103] The BHA's sensitivity to the issue induced it to survey opinion on the introduction of the test. The results supported testing provided it was administered after entry into training.[104] The Ministry of Health accepted the BHA's provisos and asked the Board of Education to offer advice and assistance in the evaluation of examination performance. The Ministry was less convinced that the GNC ought to be the sole authority responsible for administering the test. This was so particularly because the Council demonstrated deep ambivalence towards accepting the services of their inspectorate in devising the test.[105] As it transpired, the test was approved in principle by the Ministry of Health in 1935 but withdrawn in 1939 at its request, as recruitment rates failed to match demand. Throughout the negotiations the GNC had been prepared to accommodate external pressure to divide the preliminary or test examination. But it feared for incursions into its autonomy, especially where the Council was expected to devolve responsibility to 'outside' authorities.[106] This was especially threatening when considered in the context of the Council's relations with such bodies as the Royal Medico-Psychological Association (RMPA), with which the Council considered itself in competition (see Chapter 4).

CONCLUSION

Efforts to impose uniform educational standards upon nursing were effectively shattered by the alarming changes in the nursing labour market in the late 1930s. Conditions by then had deteriorated so much that they were subjected to a cascade of criticism. The Council's ambitions for selection and standardisation evaporated under pressure to capitulate to the powerful material and demographic changes which the economic recession had engendered. The twin pressures of trade union protest and unprecedented assertiveness from the nursing organisations induced the government to institute the first government-backed inquiry into nursing. This did not imply zeal on the part of government to assume greater financial responsibility for nursing services or education. Government intervention can rather be understood as a pre-emptive strategy designed to quell industrial unrest and palliate the deepening crisis in the nursing services. As in 1919, the government temporarily assumed the role of *deus ex machina*. However, it was a role assumed with only the greatest reluctance and renounced as soon as circumstances allowed.

Chapter 8

Nationalising nursing education (1939–48)

INTRODUCTION

This chapter examines nursing education policy-making from 1939 to 1948. It considers the pressures shaping the content, methods and objectives of nurse education during that period. I argue that shifts in nursing education can best be understood in the context of more general changes in health service organisation and funding. Recurrent 'crises' in nurse recruitment and preparations for the National Health Service (NHS) of necessity elevated nursing into an issue of the highest priority; experts from education and psychology were invited to join officials and leading nurses in solving the recruitment riddle. It was in this context that one of the most radical critiques of nurse recruitment and education emanated from a psychologist and civil servant, Dr John Cohen.[1] The Minority Report (1948), signed by Dr John Cohen and Mr Geoffrey Pyke, was an emphatically personal document recording the authors' commitment to the integration of health care within wider socio-political and economic changes. It denounced the 'muddling through' approach to policy-making and presented a plea for the rational organisation of nursing and health services within a planned economy. Cohen, in particular, used nursing to publicise his views on the methodological weaknesses in health service planning more generally. Indeed, debates about nursing in the early health service prefigured many of the planning problems which were to plague generations of NHS policy-makers.

By the end of the 1930s the recruitment problem in nursing had intensified; the temporary relief from crisis at the height of the Depression dissolved as the economic recovery of the later part of the decade expanded employment opportunities for women. In November 1935 the Royal College of Nursing (RCN) sent a deputation to the

Ministry of Health to request an inquiry into the nursing needs of the community. The proposal was supported by a subcommittee of the British Medical Association (BMA) and endorsed by the Federation of Medical Women.[2] Coincidentally, a separate request for an inquiry arose independently from Sir Fredrick Menzies, Medical Officer of Health to the London County Council (LCC) and Privy Council appointee to the GNC.[3] In November 1936, Dame Janet Campbell pressed the Minister for an inquiry.[4] It was no accident that six months later, the Federation of Medical Women, of which she was Vice-president, made a similar request.[5] The Federation had already established a committee on nursing with Dr Jane Walker, a campaigner for the registration of tuberculosis (TB) nursing and member of the Socialist Medical Association (SMA), as chairwoman.

Dame Janet urged the Minister to act swiftly and institute its own inquiry rather than allow the RCN to take credit for the initiative.[6] The Trades Union Congress (TUC) also provided a source of pressure. Before 1937 the TUC had focused little attention upon nursing, but by the end of the year it had convened a Joint Advisory Council for the Nursing Profession to consider improvements in organising nurses and to establish the Whitley Council machinery.[7] In June the Joint Council drew up a 'Draft Charter for the Nursing Profession' containing eleven demands related to conditions of service and training.[8]

The Charter formed the focal point for the TUC's campaign on nursing. Some TUC members maintained that the Charter should be used to exert political and economic leverage upon hospitals. It was argued that control could be exercised over voluntary hospitals which derived income from working men's funds. Sanctions could be applied to those voluntary hospitals refusing to adopt the Nurses' Charter.[9] The Charter provided a stimulus to trade union organisation by nurses.[10] Thora Silverthorne, a State Registered Nurse (SRN) at the Radcliffe Infirmary, Oxford, instituted an Association of Nurses and entered into discussions with Ernest Bevin and other trade union leaders to consider TUC affiliation.[11] Thora Silverthorne was also a member of the student Communist Party at Oxford and joined the first medical unit which was sent out to the Spanish Civil War.[12] Rival charters were produced by different union organisations in competition with each other as well as with the College.[13] This fragmentation of effort weakened overall union effectiveness. The RCN fought a determined rearguard action to wrest the political advantage from the TUC, but it was hampered in its endeavours by its apolitical stance. In a letter to branch secretaries it was declared that nursing was a 'scientific and philanthropic profession in which politics have no place, any more than colour, creed or class'.[14] The vanguard of the new militancy was provided by the Guild of Nurses, brainchild of Beatrice Drapper, the National Organising Secretary of the National Union of County Officers (NUCO).[15] As an assertive organisation it won a number of concessions from authorities sympathetic to Labour. The greatest challenge to the Guild came from its confrontation with the LCC over the abolition of the split-shift system of work and the so-called 'industrialisation' of the service.[16]

DEPRESSING PUBLICITY

National newspapers and journals lost no opportunity in publicising attacks upon hospitals where there were alleged shortages in nursing staff. Regimentation, petty rules and tyranny once again featured as impediments to recruitment.[17] Insularity and lack of opportunity to use initiative were identified as drawbacks to recruitment at a joint conference between the executive committees of the Association of Head Mistresses and the Association of Hospital Matrons (AHM) at the North London Collegiate School in February 1937.[18] Hours of work and poor salaries were also condemned.[19] The absence of a coherent educational policy, separate funding for nurse teaching, and marginalisation of nurses from the decision-making apparatus of hospital boards and government departments were deplored too.[20] Critics agreed that nursing education required radical reconstruction. The analogy between training for nurses and teachers was drawn: if training colleges could be provided by the state for teachers, why not for nurses, whose functions were no less important?[21] Moreover, it was claimed that nurses should have access to a body similar to the Burnham Committee to determine salary awards.[22]

Employers of nurses retaliated.[23] But nurses found they had many champions in the press, including such celebrities as the actress Sibyl Thorndyke and author A.J. Cronin.[24] Newspaper campaigns such as that instigated by Cronin were accompanied by public demonstrations of discontent by nurses. The Guild of Nurses, a branch of NUCO, marched down the Strand in masks to avoid victimisation in protest over the split-shift system of work. RCN representatives sought to discredit media coverage of the TUC initiatives and blamed the adverse publicity itself for the slump in recruitment.[25] In spite of mounting pressures, the government refused to intervene in a question it perceived as involving so many 'political and sociological' variables.[26] Any immediate response, however, would have suggested that the government considered that the threats confronting it were serious. In this sense stalling action could have had two main advantages: not only did it distance the government from immediate political pressures but it also provided the opportunity for any subsequent action to be represented as independent rather than reactive. Furthermore, any thorough investigation would have been likely to have significant economic implications, and unfavourable comparisons with other forms of employment could have generated pressure for state expenditure.[27]

By the summer of 1937, all interested parties were agreed that a government commission was necessary for the problems to be invested with the requisite authority. However, the prospect of providing nursing services for the military and civilian populations under wartime conditions provided an additional stimulus to action. In November 1936 the Ministry of Health had requested information from the RCN to help a subcommittee of the Committee of Imperial Defence calculate the reserves of nurses in the defence services compared with civilian strength.[28] The announcement of the Inter-departmental Committee on Nursing Services in September 1937 was welcomed as a step towards remedying recruitment.[29] The timing was designed to pre-empt a second request from the RCN for an inquiry, and to follow the election of a new GNC and a proclamation of its attitude towards recognising a separate grade of attendant. The Limitation of Hours Bill was also being debated in Parliament and it was considered prudent to forestall the establishment of the committee until Parliament had the opportunity to debate the issue.[30]

In considering the necessity of a fresh investigation the Lancet Commission was acknowledged as a comprehensive report, but its conclusions were considered out of step with the different service demands of an expanding municipal and domiciliary nursing service in the late 1930s.[31] The task for the inter-departmental inquiry was to identify recruitment and training needs in relation to projected demands on health services. The constitution of the committee was to be determined by efficiency rather than representativeness. Scotland was excluded on the grounds that it had already taken an initiative, although in practice the Scottish recommendations had been concerned chiefly with recruitment and conditions of service, rather than with training.[32] Ministry of Labour involvement was proscribed on the grounds that it was perceived as antagonising the profession. The Boards of Control and Education were consulted, but the intricate and controversial nature of the issues persuaded the Minister of Health to keep the Council small.[33]

The scope of the inquiry was to be comprehensive, encompassing questions of recruitment as well as training. Specific attention was to focus upon treating probationers as trainees rather than cheap labour. Officials were concerned that the inquiry might be perceived as criticism of the GNC's capacity to produce a progressive revision of curriculum in its existing form. They lamented the failure of the nursing profession to produce 'big and progressive personalities' as leaders, and saw this as a major impediment to reform.[34] Some officials hinted that had the GNC been discharging its functions effectively, the need for any official investigation might well have been avoided.[35] Where possible, members were selected for their multiple representational roles. As this was an investigative committee, the government claimed a free hand in determining its constitution. Members were recruited for their professional and research expertise.[36] Lord Merthyr was suggested as chairman to pacify the Welsh lobby. Five nursing representatives were proposed to embrace GNC, municipal hospital, district nursing, mental nursing and rank-and-file interests. Voluntary hospitals, hospital consultant physicians and surgeons, public health services, private medical practice, teaching and departmental representatives were also identified for inclusion.[37]

Few representatives of specialist interests were included, which provoked censure from the Board of Control.[38] Brock, now its President, criticised the representation of mental and mental deficiency nursing by a single nominee. He suggested that a representative from the Mental Hospitals Association rather than a nurse should supplement the technical advice of a doctor. This was crucial, he argued, if local authorities were to attach weight and authority to the committee's recommendations.[39] The Earl of Athlone, rather than Lord Merthyr, finally accepted the chairmanship of the committee.[40] As President of the Queen's Institute, he was perceived as having greater credibility with nurses. Dorothy Brock, who had been involved in discussions of nurse education matters with the AHM, was considered well qualified to comment upon the 'mentality' of schoolgirls entering nursing. It is possible that Dorothy Brock provided an additional source of influence for Lawrence Brock. He discussed the work of the committee with his sister and warned her of the 'scornful' opinion of committees composed mainly of doctors.

Brock concluded his advice to the committee that care should be taken to select a matron young enough to have some sympathy with the girls' point of view: he averred that 'if the choice were left to the GNC there was always the danger the kind of Matron represented on that body would be selected'.[41] Brock's attitude reflected a more widespread scepticism of the GNC's credibility by officials.

The Committee's terms of reference were ambitious. Long- and short-term demands for an institutional and domiciliary nursing service were to be assessed.[42] Interest groups agreed that the shortage was both quantitative and qualitative in kind. Current registration and wastage figures suggested a further 10,000 more registered nurses were required to meet existing demand. The total output of girls aged 16 years and over from grant-aided secondary schools in 1937 was 28,250. The total number of those who left at 17 or upwards was 10,600. A little more than 4,000 girls over 18 years had gone to universities or teachers' training colleges in 1937. The percentage of girls entering professional, commercial or clerical employment had risen from 18 per cent in 1920–1 to 40.6 per cent in 1936–7. The Board of Education concluded that recruitment for nursing could not be met by secondary schools alone. However, their method for calculating 'need' was neither disclosed nor defined.[43] The numbers of girls remaining at home and not taking up employment within those years declined from 25.8 per cent to 8.9 per cent.[44] Given these demands, it therefore seemed inevitable that a very large proportion of entrants had to be sought from girls whose full-time education had been confined to the elementary school.

LESSONS FROM EDUCATION

The key question confronting the Committee was whether nurses should be treated in parity with teachers and therefore be entitled to state aid in training. This formed part of the wider issue of whether health should receive a state subsidy on the same basis as education. A number of witnesses claimed that teaching had benefited from improved recruitment through enhanced conditions of service.[45] By contrast, nurses seemed inescapably consigned to a position of weakness in recruitment terms as long as poor conditions in the labour market prevailed. Girls who wished to remain at school were normally expected to take the higher school certificate. Inducements to stay at school could be greater if local education authorities were prepared to offer awards to prospective nurses. The attraction of such courses could be improved if the GNC were to offer some relief from training.[46] A number of pre-nursing courses which had 'split' the preliminary examination between school and hospital had been the subject of experiments in Leicester, Surrey, Kilburn and Battersea Polytechnic. A survey of the uptake and financing of such schemes, however, revealed minimal success and support.[47]

Financial impediments to providing a scheme of full-time education for prospective nurses on the scale required were formidable. It was estimated that the cost of providing full-time training for 8,000 students in each of three years would amount to £1,000,000. The general shortage of juvenile labour ensured that there was no lack of employment opportunities for girls at 16 with secondary education. Moreover, competing opportunities for girls whose parents could afford to keep them at school until 18 were many and varied. These included pharmacy, scientific, secretarial and professional careers, the Civil Service and other posts requiring success in executive examinations.[48] As a result, state-sponsored schemes enabling girls to continue their education and prepare for a nursing career were advocated. A key recruitment strategy recommended targeting recruitment at entrants disenchanted with jobs devoid of human contact.[49]

The more radical wing of nursing opinion objected to handing over the teaching of 'professional' nursing to 'unprofessional' teachers in schools.[50] Nursing education consisted of two key elements: scientific subjects (such as anatomy, physiology and hygiene) and self-discipline and etiquette. The latter were identified as crucial to the traditions determining the 'standard of correct behaviour to the medical profession and her patients'.[51] Removing nurses from hospitals for part of their training, it was argued, would deny them exposure to the environment and example necessary to develop the 'particular brand of good manners which is inseparable from a nurse'.[52] Medical complaints of nurses' educational attainments identified spelling, writing and grammatical abilities as particularly defective rather than technical knowledge. Any extra time at school, it was asserted, should be spent improving general rather than technical education.[53] Improving access to and expanding the means to 'bridge the gap' between school and hospital were key concerns for most witnesses.[54] Lowering the age at which probationers were admitted to hospital work was forcefully rejected. The Headmistresses Association argued girls of 16 or 17 were unfit for the strain of work and sight of death. Exposure to such experiences was calculated to induce callousness or acute anxiety in probationers.[55] Part-time schemes which controlled exposure to the emotional and physical strains of nursing work were the only concessions considered permissible.[56]

Broadening the basis of general training to incorporate a wider range of hospitals into a training unit received wide support.[57] Closer integration of theory and practice using the 'block' system, pioneered in Eastern Europe, was also recommended.[58] Dr Harold Balme, non-elected member of the GNC and outspoken critic of nursing education, pressed for a more scientific training, one which encouraged initiative and the exercise of critical judgement.[59] Countering the liberal view were those arguing for a reorientation of the emphasis in training. The Voluntary Hospitals Committee for London complained nurses' instruction was already saturated with theory.[60] The Royal College of Physicians and the British Hospitals Association (BHA) considered that nurses' training was already too elaborate.[61] Examination questions, according to the BMA, were weighted excessively in favour of diagnosis and medical treatment.[62]

GRANTING SUBSIDY

A common thread running through the evidence of many organisations to the Inter-departmental Committee was that nurses had failed to modernise their methods of work organisation and training. The acute labour shortage was attributed to increasing demand rather than diminishing supply of labour. Longer-term causes were identified as inadequate pay, over-exacting hours and other conditions of employment. Remedies, through improvements in pay and the establishment of salary committees analogous to the Burnham Committee, all had significant financial implications. The most radical recommendation related to government subsidy of nurse training. Government grants to all 'efficient' voluntary hospitals administered through local education authorities were recommended to meet the costs of increased salaries and reduced hours. Training grants were to be given from national funds administered by the Ministry of Health to voluntary and municipal hospitals. Improvements in employment conditions for nurses were linked, in officials' minds, to the wider question of financial assistance to voluntary hospitals. Strong pressure was brought to bear upon Ministry officials to make economic concessions to hospitals.[63] However, the argument that probationers were an asset to and not a burden upon hospitals was exploited by officials anxious to resist financial commitment to nurse training.[64]

Both the TUC and the College of Nursing claimed that the Athlone Committee legitimised many of their recommendations.[65] The nursing press was pessimistic about the prospects for radical reform. The degree to which hospitals retained their charitable ethos and nursing education depended upon subscriptions for the relief of illness; any 'revolutionary changes' were considered outside the range of practical politics.[66] The Inter-departmental Committee exploded the myth that the occupation was competing mainly in a middle-class labour market. This angered the more status-conscious organisations. The RCN welcomed most of the committee's findings but deprecated its emphasis upon elementary rather than secondary school recruitment. The feminist press condemned the conciliatory tone of the report and its concessions to what it considered to be the 'traditional' interests, attributing its weakness to the RCN matrons on the Committee.[67]

COSTING BENEFITS

Ministry of Health officials estimated the cost of adjusting nurses' salaries to those of teachers would place a further financial burden of £733,000 per year upon the voluntary hospitals. If superannuation were included this would raise the figure to approximately £770,000, or £70 per nurse.[68] Not surprisingly, there was a grave reluctance on the part of officials to endorse the analogy between teaching and nursing. The Burnham Committee was jointly constituted by teachers and local education authorities. The latter were obliged to meet only half the cost of claims and were perceived as having only a partial interest in resisting extravagant claims for remuneration. Officials surmised that if the costs of salary increases for nurses were similarly met, employing authorities (and especially those from voluntary hospitals) might lose the incentive to economise on claims.[69] The Treasury responded unsympathetically to any notion that training grants should be made available to nurses. Capitation grants to voluntary hospitals for SRNs were also considered as an option.[70] But Treasury officials were not convinced that a grant to voluntary hospitals was justified. Establishing a Burnham Committee which could lead the government to accept responsibility for maintaining the education of nurses was viewed as highly undesirable. Local education authorities already provided the incentive for the voluntary sector to follow suit and consequently no need was perceived for a government grant to 'accelerate this process'.[71] Moreover, not all voluntary hospitals were in grave financial difficulties. Some had surpluses of £1 million in their maintenance account, which they were unlikely to want to share if regional grouping were adopted.[72] Grants to voluntary hospitals were considered highly undesirable on two counts: not only were they difficult to withdraw once made but they might remove the justification for public charity.

The outbreak of war and the appointment of the Earl of Athlone as Governor-General to the Dominion of Canada provided an ideal justification for inaction.[73] The interim report of the Inter-departmental Committee was not followed by a final report. Meetings of the Committee were postponed indefinitely. The government's attitude towards nursing reflected resistance to subsidising and controlling the affairs of the voluntary hospital sector. This is consistent with Webster's scepticism of the argument for hierarchical regionalism and integration of hospital organisation, which Fox alleges commanded universal consensus in the late 1930s.[74] Webster warns against glib acceptance of the consensus argument, which exaggerates cohesion between the parties concerned.[75]

'War is a searchlight which exposes flaws in the body politic.'[76] The outbreak of war had a number of consequences for nursing and the health services, including a predictable crisis in nurse staffing. Preparation for receiving casualties had been undertaken by the Committee of Imperial Defence in 1926 and again in 1935.[77] A subcommittee on supply of nurses in war was reconstituted in 1939 under the chairmanship of Sir Arthur MacNalty, Chief Medical Officer at the Ministry of Health.[78] The Committee was charged with three tasks. First, it was to establish an emergency committee for trained nurses to work on parallel lines to those of the Emergency Committee of the BMA. Second, it was to liaise with relevant organisations, and third, to make arrangements for the supply of auxiliary and unqualified nursing staff.[79] Although 89,254 nurses were registered with the GNC, there was no information available related to reserves of unregistered but trained, or untrained, nurses. The RCN was asked to compile a register of all nurses and assistant nurses. The British Red Cross and Order of St John were to undertake a similar exercise for auxiliary nurses.

A Central Emergency Committee for nurses, similar to the Central Medical War Committee, was established in December 1938 under the chairmanship of Sir Malcolm Delevinge.[80] The Committee's functions were to draw up a register of all categories of nursing personnel, from those currently employed as registered nurses to assistant nurses and nursing auxiliaries. Each of these groups were further classified into three grades according to their mobility and employment status. For the first time, standardised rates of pay were identified for employers to follow.[81] This constituted the first step towards legitimising the status of the assistant nurse. Restrictions were placed upon entry into the Civil Nursing Reserve to prevent recruitment deficits in essential nursing services. Trained nurses in hospitals or public health, district or industrial nursing service were ineligible for registration with the more highly remunerated Civil Nursing Reserve, as were assistant nurses in public institutions. Local Emergency Committees were appointed to advise and administer the Reserve in planning the allocation of staff to areas of need. Sector matrons were attached to hospital groups as part of the Emergency Hospital Scheme. Ten sectors were identified in London and six in the provinces to facilitate the distribution of nurses.[82]

Expanding the quality, quantity and distribution of nursing and hospital services presupposed a sound information basis for planning. At the beginning of hostilities this was not available. Officials had little appreciation of the variable standard of hospital accommodation. As the Director General of the Emergency Medical Service (EMS) remarked in 1939, 'even those institutions that want to be regarded as the centres of enlightenment and teaching in our large cities are with few exceptions structurally unsafe or antiquated'.[83] In establishing the EMS the Ministry of Health had to weld together the facilities of a disparate range of resources, standards, value systems and heritages. Local authority hospitals, rather than voluntary ones, became the backbone of the EMS. The size and clinical standards of the voluntary hospitals varied enormously. Of the 700 general hospitals, more than 500 had fewer than 100 beds and 250 had fewer than 30 beds.[84] The EMS required all designated hospitals to receive casualties and brought each into a regional system of planning staffed by full-time salaried officers. Voluntary hospitals were eligible for exchequer subsidies. Surveys of hospital accommodation and staffing exposed deficiencies of distribution – that is, hospitals in many parts of the country suffered shortages while others experienced high levels of nurse unemployment. Such a situation was attributed to the movement of populations and the voluntary closure of many nursing homes at the outbreak of war.[85] Civilian institutions such as those for TB and mental and chronic illness were particularly disadvantaged.[86]

Standards in some institutions had deteriorated to such an extent that they were regarded as contributors to the rise of mortality from dysentery and TB.[87]

Short- and longer-term strategies were adopted to boost the supply of nursing labour. The 'standstill' order had been introduced in 1941 to prevent nurses of more than twelve months' service leaving their posts without the permission of the local emergency committee.[88] After the Central Emergency Committee had completed its task of organising the Civil Nursing Reserve, it was disbanded. Its executive functions were transferred to the Ministry of Health and its advisory responsibilities to a new body called the Civil Nursing Reserve Advisory Council. This was chaired by Miss Florence Horsburgh MP, Parliamentary Secretary to the Ministry of Health.[89] Regional Nursing Officers were appointed in January 1940 to promote efficiency in the organisation of nursing services in a variety of ways. By April 1941 a Nursing Division within the Ministry of Health had been created to deal with professional matters. Miss Katherine Watt, Principal of the Civil Nursing Reserve, was appointed first Chief Nursing Officer, and two Deputy Chief Nursing Officers were also appointed.[90]

Remedying the poor distribution of the nursing workforce implied rationalising payments to nurses of different grades.[91] Whilst these were standardised in the Civil Nursing Reserve, they were not universal. If 'leakage' of staff from essential areas to the Civil Nursing Reserve were to be avoided, a more permanent solution to labour mobility had to be found. Salary rises announced in April 1941 for the Civil Nursing Reserve were more generous than those of the local authorities, and considerably more generous than voluntary hospital rates. It was in this context that the government stepped in and pledged to provide a large proportion of the cost.[92]

Lord Rushcliffe reluctantly agreed to chair a committee on nursing salaries in 1941.[93] The Committee considered conditions of service as well as salary determination for all grades of nurse, including the controversial assistant nurse.[94] By the middle of 1941 both the TUC and the RCN advocated Whitleyism as the most appropriate form of machinery for the nursing profession,[95] but both were prepared to accept that, as an interim measure, the Committee should function as a Burnham Committee. The government was adamant that any scheme which did emerge should be controlled by its officials, since settlements devolved upon the national exchequer. The Committee recommended raising and standardising salary scales in its first report, published in 1943.[96] In doing so, however, it removed the differentials which had provided an inducement to recruitment in less popular areas. Grants enabling voluntary hospitals to meet the costs of salary awards were to be made available by the Treasury but administered through the BHA.[97] For the first time, grades of staff were to be defined and differentiated. The state had become much more closely involved in the administration of nursing services. Salary increases were substantial, costing a net sum of £2 million in 1943. As Webster notes, the war did more to advance nurses' pay than the previous twenty years of peace.[98]

RECONSTRUCTING NURSING

The RCN was disappointed by the disbanding of the Athlone committee and had taken steps to establish a substitute committee of inquiry.[99] Borrowing the terminology favoured at the time, a 'nurses' reconstruction' committee was established in November 1941.[100] Lord Horder was appointed its chairman. Half the members were drawn from the RCN and the other half from a range of 'interested' organisations.[101] Its aims were to consider means of implementing the recommendations of the Athlone Committee. As a matter of priority, the first part of its report in 1942 echoed Athlone in recommending official recognition of the assistant nurse.[102] This was reinforced by the inclusion of the assistant nurse grade in the Rushcliffe salary scales.

The Civil Nursing Reserve had provided the early stimulus to official recognition by defining the status of assistant nurses as those with not less than two years' hospital training, although not necessarily in a hospital recognised by the GNC.[103] Employers were keen to have the grade regularised and minimum levels of competence defined to retain assistant nurses, rather than lose them to nursing co-operatives and agencies paying higher salaries.[104] In 1943 a Nurses' Act was passed to legitimise the status of the assistant nurse and provide a separate, two-year training recognised by the GNC. Both the RCN and GNC had initially opposed official recognition of assistant nurses. Defining and limiting the activity of the assistant nurse, however, came to be perceived as having clear advantages for registered nurses. Rather than being maligned as the enemy of professionalism, the assistant nurse was transformed into an important ally in the pursuit of professional goals by registered nurses. Under the Horder arguments, the assistant nurse was represented as the key to the professionalisation of the registered nurse and an important element in achieving student status.[105] A lower grade of worker could assume the kinds of task which would allow student nurses to pursue a more intellectually demanding and stimulating form of education.

Differentiation between the 'qualified' and 'unqualified' was particularly contentious in mental nursing, where assistant nurses had often been used interchangeably with certificated and registered ones.[106] But to the radical section of nursing opinion, officially sanctioning the assistant nurse's status was anathema. Government action was described as: 'Nazism of a flagrant type, it is a return to economic slavery; it is the forbidding of self-government to a professional and most useful group; it is the degradation of the worker'.[107] With characteristic rhetorical extravagance, Mrs Bedford Fenwick mourned official endorsement of the assistant nurse as the ˙ᴗath knell to professionalism. She opined, 'now the blow has fallen and nursing as a profession for educated women may cease to exist. ... There is to be no closed profession of nursing'.[108] Legitimising the status of uncertificated workers was part of a wider movement advocated by such occupational groups as teachers.[109] In the case of assistant nurses, efforts were required to stem the unregulated flow of labour into the private agencies and to maintain staffing levels in sanatoria, mental hospitals and institutions for the chronic sick. These institutions were the most understaffed of any.[110]

Official recognition of assistant nurse status as a second portal of entry into the occupation and a second tier of labour can be conceived of as a pragmatic response to the deepening crisis in traditionally depressed forms of institutional work. The second report of the Horder Committee was devoted to education and training. Its brief was to remodel pre- and post-certificate education and suggest remedies for defects perceived in relation to the functions of the GNC.[111] The Committee concluded that a liberal and well-planned curriculum could potentially develop nursing into 'one of the great national educational movements for women'.[112]

QUALIFYING INTELLIGENCE

Intelligence tests were seized upon as the panacea for nurse selection and recruitment. Their apparent capacity to discriminate between innate talent and educational background was considered especially useful in selecting recruits of poor educational attainment but intellectual promise. Stratifying nurses into an intellectual hierarchy was also consistent with Lord Horder's wider eugenic beliefs.[113] Conflicting views were held on the need for nurses to be intelligent. The majority of nurses were identified as being drawn from a population who achieved between 60 and 70 per cent in intelligence tests.[114] Curricular discussions revealed a degree of anti-intellectualism which assumed that intelligence and practical skill in nurses were incompatible. Like teachers, it was argued, the best scholars did not always make the best practitioners. However, there were exceptions, and on occasions the best nurses could be the brightest. A distinction was drawn by one author between intelligence and intellect, arguing that the former was necessary whilst the latter was not.[115] Vestiges of anti-American feeling were also evident in Committee members' remarks. Miss Macmanus, matron of Guys Hospital and GNC member, commented: 'whilst the profession did not want the dunce with clever hands, American methods led her to consider nursing more an exploration into medicine'.[116] The adoption of American methods was repudiated on the grounds that it was feared that practical skill would be sacrificed to academic knowledge. The danger of producing a pseudo-doctor was a major impediment to importing American models of training.

The second Horder report echoed both Athlone and the second Rushcliffe report in recommending hospitals receive financial aid towards the cost of nurse training.[117] Treasury aid along the lines of the University Grants Commission, with inspection facilities but not state control, was suggested as the way forward. Horder sought to harmonise nurse training with the range of experience offered by regionalised health services.[118] To this end it was suggested that the 'block' system should predominate and a greater emphasis on social medicine should prevail.[119] A catalogue of criticisms was levelled at the GNC for its poor geographical and specialist representation, insularity, inadequate funding, inspection procedures, selection of examiners and lack of syllabus review.[120] None of these factors was addressed in the Nurses' Act of 1943 which followed the publication of the Horder recommendations. But the Committee's call for enhancing and rationalising the qualifications of sister tutors was finally recognised there. Nurses could qualify for sister-tutors' posts through a number of certificated courses: the nurse teacher's certificate at the RCN, the sister-tutor certificate at King's College of Household and Social Science, Battersea Polytechnic and Leeds University, and the Diploma in Nursing at the universities of Leeds and London.[121] Ultimately, however, beyond drawing attention to the anomalies in the employment conditions of sister-tutors and assistant nurses, the Horder Reports contributed little of substance to the reconstruction of nursing during wartime.

NATIONALISING HEALTH

The wartime emergency health services had a number of important consequences for nurses. One was the acceptance by all political parties that there could be no return to the pre-war heterogeneity of health care. The state had not only come to assume financial responsibility for health services, but also become a major co-ordinating force in the health service, including the direction and control of labour. In September 1943 the Control of Engagement Order, permitting the direction of labour in essential services, had been applied to nurses and midwives. This followed the Registration for Employment measure of April 1943, which required all persons over 17 and under 60 years, with nursing experience in the past ten years, to register.[122] Ministry of Labour and National Service staff in Appointments Offices interviewed nurses not currently engaged in nursing work, with the intention of encouraging them to accept work in an understaffed area. These areas were arranged according to a priority list headed by sanatoria and fever, maternity and mental institutions. From September 1943 all nurses and midwives were obliged to obtain their employment through an Appointments Office of the Ministry of Labour and National Service. Many opted to pursue further training to avoid direction of labour, although such a strategy did benefit hard-pressed areas such as midwifery. Surprisingly little disruption occurred to the conduct of training throughout the war; only one state examination was postponed throughout its duration.[123] Numbers entering training had increased throughout the war, but the Ministry of Labour considered it imprudent to compel any person to undertake nurse training. Centrally, a National Advisory Council for the Recruitment and Distribution of Nurses and Midwives was established jointly by the Ministries of Labour and National Service and Health. It was chaired by Mr McCorquodale MP, Parliamentary Secretary to the Minister of Labour and National Service, and contained representatives from nursing and employers' organisations. Stricter controls were introduced in April 1944 to direct nurses away from their training schools and towards one of the priority fields, with some limited effect upon distribution.[124] Nursing organisations were particularly fearful that such a policy would continue beyond the end of hostilities and that the NHS would provide the ideal excuse for the state to direct nursing labour after the war.[125]

Although the EMS has been hailed as a 'great experiment... in working a hospital system on a national basis', the post-war shortage of nurses threatened the viability of a national health service.[126] The shortage of nurses after the war was described by Aneurin Bevan, Minister of Health, as approaching a 'national disaster'.[127] In a publicity campaign launched jointly by the Ministry of Health and Labour and the Secretary of State for Scotland, an accompanying brochure on staffing the hospitals listed details of recommended conditions of service for immediate adoption by all hospitals. These included removal of the marriage bar, employment of part-time staff, hours of duty, supervision of health and the formation of representative bodies.[128] The traditional technology of the Ministry of Labour publicity campaigns – broadcasts and exhibitions – failed to attract sufficient numbers of recruits into the occupation.[129] The numerical significance of nurses led Ministry of Health officials to publicise nursing as an important resource in the new service.[130] But the rhetoric of crisis failed to translate into participation in the NHS advisory and policy-making machinery. In a speech to the RCN on the occasion of the fourth Nation's Nurses Conference, Aneurin Bevan reassured delegates that the direction of nursing labour would not be enforced in the NHS.[131] He was, however, evasive on the question of consultation on policy matters, but was subjected to little external pressure from the RCN for greater nurse representation. This contrasted markedly with the recalcitrance and assertiveness of the BMA leadership on the representation issue.[132]

TASKS OF TRAINING

Although the Horder reports helped to maintain the momentum for reform, they had little direct effect on policy outcomes. Horder himself was deeply antagonistic to the introduction of the NHS. In a speech to the convention of the American Medical Association, he charged the 'reactionaries' responsible for socialising medicine in Britain with putting back the 'progress of medicine... 100 years.... We have moved from... political clamour to... subservience to a doctrinaire Socialist adventure.'[133] The establishment of the NHS, with the anticipated expansion in facilities and demand for labour, suggested that a comprehensive review of the nursing position was required.[134] Originally this was envisaged as a task for Ministry of Health officials; staff shortages, however, militated against releasing personnel to undertake the work, and a separate team of investigators was eventually identified. The Working Party on Nurse Recruitment and Training, under the chairmanship of Sir Robert Wood, was appointed in January 1946.[135] No attempt was made to achieve representativeness of nursing groups. Officials were drawn from a range of relevant Ministries. Miss Katherine Watt, Chief Nursing Officer at the Ministry of Health, recommended Miss Elizabeth Cockayne, then matron of the Royal Free Hospital, and Miss Daisy Bridges, former tutor to the Florence Nightingale International Foundation. Both Miss Bridges and Miss Cockayne had held Rockefeller travelling fellowships, which had given them the opportunity to study and observe nursing in the USA. The report reflected the American and Canadian experience in its evidence.[136] Dr J. Cohen and Dr T.D. Inch were drawn from the Cabinet Office and Department of Health, Scotland, respectively. The Working Party was supported by a steering committee, with additional expertise drawn from the Ministry of Pensions, the Board of Control and the Ministry of Labour.[137]

The task of the Working Party was to assess the nursing force required for the future health service and make recommendations as to how such a force could best be recruited, trained and deployed.[138] The research consisted of quantitative analyses of training wastage from existing statistical evidence and qualitative explorations of 'causes' from interview and questionnaire data. Job analysis was considered crucial to determining training needs and selecting personnel. Demographic data on sources of recruitment, social composition of the workforce, educational history and pre-nursing education were all identified as appropriate for investigation. Comparative studies of different training methods, such as the 'block' versus the 'sandwich' system, were also to be considered. Morale was a priority issue and its relationship to the quality of leadership in institutions was to be examined. Social relationships between different levels of the nursing hierarchy were to be scrutinised, and discipline, use of authority and opportunities for nurses to lead a 'normal' life were regarded as particularly important.[139] The investigation was unique in its endeavour to draw international comparisons with other countries such as the USA, Finland and selected

Commonwealth countries, including Australia, Canada, New Zealand and South Africa.[140]

STATISTICAL SIGNIFICANCE

The chief impediments to efficient planning of the nursing services identified by the Working Party were the gaps, ambiguities and discrepancies in the statistical returns on the nursing workforce.[141] Drawing upon social research methods common in education and operational research, the Working Party undertook job analyses and surveys of the causes of student wastage, nurses' ability and selection procedures. The choice of a social scientific research strategy may well have been influenced by the intellectual histories of Wood and Cohen. Psychometric testing of nurses revealed a wide range of ability and scores on intelligence tests.[142] Questionnaires were supplemented with interview data and site visits to individual hospitals. The most controversial recommendations of the Working Party concerned proposals to shorten the period of training from two to three years and to reconstitute the GNC.

The report was favourably received in Ministry circles. This may in part be accounted for by the similarities between the conclusions of the report and official thinking. Symmetries of outlook between the report and earlier SMA pronouncements on nurse training can also be detected. Just as the SMA had exerted significant influence upon official thinking in relation to health centres, so it arguably informed Ministry views of nurse training.[143] This would suggest a close alignment of thinking between the Working Party membership, Ministry officials and the SMA.[144]

Many of the report's findings promised to strengthen Ministerial control over training and recruitment through the creation of a Standing Advisory Committee on Nursing to advise on national standards of training. The Nursing Division of the Ministry of Health was to be strengthened by the appointment of advisers on nursing education.[145] Training grants were to be distributed and administered by a Regional Nursing Board. It was considered essential that this Board, responsible for the standard of training, be independent of the body responsible for running the hospitals. Examinations were to be set by regional nursing boards with nursing and educational representation.

The GNC was to be reconstituted with stronger educational, geographical and specialist representation and its functions more tightly tied to examining functions.[146] It was to remain responsible for the general content of the curriculum, standard-of-training inspection of the training units, and examinations for registration.[147] The division of labour between nursing and non-nursing work was to be redrawn to improve utilisation of registered nurse labour. A cadre of orderlies was to substitute for assistant enrolled nurses. The various registers were to be more closely integrated; a common core was to be followed by six months' specialisation in a particular field. Student placements were to be more educationally oriented and training schools grouped regionally under a director of nursing rather than a matron. An interim policy designed to alleviate immediate shortages with orderlies was recommended by Ministry officials. Selection tests such as those employed by the War Office in the assessment of intelligence, character and reliability were advocated.[148] The question of whether the Department was to be responsible for nurse training was regarded with more caution, but early legislation on reconstituting the GNC and setting up the new training system was expected.[149]

REPORTED RECEPTION

The views of interested bodies were requested for consultation. Whilst many nursing organisations were not directly involved in framing recommendations, they welcomed the Majority Report as an important 'scientific' addition to the framing of future developments. However, a number of organisations were hostile and criticised conclusions which operated to their disadvantage.[150] The danger of valuing 'science' over 'sentiment' was attacked in the medical press.[151] The RCN objected to the reduction in training, the phasing out of assistant nurses, and the prejudice against repetitive tasks in learning. The GNC were outraged at the prospect of their diminished role and authority. The prospect of training units being under the control of independent directors rather than matrons was anathema.[152] The Wood Committee had challenged the competence of the GNC to lay down and implement an educational policy for nursing. Unlike its medical counterpart, the General Medical Council (GMC), the nursing council was particularly vulnerable, since it had little educational or academic representation. The predominance of matrons from the London voluntary hospitals over municipal and public health interests was faulted.[153] The Ministry's acceptance in principle of the Working Party's recommendations reflected its deep-seated scepticism of the GNC's capacity to effect reform.

IMPLEMENTING REFORM

Cries of 'statism' and opposition from the nursing organisations seem to have diluted the radicalism of the legislative package which followed the Working Party's report.[154] Provision was made in 1949 for reconstituting the GNC with a strengthened rank-and-file, regional and educational element. The approval of experimental schemes of training was also an attempt to introduce innovation. Area nurse training committees were to be established in regional hospital boards to promote research and improvements in various aspects of training. They were charged with defraying the expenses of training, which translated into tutorial and clerical salaries. Training allowances continued to be paid by hospitals, which perpetuated the service–education conflict.[155] As in 1919, the legislation for nurses adapted the service and educational bodies to the existing structures. It was assumed that nursing policy would be determined by, rather than determine, health care policy.[156]

The Working Party did not complete its reappraisal without controversy. Dissension split it into two uneven camps, leading to the production of majority and minority reports.[157] What had originally been conceived of as an efficient task-force inquiry was converted into an embarrassing exposé of the government's incapacity to perform vital planning functions. Cohen refused to sign the Majority Report and prepared a Minority Report with assistance from a colleague, Geoffrey Pyke. Cohen was resolute that thorough diagnosis and radical treatment alone could remedy the ills of the nursing service.[158] His objections reflected more than methodological scruple: they were fundamentally opposed to the political expediency to which he considered the Working Party had succumbed in their analyses.

What Cohen advocated was a more scientific approach to government in general. He was committed to a positivistic view of social and political science.[159] But his divergence from the views of the Working Party were partly political. He implied that they had toned down their representation of the negative aspects of nursing conditions.[160] Central to his critique was the conviction that traditional committee methods of policy-making had failed to address the intractable problems of nursing. New conclusions required more specifically, new methods; opinion was no substitute for the 'scientific method'.[161] Cohen characterised the current intellectual effort involved in health service planning as 'pre-scientific'.[162] His training as a quantitative psychologist at the Psychological Laboratory, University College London, had arguably exposed him to the influence of Cyril Burt, who was appointed to the chair of psychology at University College, London, in 1931.[163] Moreover, Cohen's research interests reflect the eugenic orientation of inter-war psychology and its confidence in the application of scientific methods of measurement to the solution of social problems.[164] Nursing problems, he asserted, could only ever be amenable to solution if examined in the context of wider health service developments. An integrated and comprehensive approach to health service, social and economic planning was fundamental to the optimum use of man- and woman-power. Health was to be co-ordinated within the master plan of the national economy.[165]

Cohen was aided in his investigation by Geoffrey Pyke, who exerted considerable influence over Cohen's thinking.[166] Pyke, however, tragically committed suicide during the conduct of investigations.[167] Throughout their deliberations, Cohen and Pyke exposed the arbitrary nature of estimates of 'need' for hospital accommodation by different authorities.[168] Lack of attention to long-term planning threatened to leave nursing and other services built upon inadequate foundations. Poor quality data were perceived as the major impediment to long-term reconstruction of the nursing services. In the short term Cohen argued for the establishment of an organisation for research within the Ministry of Health. Prevailing methods of investigation utilised in the Ministry were decried by Cohen as reminiscent of 'scholastic disputation'.[169] Statistical resources there he condemned as 'lamentably defective'.[170] In the longer term he recommended the establishment of a social research council analogous to the Medical Research Council to service all government departments.[171]

Cohen's view of the functioning of institutions was organic and anticipated many of the critiques promulgated by systems and human relations theorists in health care. His appraisal of the social aspects of nursing centred upon its conventual discipline, insularity and narrow conception of citizenship.[172] Senior staff were chastised for their resistance to change and 'institutional stereotypy'.[173] Outworn traditions, authoritarian discipline and poor-quality human relations were held responsible for low morale and commitment to the work.[174] However, Cohen was convinced that an understanding of the emotional and social factors in human behaviour was crucial to understanding the dynamics of change more generally.

ENGENDERING EFFICIENCY

In attempting to measure the effectiveness of nursing care, Cohen took the novel criterion of patients' length of stay as an outcome variable. Consequently he was one of the first to propose empirical study of the relationship between length of stay and nursing skill mix.[175] His theorising on productivity in nursing reflected the wider research tradition of industrial psychology.[176] By analogy with industry, improving human relations in hospitals, it was hoped, would enhance productivity as it had in factories.[177] Training effectiveness and retention of staff could therefore be improved by enriching training and reshaping the division of labour. Underlying Cohen's contentions was a faith in scientific management as the key to efficiency. Such concepts could appeal simultaneously to Ministry officials, nurse leaders and 'experts' in efficiency, although for very different reasons. Ministry officials welcomed the opportunity to streamline trained labour. Nurse leaders applauded the clearer division between 'qualified' and 'non-qualified' staff. The 'good housekeeping' overtones promised to strengthen the matron's domain. The efficiency movement legitimised the authority of psychologists to measure, design and determine nursing work. A leaner but intellectually more demanding form of training and work organisation promised greater satisfaction for rank-and-file nurses. Scientific management could simultaneously justify the adoption or eradication of 'functional' or task allocation. It could imply greater control and autonomy over nursing work and was therefore imbued with a strong emancipatory appeal to those committed to professionalism. The 'efficiency' movement originated in America and infiltrated American nursing much earlier than British.[178] Cohen's report bears the imprint of influence from psychometric studies drawn from occupational psychology and management theory, whose origins could be located across the Atlantic.

The Minority Report was welcomed by the nursing press for its 'fresh approach' and as a 'sincere and serious contribution' to the analysis of nursing problems.[179] Much of the commentary, however, consisted in bland summaries of key findings and recommendations.[180] The fundamental differences declared by Cohen had raised expectations of a bombshell shattering the nursing world.[181] The findings were less radical and the tone milder than some anticipated, and the report was praised for its cogency and compelling conclusions. In particular, the proposals for improving research facilities within nursing and developing a social and psychological research unit in the Ministry of Health were applauded.[182] Cohen's contention that patients' length of stay was associated with the quality of trained staff and represented a valid measurement of the effectiveness of nursing care was commended. The proposal that patient recovery depended upon the calibre of nursing staff was welcomed by those anxious to improve training methods.[183] The RCN expressed its support for Cohen by inviting him to address its specialist meetings and to comment in the *Nursing Times*, now the official organ of the College.[184] The national press condoned Cohen's call for a proper diagnosis and radical treatment of nursing services rather than any 'first aid' approach.[185] The need for a scientific analysis of nursing work as the key to matching the proper role of the nurse with the needs of a comprehensively planned health service was also supported.[186] A number of commentators focused upon the outworn attitudes, 'continual nagging' and Victorian forms of discipline which allegedly inhibited retention of labour.[187]

Some took exception to Cohen's recommendation that training should be directed towards occupational efficiency in terms of both patient and nursing outcomes.[188] Others challenged his methodology, arguing that the patient's length of stay was influenced by such factors as treatment and convalescent facilities and the pressure on waiting lists as well as nurse staffing.[189] Although it was agreed that a broad view needed to be taken of nursing, confining it to a 'totalitarian economy' was considered as having a deleterious effect upon motivation to enter it.[190] According to some, nursing was at risk of being reduced from the 'dignity of a self-governing profession' to a 'State directed industry, in which so-called nurses are to be but technicians trained to fill a presumed social order'.[191]

CONCLUSION

Cohen was one of the first to analyse the relationship between nurse staffing skill mix and patient outcome. His exhortations to develop a more systematic and scientific approach to policy-making were to haunt politicians grappling with the escalating expenditure of the early NHS. Nursing exposed the weakness in NHS planning apparatus. The substantial contribution of nurses' salary rises to increases in the health expenditure revealed the contribution of nursing to the total NHS budget.[192] Paradoxically Bevan, as Minister of Health, was compromised in his defence of NHS spending by the lack of 'scientific' statistical and research data and expertise at his disposal. Nursing services and education occupied a central and sensitive position in the politics of the early NHS. Cohen's report exposed the ramshackle edifice of health care policy-making. In doing so it anticipated many of the methodological challenges with which generations of NHS policy-makers had to contend in quantifying care. To the degree that the Minority Report provided a comprehensive blueprint for action and therefore may be considered more significant than the Majority Report, an analogy can be drawn with the Minority Report of the Poor Law Commission of 1909.[193] However, despite its prescience and appropriateness, it is doubtful whether Cohen's analysis was ever taken seriously by the planners of the new service or by nursing organisations in pressing for research resources. Indeed the political and economic importance of nurses to health care was never exploited by nurse leaders to attract the resources necessary to a high-quality service and long-term career. The history of the early NHS revealed that the traditional relationship between services and education remained intact. Longer-term goals were sacrificed to the short-term gains of political expediency.

Conclusion

I have argued that policy-making in nursing education, and the political strategising associated with it, often occurred by analogy; that is, nurse leaders and policy-makers borrowed ideas and action plans developed by groups and institutions that they perceived as being already successful. As the campaign against Sarah Gamp and the nurses' registration debate illustrate, nurse reformers often adopted strategies pioneered by medical reformers. Indeed medicine's influence upon nursing extended beyond the clinical environment: it provided a model for emulation in the propagation of a populist professional politics. The symmetry between nursing and medical registration was symbolised by the careers, characters and accomplishments of their radical leaders. At the same time, though, it was during the nurses' registration debate that certain contradictions implicit in the analogy between nursing and medical registration finally came to the surface.

Historians have tended to underestimate the importance of arguments about education in the controversies surrounding the nurses' registration debate. For example, the application of such terms as 'technical' and 'scientific' to nurse training inflamed those who were committed to the education of 'character'. Furthermore, arguments against an intellectually demanding form of nurse training received a boost from developments in evolutionary biology. Hereditarian medical members of the Royal British Nurses' Association (RBNA), for example, publicised physiological justifications against higher education for women.

The pursuit of registration by nurses also needs to be understood as part of a wider international movement towards state-backed credentials; in particular, support for nurses' registration in Britain was shaped by contact between British and American nurses in a network reminiscent of an invisible college. The example of Mrs Bedford Fenwick is a case in point. Following the breakdown of relations between her and the RBNA, Mrs Bedford Fenwick looked to America for intellectual and moral support to carry registration in Britain forward. American nurses had organised autonomously from the start. By contrast, British nurses had tended to forge alliances with medical men and women who already had position and prestige, as well as seeking royal patronage. It was only when a pluralist model of organisation failed to fulfil the radical reformers' objectives that British nurses began to organise along American lines.

At the same time, however, the battle for nurses' and medical registration disguised a deeper struggle concerning independent practitioners' desire for control over their activities in opposition to the monopolistic tendencies of elite institutions. Indeed, in many ways the private nurse was analogous to the mid-nineteenth-century general practitioner. Both groups perceived that they needed protection from prestigious institutions which controlled important areas of the nursing and medical markets. The fact that some doctors supported emancipatory strategies of nurses may seem contradictory. The apparent contradiction can be explained, however, by the potential such support offered doctors to strengthen their medical control over the affairs of organised nurses. In other words, doctors' support for nurses may well have been strategic in so far as it was a means to doctors' – as opposed to nurses' – empowerment. It is also possible that the nurses' registration debate disguised deeper jealousies between medical men, who resented the exclusion from the economic rewards which were associated with appointments to institutions with private practices. The separate achievement of registration for midwives in 1902 was the first defeat for the assimilationist medical model of registration proposed by Mrs Bedford Fenwick. Her disdain for 'specialists' corresponded to initial medical prejudice against specialisation. The parallel between medicine and nursing came under severe pressure when, in the early 1900s, the process of professionalisation meant that 'specialism' in medicine was transformed from a term of disapprobation to one of approbation.

Historians of nursing have also tended to underestimate the importance of government policy and, by implication, have instead assigned priority to nurse leaders in reforming nurse education. Consideration of government policy reveals not only the limited extent to which internal reform within nursing can be achieved without government support, but also that initiative does not necessarily reside with the occupational leadership. The Nurses' Registration Act in 1919 was a corollary to the government's post-World War I social reconstruction package. Robert Morant, chief architect of the 1902 Education Act and Permanent Secretary to the new Ministry of Health, applied an analogical pattern of reasoning from the organisation of education to that of health services and nurse training. In the latter case, it was envisaged that grants would be administered by the Board of Education even after the General Nursing Council (GNC) had been created. Government scepticism of the Council's capacity to place public before professional concerns was reflected in the reduced powers of the Council. Official doubt seemed to be vindicated when the collapse of the Caretaker Council revealed the lukewarm support for state registration by moderates. To the degree that training schools were to be treated as voluntary hospitals, subsidised by government grant, the GNC can be perceived as the equivalent of the British Hospitals Association (BHA), and as such an additional barrier to government intervention. The analogy between the GNC and the BHA is strengthened when one considers that both organisations cherished plans to organise hospitals according to their own schemes of 'hierarchical' grouping. Yet both failed to attract and secure the level of resources needed to realise their schemes and ambitions.

Officials such as Robert Morant and Lawrence Brock represented an administrative elite committed to resolving social problems by bureaucratic expertise. Harold Perkin argues that they were motivated by the professional ideal of an elitist society run by professional experts.[1] In such arguments Morant is represented as a bureaucratic socialist, committed to harnessing those ideals in the service of social efficiency.[2] Gillian Sutherland argues that political patronage persisted in certain quarters of the civil service until after World War I. Most examiners and inspectors of education, for example, were recruited from Oxford and Cambridge. Moreover, even after open competition for examinations was introduced, it was the upper classes who excelled, since it was they who had access to the kind of education thought necessary for success in open competition.[3] Steven Stacey has argued that the inter-war period marked the apotheosis of the higher civil service in Britain, in terms of its corporate influence.[4] Official interest in nursing and nurse training needs to be seen in the context of this growth of bureaucratisation of government and its extension into areas not previously contemplated.[5] Morant provided the impetus for assimilating nursing functions and services within state control, and the GNC's educational proposals reflected the spirit as well as the letter of Morant's vision of technical education for nurses within a unified health service. But this too was an unfortunate analogy for the meaning and policy status of responsibility, for technical education remained ambiguous throughout the inter-war period.[6]

Exclusionary tactics used by the Council against Board of Education appointees to the Education and Examinations Committee of the GNC reduced opportunities for the introduction of external expert advice into the Council's educational deliberations. Cross-membership between nursing organisations resulted in a 'circulating' elite which was epitomised in the dual chairmanship exercised by Alicia Lloyd Still of the GNC Education and Examinations Committee and the College of Nursing Education Committee. The overlapping nature of appointments arguably reduced opportunities for innovation.

The oligarchic politics of the GNC were doubly difficult to break since appointments could depend upon pragmatics as well as on position. Only the large, well-endowed institutions had the staff resources to afford matrons the opportunities to attend policy meetings. Similarly, candidates for election from prestigious institutions were more likely to be elected than those of obscure origin. Few nurses were wealthy enough to buy a nursing journal and pursue nursing politics full-time – as Mrs Bedford Fenwick did. Recurrent crises in nurse recruitment and demonstrations of industrial militancy by nurses forced the Council to lower the sights of its educational ambitions. By the mid-1930s it was under pressure to collaborate with local education authorities. It was forced to split the preliminary examination and devolve some of its responsibilities to secondary schools and local education authorities. Its reference point therefore changed from post-secondary technical education to secondary school education. Criticism of the Council's role in regulating nurse education was crystallised in the reports of the Lancet Commission and Athlone Committee. Reservations about the Council's credibility and competence culminated in the Wood report's recommendation in 1947 to consign the GNC to a figurehead rather than key policy-making role in the new National Health Service (NHS).

Throughout the period under discussion, nursing education proved a chronic problem, which fluctuated in public importance. However, during episodes of crisis there was no single solution and little evidence of obvious forward movement. Nurses were only ever one of a number of groups ambitious to reform training; furthermore, they were not necessarily the first or the only group to take the initiative. Nurse education policy was more the product of conflict than of consensus, and its implementation was predicated predominantly upon political and economic contingencies. In this respect I have argued in this book that it is in the context of convergence between government and occupational priorities that the implementation of nurse education policy can best be understood. At the same time, though, I have acknowledged other social forces, such as class and gender politics, that also need to be taken into account. However, the manner in which class and gender politics intersect is complex and cannot be captured by any single explanation or study. The pioneering work of Davies, Maggs, Carpenter, Simnet and Summers has explored the various ways in which nursing work, training, reform and political identity were constructed by the gender and class composition of the occupation.[7]

Recent sociological analyses have added a further twist of sophistication to our understanding of the vexed relationship between nursing and professionalism.[8] Commentators such as Anne Witz and Celia Davies have pointed out that professions, as crucibles of prestige and privilege in society, are gendered institutions, organised around male patterns of career development and priorities. Nursing, as a female-dominated occupation, does not fit easily into the traditional mould within which the archetypal professions have been cast.[9] Moreover, nursing itself is caught in a contradiction in so far as it provides the necessary support for medicine to maintain its dominance, thereby perpetuating the subordination of nursing to medicine. Thus the question has to be asked: to what extent can or should a female-dominated occupation strive to become a profession, especially if that occupation can never, by its very nature, 'arrive' at the state of full professionalism? Furthermore, to what extent is the notion of 'profession' incompatible with the career patterns and lifestyle opportunities of women? Indeed, is the idea of a female-dominated profession a contradiction in terms?

Anne Witz has elaborated our understanding of the complexities surrounding the 'female professionalising project' by pointing to the strategies by which women created variants of prototypical professional models in response to male occupational closure.[10] Celia Davies's brilliant exegesis of gender and nursing illustrates how gender serves to undermine the contribution of nursing to the calculus of care. Her analysis of gender as a political tool fleshes out our fragmentary understanding of the particular predicament that the pursuit of professionalism presents for nursing.[11] Yet notwithstanding the insights derived from two decades of scholarship, our understanding of the role that knowledge and education play in mediating the power relations between different status groups within health care remains incomplete, if not inchoate. What is needed is a historical sociology of nursing knowledge to take the analytic and, I would argue, political project for nursing forward.

But where should we turn for inspiration? Where can we find appropriate models for analysis? Recent commentators have clutched at what is called critical social science in the hope that its holy trinity of enlightenment, empowerment and emancipation may provide a convenient exit for nurses caught in the knowledge/power trap.[12] Susan Reverby describes the dilemma of nursing as being the duty to care in a society that refuses to value caring. But that dilemma extends beyond the contours of caring; it infiltrates and informs the very essence of what it means to be a discipline. In so doing it creates a double-edged dilemma of disciplinary development. But what should we take as our reference in analysing the intellectual development of nursing?

The sociology of knowledge and professions has provided an important stimulus to analyses of the political role that knowledge plays in institutionalising the power relations between groups of different status and power. By that I mean the manner in which ideas, individuals and institutions interact to shape the knowledge base of nursing at any given time. Unfortunately such studies have tended to obscure or ignore the fine-grain detail of how different groups mobilise 'epistemologies of esteem' to legitimise their claims to expertise. What we still need to develop is a vocabulary with which to articulate the processes by which the micro- and macro-politics of knowledge production and utilisation contribute to discipline building and, in turn, the creation and consolidation of disciplinary hierarchies. Any future agenda for research should include more comparative studies of professions and learned disciples.[13] Disciplinary histories to date have tended to treat disciplines as separate from each other, through a single- rather than multi-focus lens. Crucial though such studies might be to exploring the genesis and genealogy of disciplinary development, they are not in themselves sufficient to illuminate the processes by which cognitive and institutional identity shape professional identity. So what kinds of study are available to help us explore nursing as an academic discipline and intellectual endeavour?

In her analysis of the development of social science in America, Dorothy Ross has pointed to the symbiosis between professional expertise and the authority of science.[14] Sociologists of science have referred to the role that scientifically inclined intellectuals assigned to scientific reason in claiming special authority, status and rewards in society.[15] Other commentators have referred to the use of 'science' to advance the interests of intellectual parvenus.[16] Ross elaborates this point by arguing that the intellectual gentry in the nineteenth century drew upon the authority of science to gain an entrée into secular forms of political power from which they had been hitherto been excluded.[17] Nursing has invested much of its intellectual identity in science, although social rather than 'natural' science. Nursing's intellectual alignment with social science has partly been defined in opposition to the alleged positivistic and technocratic values of medicine. But this identification is also a response to medicine's appropriation of the intellectual high ground of science – it is part of a desire to cleave a cognitive course which distances nursing from medicine. Thus nursing's alignment with social science can be read as a strategic attempt to circumnavigate the intellectual hegemony of medicine. But while social science may provide one form of escape route from medical dominance, it by no means eliminates the epistemological web in which nursing is enmeshed in health care. Nursing is at times sandwiched between, and at times encapsulated by, the workers who surround it in the division of labour. Nursing's future as a discipline may depend upon the extent to which it can create space to manoeuvre in clinical and academic environments. Thus nursing's freedom to expand intellectually and, I would argue, politically hinges upon its power relations with kindred disciplines, such as medicine and social work, as well as its wider social attitudes towards class, gender and mind/manual labour.

As with any discipline, including that of medicine, nursing's identity is not 'pure' but the product of a mixed marriage. Eclecticism is arguably something to be embraced rather than eschewed as a source of embarrassment.[18] Systems of economic support, and the values that structure the reward systems and career choice of members of an intellectual community, all come into play in delineating the boundaries and organisation of a discipline.[19] Moreover, short-term crises of confidence should not be confused with a state of chronic instability. Disciplines of knowledge, by their very nature, are self-critical: they interrogate themselves, police their borders and boundaries, and experience periodic episodes of catharsis. English literature, history, public health, sociology and anthropology have all had to struggle with challenges to their legitimacy. Episodic self-doubt and evaluation are a natural process and a healthy consequence of the politics of knowledge growth and intellectual specialisation.[20]

But the question of whether or not nursing can be considered a discipline is a contested one.[21] If we accept Josephine Guy's and Ian Small's definition that a discipline is defined by social utility and specialisation, then nursing undoubtedly qualifies by the first criterion, but the second is much more dubious.[22] Nursing has none of the intellectual specialisation of medicine; for example, we have no chairs in molecular, cardiovascular, endocrinological or neurophysiological nursing. Indeed, there is a sense in which the drive for social utility and the development of means–ends relationships in 'applied' disciplines may undermine opportunities for specialisation. It truncates the pursuit of knowledge for anything other than such a relationship. Moreover, the relatively short history of nursing's association with research and university education means that it has had to establish itself as a generic discipline first, before branching out into more focused areas of development. Perhaps there is also more than a 'trace element' here of nursing rejecting a medical model of academic organisation. However, appointments to chairs in psychiatric nursing, health care of the elderly and community nursing suggest that to some extent nursing has adopted this traditional mode of organisation, where it has the opportunity to do so and where the academy is receptive.

But what are the criteria or standards by which we can evaluate the achievements of nursing as a discipline? What kind of yardstick can we use? Before we even begin to confront this question, we should avoid falling into the same trap as we did with professionalisation. That is, we should not attempt to measure the success or otherwise of nursing by some *a priori* criteria about what a profession or learned discipline should ideally be. Nursing's youth in academe means that any comparison between nursing and any established academic disciplines can hardly be conducted on a level playing field.[23] This would suggest that any insights we may draw from those disciplinary domains must necessarily remain tentative. Lemaine's collection of essays provides a useful 'map' for reading the intellectual landscape of emerging disciplines.[24] But the exclusion of gender, race and class from analyses suggests that caution must be exercised in eliciting and applying lessons that any such studies might have for disciplines such as nursing. Without factoring race, class and gender into the equation, it is impossible to account for the intellectual and social subordination of nursing to disciplines such as medicine, and indeed of the historical stratification and segmentation of nursing more generally. Crucially for nursing, such studies raise the more fundamental question of the extent to which nursing can, in any context, be considered as an analogue of (or anomaly in relation to) other learned disciplines and professions.[25]

If anything, then, this book has used the politics of nursing education to highlight the paucity of research into nursing knowledge, its derivation and differentiation from medicine and other disciplines. For too long this has remained a neglected subject in the history and sociology of health care. What is needed for a future agenda in research is a historical sociology of nursing knowledge, one which takes account of the micro- as well as the macro-politics within which the cognitive and institutional boundaries between disciplines of differential status are negotiated. How are knowledge and access to knowledge controlled by different groups in legitimising claims to authority and in demarcating professional boundaries between rival contestants to occupational turf? The sociology of knowledge and the professions has been articulate about the rise of professional dominance, and medicine is often taken as the paradigmatic example.[26] Lacunae lie, however, in explaining not only what might be called the gendered stratification of cognate health care labour, but the precise historical and political micro-processes by which that intellectual subordination comes about. While we may accept the neo-Weberian view that credentials are the key to commanding social closure for dominant occupations, that 'esoteric knowledge' or 'cognitive exclusiveness' and 'mastery of the indeterminate' are central features of the control of expertise, these explanations, while necessary, are not in themselves sufficient to account for the processes by which such strategies are used in the subordination of other groups.[27] Carpenter argues that the critical theoretical framework within which nursing has traditionally been analysed has concentrated upon the impact of structures of power to the neglect of the processes involved in subordination.[28] However, there still remains only a handful of empirical studies which indicate that the operation of the power balance between nursing and medicine is much more textured and nuanced than conventional assumptions might allow. Such studies, most notably those of the so-called 'new nursing', demonstrate that certain configurations of power relations are not inevitable, but are susceptible to challenge and renegotiation.[29] Translated into disciplinary terms, it is clear that the boundaries of knowledge or practice between different disciplines are fluid rather than fixed, and are historically and socially constructed by the complex interplay that characterises the power relations between different groups. Oral history, supplemented by ethnographic research tailored to explore the 'negotiated order' of clinical practice and expertise, will help to shed light on the micro-dynamics that characterise the ebb and flow of knowledge exchange between groups at different levels in the health care hierarchy.

In his discussion of how to take disciplinary research forward, Charles Rosenberg suggests that in accounts of the institutionalisation of knowledge, both the consumers and the transmitters of academic and professional learning should be studied, their backgrounds evaluated and the formal accounts of their ideas retrieved.[30] Drawing a parallel with the ethnologist, Rosenberg argues that historians of knowledge must integrate formal intellectual content with social and institutional organisation, systems of economic support, and the values that sanction and reward the career choice of members of a particular intellectual subculture.[31] But any further study which attempts to apply insights from the sociology of knowledge to nursing must also include issues of race, class and gender in the analysis.[32] Class prejudice, misogyny and racist perceptions of educability have all at times constrained the development of nursing as an academic project.

There is, however, the danger that, in concentrating upon knowledge as the key to power, one is missing the target by focusing upon the superstructure rather than the substance of power. Any strategy for radical change must be multi-focal, multi-purpose and multi-stranded. It must be prepared to rethink the structure and provision of health services and education from the foundations up in a manner that challenges the categorical ordering of power relations between institution/community, male/female, science/sentiment, professional/lay. What other models of occupational and educational organisation could nurses draw upon in building a positive future grounded in the principles of social justice for society in the future? What role might a generic, multi-disciplinary education for all health workers play in creating a workforce flexible enough to contribute to that future? This book has considered the pressures shaping ideas about nurses' educability, the content of curricula and the implementation of education policy from the late nineteenth century to the mid-twentieth century in England and Wales. It has sought to go some small way to preparing the ground for a historical sociology of nursing education, which has a politics of nursing knowledge at its heart and in its mind.

Notes

INTRODUCTION

1 S. Reverby, *Ordered to Care: The Dilemma of American Nursing 1850–1945*, Cambridge, Cambridge University Press, 1987, p. 1.
2 C. Davies, 'Professional Power and Sociological Analysis: Lessons from a Comparative Historical Study of Nursing in Britain and the USA', University of Warwick, PhD thesis, 1981; B. Abel-Smith, *A History of the Nursing Profession*, London, Heinemann, 1960.
3 A. Summers, *Angels and Citizens: British Women as Military Nurses, 1854–1914*, London, Routledge, 1988; A. Summers, 'The Mysterious Demise of Sarah Gamp: The Domiciliary Nurse and her Detractors', *Victorian Studies*, 1989, vol. 32, pp. 365–86; C. Maggs, *The Origins of General Nursing*, London, Croom Helm, 1983.
4 R. Dingwall, A.M. Rafferty and C. Webster, *An Introduction to the Social History of Nursing*, London, Routledge, 1988.
5 C. Rosenberg, *The Care of Strangers: The Rise of America's Hospital System*, New York, Basic Books, 1987; Reverby, *Ordered to Care*.
6 B. Melosh, *The Physician's Hand: Work, Culture and Conflict in American Nursing*, Philadelphia, Temple University Press, 1982.
7 Summers, 'Mysterious Demise'.
8 M. Baly, *Florence Nightingale and the Nursing Legacy*, London, Croom Helm, 1986; J. Prince, 'Florence Nightingale's Reforms of Nursing 1860–1887', University of London, PhD thesis, 1986.
9 C. Davies, 'Professionalising Strategies as Time and Culture-bound: American and British Nursing circa 1893', in E. Condliffe Lagemann (ed.), *Nursing History: New Perspectives, New Possibilities*, New York, Teachers College Press, 1983, pp. 47–64; N. Tomes, 'The Silent Battle: Nurse Registration in New York State 1903–1920', in E. Condliffe Lagemann (ed.), *Nursing History: New Perspectives, New Possibilities*, New York, Teachers College Press, 1983, pp. 107–32.
10 A.M. Rafferty, 'Art, Science and Social Science in Nursing: Occupational Origins and Disciplinary Identity', *Nursing Inquiry*, 1995, vol. 2, pp. 141–8.

1 REFORMATORY RHETORIC

1 A. Summers, 'The Mysterious Demise of Sarah Gamp: The Domiciliary Nurse and her Detractors', *Victorian Studies*, 1989, vol. 32, pp. 365–86.
2 Ibid.
3 For a more general discussion on representations of nurses in novels see C. Maggs, *The Origins of General Nursing*, London, Croom Helm, 1983, pp. 174–200.
4 C. Dickens, *Martin Chuzzlewit*, Oxford, Oxford University Press, 1984, p. 265. For hospital reformers' views see K. Williams, 'From Sarah Gamp to Florence Nightingale: A Critical Study of Hospital Nursing Systems from 1840–1897', in C. Davies (ed.), *Rewriting Nursing History*, London, Croom Helm, 1980, pp. 41–75.
5 Summers, 'Mysterious Demise', p. 365; A. Summers, 'Hidden from History?: The Home Care of the Sick in the Nineteenth Century', *History of Nursing Journal*, 1992/3, vol. 4, pp. 227–43; E.H. Sieveking, 'Training Institutions for Nurses', *Englishwoman's Magazine*, 1852, vol. 7, p. 294. Dr Edward Sieveking was active in sanitary reform organisations such as the Epidemiological Association, which he used to form a committee to press for training provision in home nursing for female workhouse inmates: see Summers, 'Hidden from History?'.
6 As was the 'trained' nurse who replaced her and, according to Maggs, competed with the general practitioner for patients: see Maggs, *Origins*, p. 2.
7 Ibid., pp. 178–9.
8 See Summers, 'Mysterious Demise', p. 367; for the growth of the hospital system in England and Wales see B. Abel-Smith, *The Hospitals 1848–1948*, London, Heinemann, 1964, and its companion volume by R. Pinker, *English Hospital Statistics 1861–1938*, London, Heinemann, 1966; L. Granshaw and R. Porter (eds), *The Hospital in History*, London, Routledge, 1989; J. Woodward, *To Do the Sick No Harm: A Study of the British Voluntary Hospital System to 1875*, London, Routledge and Kegan Paul, 1974. For American trends see C. Rosenberg, *The Care of Strangers: The Rise of America's Hospital System*, New York, Basic Books, 1987; R. Stevens, *In Sickness and in Wealth: American Hospitals in the Twentieth Century*, New York, Basic Books, 1989.
9 For an account of pre-reform nurses in novels see the illuminating discussion by Maggs, *Origins*, pp. 174–200.
10 Ibid., p. 189.
11 A.T. Thompson, *The Domestic Management of the Sick Room: Necessary, in Aid of Medical Treatment for the Cure of Disease*, London, Orme, Brown, Green, Longman, 1841, p. 123.
12 Ibid.
13 Ibid., p. 124.
14 Ibid., p. 483.
15 Ibid., pp. 482–3.
16 Ibid., p. 483.

17   William Gairdner, lecturer in medicine at the University of Edinburgh, argued only the quack would pander to the excesses of public opinion: see W. Gairdner, *On Medicine and Medical Education: Three Lectures with Notes and an Appendix*, Edinburgh, Sutherland and Knox, 1858, p. 43.

18   See C. Davies, 'Professionalising Strategies as Time and Culture-bound: American and British Nursing circa 1893', in E. Condliffe Lagemann (ed.), *Nursing History: New Perspectives, New Possibilities*, New York, Teachers College Press, 1983, pp. 47–64; C. Davies, *Gender and the Professional Predicament in Nursing*, Buckingham, Open University Press, 1995; E. Freidson, *Professionalism Reborn: Theory, Prophecy and Policy*, Chicago, University of Chicago Press, 1994; T. Gelfand, *Professionalising Modern Medicine: Paris Surgeons and Medical Science and Institutions in the Eighteenth Century*, Westport, CT, Greenwood Press, 1980; R. Hugman, *Power in Caring Professions*, London, Macmillan, 1991; G. Larkin, *Occupational Monopoly and Modern Medicine*, London, Tavistock, 1983; T. Johnson, G. Larkin and M. Saks (eds), *Health Professions and the State in Europe*, London, Routledge, 1995; N. Parry and J. Parry, *The Rise of the Medical Profession*, London, Croom Helm, 1980; M.J. Petersen, *The Medical Profession in Mid-Victorian England*, London, Croom Helm, 1978; A. Witz, *Professions and Patriarchy*, London, Routledge, 1992.

19   B. Bynum and R. Porter (eds), *Medical Fringe and Medical Orthodoxy*, London, Croom Helm, 1987, pp. 1–4.

20   Cross-membership between temperance and evangelical organisations is discussed by B. Harrison, 'State Intervention and Moral Reform', in P. Hollis (ed.), *Pressure from Without in Early Victorian England*, London, Arnold, 1974, pp. 289–322.

21   P. Abrams, *The Origins of British Sociology 1834–1914*, Chicago, University of Chicago Press, 1968, p. 39.

22   No comprehensive history of the NAPSS's activities exists but its effects upon social policy are discussed by E. Yeo, 'Social Science and Social Change: A Social History of Some Aspects of Social Science and Social Investigation in Britain 1830–1890', University of Sussex, D. Phil thesis, 1972; the Association's participation in debates on women's education are discussed by S. Fletcher, *Feminists and Bureaucrats: A Study of Girls' Education in the Nineteenth Century*, Cambridge, Cambridge University Press, 1980, pp. 14–19.

23   F.B. Smith, *Florence Nightingale: Reputation and Power*, London, Croom Helm, 1982, pp. 132–42.

24   For details of the early history of the British Association for the Advancement of Science see J. Morrell and A. Thrackray, *Gentlemen of Science: Early Years of the British Association for the Advancement of Science*, Oxford, Clarendon Press, 1981.

25   Smith, *Florence Nightingale*, pp. 132–3.

26   Ibid., p. 134.

27   M. Dean and G. Bolton, 'The Administration of Poverty and the Development of Nursing Practice in Nineteenth Century England', in Davies, *Rewriting*, pp. 76–101.

28 Smith, *Florence Nightingale*, pp. 169–70.
29 *The Times*, 30 October 1869; see also commentary by M.M. Gordon, 'The Double Cure or What is a Medical Mission?', *Theological Pamphlets*, 1869, vol. 27, pp. 68–9. Hospital nursing provided a prime target for reformers' strictures: see B. Abel-Smith, *A History of the Nursing Profession*, London, Heinemann, 1960; R. White, *Social Change and the Development of the Nursing Profession: A History of the Poor Law Nursing Service 1848–1948*, London, Henry Kimpton, 1973.
30 J. Higgins, 'The Improvement of Nurses in the County Districts', *Transactions of the National Association for the Promotion of Social Science*, London, Parker, 1861, pp. 574–7.
31 See M. Barfoot, 'Brunonionism Under the Bed: An Alternative to University Medicine in the 1780's', *Medical History*, 1988, Supplement No 8. p. 22.
32 Anon., 'Hospital Nursing without Alcoholic Drinks', *Pamphlets on Temperance*, 1882, vol. 24, pp. 2–16.
33 Ibid., p. 12.
34 Ibid., p. 2.
35 Ibid., p. 3.
36 Ibid., p. 4.
37 B. Harrison, *Drink and the Victorians: The Temperance Question in England, 1815–1872*, London, Faber and Faber, 1983, pp. 37–8.
38 Ibid., p. 40; E.P. Thompson 'Time, Discipline and Industrial Capitalism', *Past and Present*, 1967, vol. 38, pp. 56–97.
39 Little has been written about male nurses generally, although more is known about their involvement in trade unionism and mental health nursing respectively: see M. Carpenter, *Working for Health: The History of the Confederation of Health Service Employees*, London, Lawrence and Wishart, 1988; P. Nolan, *A History of Mental Health Nursing*, London, Chapman Hall, 1993. For a brief review of the 'marginalisation' of men from the history of general nursing see K. Robinson and A.M. Rafferty, *The Nursing Workforce*, London, Polytechnic of the South Bank, 1988, pp. 48–51.
40 Anon., 'Hospital Nursing', pp. 4–5.
41 Thompson, *Domestic Management*, p. 6.
42 Ibid., p. 7.
43 Ibid., p. 9.
44 Ibid., p. 11.
45 Ibid., p. 130.
46 Barfoot, 'Brunonionism Under the Bed', p. 24.
47 See National Temperance League, *Alcohol in Hospital Practice*, London, National Temperance League, 1934, pp. 8–9.
48 See Public Record Office, Kew, London, T161/1056, *Grant In Relief of Duty Paid on Spirits etc Used For Medical and Surgical Purposes*.
49 G. Stedman Jones, *Outcast London: A Study of the Relationship between Classes in Victorian Society*, Oxford, Oxford University Press, 1971, p. 289.

50   L. Chevalier, *Labouring Classes and Dangerous Classes in Paris during the First Half of the Nineteenth Century*, London, Routledge and Kegan Paul, 1973.

51   For a study of the evolution of technical terminology used to describe social class in the early to mid-nineteenth century see A. Briggs, 'The Language of Class in Early Nineteenth Century England', in A. Briggs and J. Saville (eds), *Essays in Labour History in Memory of G.D.H. Cole*, London, Macmillan, 1960, pp. 43–73.

52   Mrs Trimmer, *The Oeconomy of Charity, or an Address to Ladies, Adapted to the Present State of Charitable Institutions in England with a Particular View to the Cultivation of Religious Principles among the Lower Orders of Society*, London, J. Johnson and F.C. Rivington with G.G. and J. Robinson and Longman and Rees, 1801, pp. 6–7.

53   See M. Baly, 'The Nightingale Nurses and Hospital Architecture', *Bulletin of the History of Nursing Group*, 1986, vol. 2, pp. 1–6; J. Thompson and G. Goldin, *The Hospital: A Social and Architectural History*, New Haven, Yale University Press, 1975.

54   S. Pollard, *The Genesis of Modern Management*, London, Edward Arnold, 1965.

55   F. Nightingale, *Notes on Nursing: What it Is and What it Is Not*, London, Harrison, 1860, pp. 50–1.

56   M. Baly, *Florence Nightingale and the Nursing Legacy*, London, Croom Helm, 1986, p. 57, notes that misconduct was one of the most frequently recorded reasons for dismissal of probationers at the Nightingale Training School.

57   D. Armstrong, *Political Anatomy of the Body: Medical Knowledge in Britain in the Twentieth Century*, Cambridge, Cambridge University Press, 1983; M. Foucault, *Discipline and Punish: The Birth of the Prison*, New York, Pantheon, 1971.

58   H. Braverman, *Labour and Monopoly Capital: The Degradation of Work in the Twentieth Century*, New York, Monthly Review Press, 1974, pp. 67–9.

59   This usage is ascribed to the *Westminster Gazette*, 16 August 1909, in the *Oxford English Dictionary*, 2nd edn, Oxford, Oxford University Press.

60   Abel-Smith, *Hospitals*, p. 43, contains rules governing behaviour of patients; further details are included in *The Old Statutes and Rules For the Government of the General Hospital near Nottingham open to the Sick and Lame Poor of any County*, Nottingham, 1783, pp. 34–6.

61   Abel-Smith, *Hospitals*, p. 11. These rules demonstrate that the 'dependency' of patients was considerably less than that of patients today.

62   Baly, *Nursing Legacy*, pp. 47–8.

63   See Summers, 'Mysterious Demise', p. 371; for discussion of the class bias in the production of literature and the relationship between literature and working-class culture see M. Vicinus, *The Industrial Muse: A Study of Nineteenth Century British Working Class Literature*, London, Croom Helm, 1974; R. Williams, *Culture and Society 1780–1950*, London, Chatto and Windus, 1958.

64   Higgins, 'Improvement of Nurses', pp. 574–7.

65 For a discussion of the principles of caricature in art, see E. Kris and E. Gombrich, 'The Principles of Caricature', *Journal of Medical Psychology*, 1937, vol. xvii, pp. 319–42.
66 Summers, 'Mysterious Demise', p. 372.
67 S. Monod, *Martin Chuzzlewit*, London, Allen and Unwin, 1985, p. 68.
68 L. Jordonova, 'Natural Facts: A Historical Perspective on Science and Sexuality', in C. MacCormack and M. Strathern (eds), *Nature, Culture and Gender*, Cambridge, Cambridge University Press, 1983, pp. 42–69.
69 Ibid., p. 44.
70 See A. Summers, 'The Costs and Benefits of Caring: Nursing Charities, c.1830–c.1860', in J. Barry and C. Jones (eds), *Medicine and Charity Before the Welfare State*, London, Routledge, 1991, pp. 133–48; C. Helmstadter, 'The First Training Institution for Nurses: St John's House and 19th Century Nursing Reform Part II', *History of Nursing Journal*, 1994/5, vol. 5, pp. 3–18.
71 A. Summers, 'Pride and Prejudice: Ladies and Nurses in the Crimean War', *History Workshop Journal*, 1983, vol. 6, pp. 33–56; Summers, 'Costs and Benefits of Caring'.
72 Maggs, *Origins*, p. 16.
73 Ibid., p. 14.

2 THE CHARACTER OF TRAINING AND THE TRAINING OF CHARACTER

1 S. Pollard, *The Genesis of Modern Management*, London, Edward Arnold, 1965, pp. 255–6.
2 For details of girl's educational provision in mechanics institutes see J. Purvis, *Hard Lessons: The Schooling of Working Class Girls*, Cambridge, Polity Press, 1989, pp. 109–15.
3 S. Rothblatt, *The Revolution of the Dons: Cambridge and Society in Victorian England*, London, Faber and Faber, 1968, addresses male dons only; see also J. Purvis, 'Working-class Women and Adult Education in Nineteenth-century Britain', *History of Education*, 1980, vol. 9, pp. 193–212; E.Gomersall, 'Ideals and Realities: The Education of Working-Class Girls, 1800–1870', *History of Education*, 1988, vol. 17, pp. 37–53; P. Horn, 'The Education and Employment of Working-class Girls, 1870–1914', *History of Education*, 1988, vol. 17, pp. 71–82.
4 F. Hunt (ed.), *Lessons for Life: The Schooling of Girls and Women 1850–1950*, Oxford, Blackwell, 1989. Accounts concerned with the history of education in the working classes devote little attention to girls: see J.S. Hurt, *Elementary Schooling and the Working Classes 1786–1918*, London, Routledge and Kegan Paul, 1979; B. Simon, *Education and the Labour Movement 1870–1920*, London, Lawrence and Wishart, 1965; H. Silver, *The Concept of Popular Education: A Study of Ideas in and Social Movements in the Nineteenth Century*, London, Methuen, 1977; H. Silver, 'Aspects of Neglect: The Strange Case of Victorian Popular Education', in *Education as History*, London, Methuen, 1983, pp. 17–34.

5   J. Kamm, *Hope Deferred: Girls' Education in English History*, London, Methuen, 1965; J.B.S. Pedersen, 'The Reform of Women's Secondary and Higher Education: A Study in Elite Groups', University of California, PhD thesis, 1974; J. Burstyn, *Victorian Education and the Ideal of Womanhood*, London, Croom Helm, 1980; C. Dyhouse, *Girls Growing Up in Late Victorian and Edwardian England*, London, Routledge and Kegan Paul, 1981; G. Sutherland, 'The Movement for the Higher Education of Women: Its Social and Intellectual Context in England c.1840–80', in P. Waller (ed.), *Politics and Social Change in Modern Britain: Essays presented to A.F. Thomson*, Brighton, Harvester, 1987, pp. 91–116. A compact and comprehensive summary of women and higher education is provided by J. Howarth in E. Davies, *The Higher Education of Women: A Classic Victorian Argument for the Equal Education of Women (1866)*, London, Hambleton, 1988, pp. vii–liii; D. Bennett, *Emily Davies and the Liberation of Women*, London, Andre Deutsch, 1990.

6   C. Maggs, *The Origins of General Nursing*, London, Croom Helm, 1983, pp. 73–101; A. Simnet, 'The Pursuit of Respectability: Women and the Nursing Profession, 1860–1900', in R. White (ed.), *Political Issues in Nursing: Past, Present and Future*, Chichester, John Wiley, 1986, pp. 1–24. Social classification and nursing employment are also discussed by C. Davies, 'Making Sense of the Census', *Sociological Review*, 1980, vol. 28, pp. 595–609; K. Robinson and A.M. Rafferty, *The Nursing Workforce*, London, Polytechnic of the South Bank, 1988, pp. 34–43.

7   F.B. Smith, *Florence Nightingale: Reputation and Power*, London, Croom Helm, 1982; M. Baly, *Florence Nightingale and the Nursing Legacy*, London, Croom Helm, 1986; A. Summers, *Angels and Citizens: British Women as Military Nurses, 1854–1914*, London, Routledge, 1988, pp. 29–66.

8   B. Abel-Smith, *The Hospitals 1848–1948*, London, Heinemann, pp. 43–5; M.J. Peterson, *The Medical Profession in Mid-Victorian England*, London, Croom Helm, 1978, pp. 14–15.

9   J. Berlant, *Profession and Monopoly: A Study of Medicine in the United States and Britain*, Berkeley, CA, University of California Press, 1975, pp. 145–65; C. Newman, *The Evolution of Medical Education in the Nineteenth Century*, Oxford, Oxford University Press, 1957. Lawrence's research is one of the few pieces to have investigated clinical teaching, but is concerned predominantly with the period 1750–1815: see S. Lawrence, 'Science and Medicine at the London Hospitals: The Development of Teaching and Research, 1750–1815', University of Toronto, PhD thesis, 1985; I.S.L. Loudon, *Medical Care and the General Practitioner 1750–1850*, Oxford, Clarendon Press, 1986; L. Rosner, *Medical Education in the Age of Improvement*, Edinburgh, Edinburgh University Press, 1991; P. Underhill, 'Science, Professionalism and the Development of Medical Education in England: An Historical Sociology', University of Edinburgh, PhD thesis, 1987. For more recent appraisal see A. Wear, J. Geyer-Kordesh and R. French (eds), *Doctors and Ethics: The Earlier Historical Setting of Professional Ethics*, Clio Medica, Amsterdam, Rodopi, 1993, vol. 24.

10 For the American hospital system and its impact upon nursing see S. Reverby, *Ordered to Care: The Dilemma of American Nursing*, Cambridge, Cambridge University Press, 1987, pp. 212–36; C. Rosenberg, *The Care of Strangers: The Rise of America's Hospital System*, New York, Basic Books, 1987, pp. 166–89. For a sociological analysis of British nurses see E. Gamarnikov, 'Women's Employment and the Sexual Division of Labour: The Case of Nursing 1860–1923', University of London, PhD thesis, 1985; E. Gamarnikov, 'Nurse or Woman: Gender and Professionalism in Reformed Nursing 1860–1923', in P. Holden and J. Littlewood (eds), *Anthropology and Nursing*, London, Routledge, 1991, pp. 110–29.

11 Summers, *Angels and Citizens*, p. 21. Nurses in hospitals can be considered the 'medical' equivalent of deference givers: see E. Goffman, 'The Nature of Deference and Demeanour', *American Anthroplogist*, 1956, vol. 58, pp. 473–512.

12 Women workers generally were cheaper and bedside nursing was already established as 'gendered' work. Women were consistently paid less for the same work as men. See S. Allen, 'Gender Inequality and Class Formation', in A. Giddens and G. MacKenzie (eds), *Social Class and the Division of Labour: Essays in Honour of Ilya Neustadt*, Cambridge, Cambridge University Press, 1982, pp. 137–47; S. Hogg, 'The Employment of Women in Great Britain 1891–1921', University of Oxford, DPhil thesis, 1967; J. Lewis, *Women in England 1870–1950: Sexual Divisions and Social Class*, Brighton, Wheatsheaf, 1984.

13 S. Jex-Blake, *Medical Women: A Thesis and a History*, Edinburgh, Oliphant, Anderson and Ferrier, 1872; R. Morantz Sanchez, *Sympathy and Science*, Oxford, Oxford University Press, 1985; M. Barfoot, ' "To Do Violence to the Best Feelings of their Nature": The Controversy Over the Clinical Teaching of Women Medical Students at the Royal Infirmary of Edinburgh', Edinburgh, Lothian Health Board Medical Archives Centre, 1992. Evidence of a fluid rather than fixed division of labour between medical students, dressers, clerks and nurses is provided by G. Risse, *Hospital Life in Enlightenment Scotland*, Cambridge, Cambridge University Press, 1986.

14 See Rosenberg, *Care of Strangers*, pp. 122–41. Florence Nightingale's crusade was waged against this so-called evil.

15 I. Pinchbeck, *Women Workers and the Industrial Revolution 1750–1850*, London, Virago, 1985, pp. 194–201.

16 The role of economic interests in the calculus of reformed nursing care is most clearly articulated by C. Maggs, 'Profit and Loss and the Hospital Nurse', in C. Maggs (ed.), *Nursing History: The State of the Art*, London, Croom Helm, 1987, pp. 176–89.

17 For the contradictory expectations imposed upon women see E. Trudgill, *Madonnas and Magdalens: The Origins and Development of Victorian Sexual Attitudes*, London, Heinemann, 1976.

18 For the origins of the so-called domestic ideology see C. Hall, 'The Early Formation of Victorian Domestic Ideology', in S. Burman (ed.), *Fit Work for Women*, London, Croom Helm, 1979, pp. 15–32; J. Lewis

(ed.), *Labour of Love: Women's Experience of Work and the Family*, Oxford, Blackwell, 1986. For an authoritative analysis of the emergence and consolidation of middle-class attitudes to domesticity see especially L. Davidoff and C. Hall, ' "The Nursery of Virtue": Domestic Ideology and the Middle Class', in L. Davidoff and C. Hall, *Family Fortunes: Men and Women of the English Middle Class 1780–1850*, London, Hutchinson, 1987, pp. 149–92.

19 The notion of a sharp division between the private world of the family and the public world of work for many women was a fantasy they could not afford: see Lewis, *Women in England*, p. 145; L. Davidoff and C. Hall, ' "The Hidden Investment": Women and the Enterprise', in *Family Fortunes*, pp. 272–315.

20 For details of probationer duties and expectations regarding conduct see Baly, *Nursing Legacy*, pp. 230–2.

21 For comments on marriage and morality in nursing see Reverby, *Ordered to Care*, pp. 11–21. For details of the changing age and marital profile of 'sick nurses' from nineteenth century census data see Robinson and Rafferty, *Nursing Workforce*, pp. 30–8.

22 For a review of nursing 'systems' which predated Florence Nightingale see K. Williams, 'From Sarah Gamp to Florence Nightingale: A Critical History of Hospital Nursing Systems from 1840–1897', in C. Davies (ed.), *Rewriting Nursing History*, London, Croom Helm, 1980, pp. 41–75.

23 Baly's demythologising account of the politics of the Nightingale fund is a more tempered revisionist account than Smith's iconoclasm: see Baly, *Nursing Legacy*; Smith, *Florence Nightingale*.

24 The ideological function of Florence Nightingale as a 'heroine legend' is explored by E. Whittaker and V. Olesen, 'The Faces of Florence Nightingale: Functions of the Heroine Legend in an Occupational Sub-culture', *Human Organisation*, 1964, vol. 23, pp. 123–30. For a literary treatment of the female hero in fiction see C. Pearson and K. Pope, *The Female Hero in American and British Literature*, New York, Bowker, 1981; see also W.J. Bishop and S. Goldie, *A Bio-bibliography of Florence Nightingale*, London, Dawsons of Pall Mall for the International Council of Nurses and Florence Nightingale International Foundation, 1962.

25 Baly, *Nursing Legacy*, p. 266.

26 See R. Wilkinson, 'The Gentleman Ideal and the Maintenance of a Political Elite. Two Case-Studies: Confucian Education in the Tang, Sung, Ming and Ching Dynasties and the Late Victorian Public Schools 1870–1914', in P. Musgrove (ed.), *Sociology, History and Education*, London, Methuen, 1970, pp. 126–42. Interpretations of 'liberal' education were controversial and the subject of debate on the reform of the university system in the 1860s and 1870s. For details see T. Heyck, *The Transformation of Intellectual Life in Victorian England*, London, Croom Helm, 1982, pp. 155–89.

27 C. Rosenberg, 'Florence Nightingale on Contagion: The Hospital as Moral Universe', in C. Rosenberg (ed.), *Healing and History: Essays for*

George Rosen, New York, Dawson, Science History Publications, 1979, pp. 116–36.

28 For discussion of the impact of biological metaphors upon political theorising see R. Cooter, 'The Power of the Body in the Early Nineteenth Century', in B. Barnes and S. Shapin (eds), *Natural Order: Historical Studies of Scientific Culture*, London, Sage, 1979, pp. 73–96. Paul Weindling has explored the relationship between organicist ideology and social structure in imperial Germany: see P. Weindling, 'Theories of the Cell State in Imperial Germany', in C. Webster (ed.), *Biology, Medicine and Society 1840–1940*, Cambridge, Cambridge University Press, 1981, pp. 96–156.

29 Rosenberg, 'Moral Universe', pp. 116–36.

30 C. Rosenberg, 'Florence Nightingale and Contagion: The Hospital as Moral Universe', in *Explaining Epidemics and Other Studies in the History of Medicine*, Cambridge, Cambridge Univeristy Press, 1992, pp. 90–108.

31 Ibid., p. 92.

32 For an intellectual biography of Farr and his views on 'zymosis' see J. Euler, *Victorian Social Medicine: The Ideas and Methods of William Farr*, Baltimore, Johns Hopkins University Press, 1979, pp. 97–122. For the debate on the 'germ' theory and the definitional challenge posed by theories of fever causation see M. Pelling, 'Contagion/Germ Theory/Specificity', in W. Bynum and R. Porter (eds), *Companion Encyclopedia of the History of Medicine*, London, Routledge, 1994, vol. 1, pp. 309–34. Rosenberg reveals that Farr shifted some ground under pressure from contagionists and that Farr's relationship with Florence Nightingale also changed: see Rosenberg, *Explaining Epidemics*, pp. 97–8; Z. Cope, *Florence Nightingale and the Doctors*, London, Museum Press, 1958.

33 Showalter argues for a more sympathetic treatment of Florence Nightingale's attitude towards 'feminism' than she has traditionally received at the hands of historians: see E. Showalter, 'Florence Nightingale's Feminist Complaint: Women, Religion and *Suggestions for Thought*', *Signs*, 1981, vol. 6, pp. 395–412.

34 R. Quain (ed.), *A Dictionary of Medicine: Including General Pathology, General Therapeutics, Hygiene, and the Diseases Peculiar to Women and Children*, London, Longman, Green, 1882, vol. 2, p. 1043. The entry on nursing was written by Miss Nightingale.

35 For analysis of the social origins and functions of etiquette texts see L. Davidoff, *The Best Circles: Society, Etiquette and the Season*, London, Croom Helm, 1974; M. Quinlan, *Victorian Prelude: A History of English Manners 1700–1830*, London, Cassell, 1941.

36 Early professional codes of conduct have received little attention from researchers. For a rare glimpse see I. Waddington, 'The Development of Medical Ethics – A Sociological Analysis', *Medical History*, 1975, vol. 19, pp. 36–51; V. Nutton and R. Porter (eds), *The History of Medical Education in Britain*, Oxford, Pergamon, 1995, vol. 30.

37 In so far as ethical writings and tracts were concerned with conduct they were often conflated with discipline: see M. Tufts, 'Hospital Discipline

and Ethics', *Nursing Times*, 1917, vol. 17, 20 October, pp. 1231–2, 24 November p. 1338–9, and 1 December, pp. 1422–5. The relationship between these two factors was still being expressed as late as 1960: see H. Way, 'Authority and Discipline', *Nursing Times*, 1960, vol. 29, April, pp. 545–6.

38   Z. Veitch, *Handbook for Nurses for the Sick*, London, Churchill, 1870, p. 43.

39   This must be one of the earliest recorded instances of nurse physician substitution and the expanding role of the nurse: ibid., p. 44.

40   C. Childe, *Operative Nursing and Technique: A Book for Nurses, Dressers, House Surgeons*, London, Balliere, 1916.

41   R. Barwell, *The Care of the Sick: A Course of Practical Lectures Delivered at the Working Women's College, London*, London, Chapman and Hall, 1857, p. 102.

42   R. Johnson, 'Education Policy and Social Control in Early Victorian England', *Past and Present*, 1970, vol. 49, pp. 96–119.

43   Veitch, *Handbook*, p. v.

44   Ibid.

45   H. Martineau, *Life in the Sickroom: Essays by an Invalid*, London, Moxon, 1844, pp. 138–140; Barwell, *Care of the Sick*, p. 101.

46   Martineau, *Life in the Sickroom*, p. 27. For details of selected correspondence between Harriet Martineau and Florence Nightingale see M. Vicinus and Bea Nergard (eds), *Ever Yours, Florence Nightingale: Selected Letters*, London, Virago, 1989, pp. 24, 202–4, 226–8, 259–61; M. Baly (ed.), *As Miss Nightingale Said*, London, Scutari Press, p. 117.

47   Mrs Ranyard, *The Missing Link, or Bible Women in the Homes of the London Poor*, London, James Nisbet & Co., 1859, p. 24. For further details of the activities of the Bible Nurses see F. Prochaska, 'Body and Soul: Bible Nurses and the Poor in Victorian London', *Historical Research*, 1987, vol. 60, pp. 336–48.

48   British Nurses Association, *First Annual Report*, London, British Nurses Association, 1889, p. 15.

49   Martineau, *Life in the Sick Room*, p. 138.

50   Barwell, *Care of the Sick*, p. 102.

51   Ibid.

52   J. Barnes, *Notes on Surgical Nursing: Being a Short Course of Lectures on Surgical Nursing delivered at the School for Nurses in Connection with the Liverpool Workhouse*, London, Churchill, 1865, p. 6.

53   R. Brudenell Carter, *On the Influence of Education and Training in Preventing Diseases of the Nervous System*, London, Churchill, 1855, p. 295.

54   Ibid., p. 296.

55   Barnes, *Surgical Nursing*, p. 8.

56   Ibid., p. 15.

57   Anon., *The Nurse and the Nursery: Being a Digest of Important Information by a Physician*, London, Hope, 1854, p. i.

58   Barnes, *Surgical Nursing*, p. 9.

59   Ibid., p. 8.

60   Ibid., p. 16.

61 Ibid., p. 10.
62 Quain, *Dictionary*, p. 1040.
63 For details of Miss Nightingale's uneasy relationship with some doctors see Cope, *Florence Nightingale*; Smith, *Florence Nightingale*. Miss Nightingale attached great importance to the articles she wrote for Quain's *Dictionary*. She sought the advice of Francis Galton to ensure they were sufficiently 'technical' and 'professional': see Bishop and Goldie, *Bio-bibliography*, pp. 23–4.
64 E. Lankester, *Sanitary Defects and Medical Shortcomings: A Lecture by E. Lankester before the Ladies' Sanitary Association*, London, Jarrold and Sons, 1883, pp. 7–8.
65 F. Nightingale, *Notes on Nursing: What it Is and What it Is Not*, London, Harrison, 1860. Although it is debatable how many probationers read *Notes on Nursing* as part of their studies, it was an immediate success, selling more than 15,000 copies in the first two months of publication: see Bishop and Goldie, *Bio-bibliography*, p. 16.
66 J. Croft, *Notes of Lectures St Thomas's Hospital*, London, Blades & Co., 1863. For the most comprehensive, critical and compelling evaluations of the Nightingale Fund's experiment in nurse training see Baly, *Nursing Legacy*; J. Prince, 'Florence Nightingale's Reform of Nursing, 1860–1887', PhD thesis, London School of Economics, 1982.
67 M. Baly, 'The Nightingale Nurses: The Myth and the Reality', in C. Maggs (ed.), *Nursing History: The State of the Art*, London, Croom Helm, 1987, pp. 33–59.
68 M. Baly, 'The Influence of the Nightingale Fund from 1855 to 1914 on the Development of Nursing', University of London, PhD thesis, 1984, p. 260.
69 F. Nightingale, *Notes on Hospitals*, London, Longmans, Green, Longman, Roberts and Green, 1883, p. 18.
70 See J. Thompson and G. Goldin, *The Hospital: A Social and Architectural History*, New Haven, Yale University Press, 1975, p. 40; M. Foucault, *Discipline and Punish: The Birth of the Prison*, New York, Pantheon, 1979.
71 M. Baly, 'The Nightingale Nurses and Hospital Architecture', *Bulletin of the History of Nursing Group*, 1986, vol. 2, pp. 1–7.
72 See A. Summers 'Ministering Angels', *History Today*, 1989, vol. 39, pp. 31–7. For a discussion of interdenominational disputes see R. Martin, 'The Pan-Evangelical Impulse in Britain 1795–1830 with Special Reference to Four London Societies', University of Oxford, DPhil thesis, 1974.
73 Quain, *Dictionary*, p. 1040.
74 Ibid.
75 Baly, *Nursing Legacy*, p. 172.
76 See Showalter, 'Feminist Complaint'.
77 S. Reverby, 'A Caring Dilemma: Womanhood and Nursing in Historical Perspective', *Nursing Research*, 1987, vol. 36, pp. 13–17.
78 For a sociological analysis of the differential representation of Florence Nightingale in university- and hospital-based schools of nursing, see Whittaker and Olesen, 'Faces of Florence Nightingale', pp. 123–30.

79 F. Nightingale, *Cassandra as an Appendix to Suggestions for Thought for the Searchers after Truth of the Artizans of England*, 3 vols, London, Eyre and Spottiswoode, 1860, published in R. Strachey, *The Cause: A Short History of the Women's Movement in Great Britain*, London, G. Bell and Sons, 1928, pp. 401–4.

80 Bishop and Goldie, *Bio-bibliography*, p. 106; L. Hektor, 'Florence Nightingale and the Women's Movement', *Nursing Inquiry*, 1995, vol. 1, pp. 38–45.

81 Showalter, 'Feminist Complaint', p. 407.

82 F. Nightingale, *Suggestions for Thought for the Searchers after Truth of the Artizans of England*, 3 vols, London, Eyre and Spottiswoode, 1860.

83 Strachey, *The Cause*, pp. 401–4.

84 Hektor, 'Florence Nightingale', p. 42.

85 The correspondence between Jowett and Miss Nightingale has been collated by E. Quinn and J. Prest, *Dear Miss Nightingale: A Selection of Benjamin Jowett's Letters 1860–1893*, Oxford, Clarendon Press, 1987. The correspondence is largely unilateral since Jowett, out of deference to Miss Nightingale's request, destroyed the bulk of her letters to him. None the less this collection offers a unique glimpse of some of Miss Nightingale's less well-publicised political and philosophical views.

86 Baly, *Nursing Legacy*, p. 193. The 1882 Married Women's Property Act gave married women the same property rights as those enjoyed by men and single women: see M. Shanley, *Feminism, Marriage and the Law in Victorian England*, London, Tauris, 1989. Shanley's account is a more restrained evaluation of the Act's political importance than Holcombe's claim that it was the greatest achievement of the Victorian women's movement: see L. Holcombe, *Wives and Property: Reform of the Married Women's Property Law in Nineteenth Century England*, Newton Abbott, David and Charles, 1983.

87 See Bishop and Goldie, *Bio-bibliography*, p. 110, and Baly, *As Miss Nightingale Said*, pp. 55–62, for details of Miss Nightingale's attitude towards women, her views on suffrage and the 'woman' question.

88 For biographical details of Elizabeth Blackwell see J. Manton, *Elizabeth Blackwell: England's First Female Physician*, London, Methuen, 1987.

89 The imagery was, however, highly ambivalent. For details of medical and literary representation of mental illness in women see E. Showalter, *The Female Malady: Women, Madness and English Culture, 1830–1980*, London, Virago, 1987; see also L. Jordonova, *Sexual Visions: Images of Gender in Science and Medicine between the Eighteenth and Twentieth Centuries*, Hemel Hempstead, Harvester Wheatsheaf, 1989.

90 K. Thomas, 'The Double Standard', *Journal of the History of Ideas*, 1959, vol. 20, pp. 195–216.

91 Nicholson attributes the notion of separation of the public and private spheres to John Locke's dualistic vision of political authority vested in the state and familial authority: see L. Nicholson, *Gender and Society: The Limits of Social Theory in the Age of the Family*, New York, Columbia University Press, 1986, pp. 133–66.

92 J. Finch and D. Groves (eds), *A Labour of Love: Women, Work and Caring*, London, Routledge, 1983.

93　A. Davin, 'Imperialism and Motherhood', *History Workshop Journal*, 1978, vol. 5, pp. 9–66; J. Lewis, *The Politics of Motherhood: Child and Maternal Welfare in England, 1900–1939*, London, Croom Helm, 1980.

94　S. Pennington and B. Westover, *A Hidden Workforce: Homeworkers in England 1850–1939*, Basingstoke, Macmillan, 1989.

95　L. Davidoff and B. Westover, 'From Queen Victoria to the Jazz Age: Women's World in England 1880–1939', in L. Davidoff and B. Westover (eds), *Our Work, Our Lives, Our Words: Women's History and Women's Work 1880–1939*, Basingstoke, Macmillan, 1986, pp. 1–36; Lewis, *Women in England*.

96　Purvis, *Hard Lessons*, pp. 25–6.

97　A. John, *Unequal Opportunities: Women's Employment in England 1800–1918*, Oxford, Blackwell, 1986.

98　Pinchbeck, *Women Workers*, p. 307.

99　For opposition to the education of the poor see A. Digby, *Pauper Palaces: Studies in Economic History*, London, Routledge and Kegan Paul, 1978, pp. 189–96.

100　For assessments of the impact of the domestic ideology upon educational provision for women in Victorian England see Burstyn, *Victorian Education*; J. Purvis, ' "Women's Life is Essentially Domestic, Public Life being Confined to Men" (Comte): Separate Spheres and Inequality in the Education of Working Class Women, 1854–1900', *History of Education*, 1981, vol. 10, pp. 227–43.

101　C. Dyhouse, 'Towards a "Feminine" Curriculum for English School-girls: The Demands of Ideology 1870–1963', *Women's Studies Quarterly*, 1978, vol. 1, pp. 298–9; C. Dyhouse, *Girls Growing Up*.

102　*Report of the Schools Inquiry Commission, PP 1867–8 Vol. XXVIII*, London, HMSO, Cmnd 3966, q. 550.

103　S. Benton, *Nurses and Nursing*, London, Henry Kimpton, 1877, p. 6.

104　Barwell, *Care of the Sick*, p. 101.

105　Gamarnikov, 'Nurse or Woman', pp. 110–29.

106　Jex-Blake, *Medical Women*; Manton, *Elizabeth Garrett Anderson*; C. Blake, *The Charge of the Parasols: Women's Entry to the Medical Profession*, London, Women's Press, 1990; Morantz Sanchez, *Sympathy and Science*; A. Witz, 'Gender and Medical Professionalisation', in *Professions and Patriarchy*, London, Routledge, 1992, pp. 73–103.

3 REGISTRATION REVISITED

1　See R. Wilkinson, 'The Gentleman Ideal and the Maintenance of a Political Elite. Two Case-Studies: Confucian Education in the Tang, Sung, Ming and Ching Dynasties and the Late Victorian Public Schools 1870–1914', in P. Musgrove (ed.), *Sociology, History and Education*, London, Methuen, 1970, pp. 126–42.

2　Neé Ethel Gordon Manson, Mrs Bedford Fenwick was the daughter of a wealthy Scottish farmer and stepdaughter of an MP. From 1881 to 1887 she was matron at St Bartholomew's Hospital, resigning on her marriage to Dr Bedford Fenwick, consultant gynaecologist and medical politician at the London Hospital where Mrs Bedford Fenwick had worked as a sister. Apart from being the most articulate nurse leader in the campaign for registration, Mrs Bedford Fenwick was also an active campaigner for women's suffrage and founder of the International Council of Nurses: see W. Hector, *The Life of Mrs Bedford Fenwick*, London, Royal College of Nursing, 1973; S. McGann, *The Battle of the Nurses: A Study of Eight Women Who Influenced the Nursing Profession 1880–1930*, London, Scutari Press, 1992, pp. 35–57.

3   For a review of the contradictions inherent in the reform of women's educational provision during the last quarter of the nineteenth century see C. Dyhouse, 'Storming the Citadel or Storm in a Teacup?: The Entry of Women into Higher Education 1860–1920', in S. Acker and D. Warren Piper (eds), *Is Higher Education Fair to Women?*, Guildford, Warren Piper, 1984, pp. 51–64.

4   P. Underhill, 'Science, Professionalism and the Development of Modern Medical Education in England: An Historical Sociology', University of Edinburgh, PhD thesis, 1987; I. Waddington, *The Medical Profession in the Industrial Revolution*, Dublin, Gill and Macmillan, 1984, pp. 128–9; I.S.L. Loudon, *Medical Care and the General Practitioner 1750–1850*, Oxford, Clarendon Press, 1986, pp. 296–301.

5   For a review of medical historiography see C. Webster, 'Historiography of Medicine', in P. Corsi and P. Weindling (eds), *Information Sources in the History of Science, Medicine and Technology*, London, Butterworth Scientific, 1983, pp. 29–43.

6   Little has been written on the historiography of British nursing. See the useful review by J. James, 'Writing and Rewriting Nursing History: A Review Essay', *Bulletin of the History of Medicine*, 1982, vol. 58, pp. 568–84; the source book with historiographical comment by C. Maggs and M. Newby (eds), *Sources for the History of Nursing in Great Britain*, London, King's Fund Centre, 1984; A.M. Rafferty, 'Historical Knowledge', in K. Robinson and B. Vaughan (eds), *Knowledge for Nursing*, London, Butterworth Heinemann, 1992, pp. 25–41.

7   B. Abel-Smith, *A History of the Nursing Profession*, London, Heinemann, 1960, pp. 81–113; C. Davies, 'A Constant Casualty: Nurse Education in Britain and the USA to 1939', in C. Davies (ed.), *Rewriting Nursing History*, London, Croom Helm, 1980, pp. 102–22; A. Summers, *Angels and Citizens: British Women as Military Nurses, 1854–1914*, London, Routledge, 1988, pp. 271–90.

8   Abel-Smith, *Nursing Profession*, p. 61.

9   See A.M. Carr-Saunders and P. Wilson, *The Professions*, Oxford, Clarendon Press, 1933; G. Baron, 'The Teachers' Registration Movement', *British Journal of Educational Studies*, 1954, vol. 2, pp. 133–44; F. Widdowson, *Explorations in Feminism: Going Up to the Next Class: Women and Elementary School Teaching, 1840–1914*, London, WRRC, 1980; E. Ellsworth, *Liberators of the Female Mind: The Shireff Sisters, Educational Reform and the Women's Movement*, Westport, CT, Greenwood Press, 1979, pp. 204–15; C. Maggs, *The Origins of General Nursing*, London, Croom Helm, 1983, pp. 135–7.

10   Acland wrote the preface to a handbook for hospital sisters written by Florence Lees, an early probationer in the Nightingale Fund 'training' scheme at St Thomas's: see F. Lees, *A Handbook for Hospital Sisters*, London, Isbister, 1874. For biographical and career details of Florence Lees see M. Baly, *Florence Nightingale and the Nursing Legacy*, London, Croom Helm, 1986, pp. 128–30; M. Baly, 'Profiles of Pioneers: Florence Lees', *History of Nursing Society Journal*, 1990, vol. 2, pp. 79–84.

11   Bodleian Library, Oxford, Acland Papers, MS Acland d.70, letter from Miss Nightingale to Sir Henry Acland, 20 July 1869 f.15.

12   Letter from Miss Nightingale to Sir Henry Acland, MS Acland d.70 20 July 1869 f.10. Sir Henry Acland later submitted a memorandum concerning the medical education of women, which reviewed the contemporary position in 1884: see H. Acland, *Memorandum concerning Medical Education of Women in reply to Communication through Lord President, from Earl Granville and the Russian Ambassador at the Court of St James by the President of the Medical Council*, London, 1884.

13   Letter from Miss Nightingale to Sir Henry Acland, MS Acland d.70, 20 July 1869 f.10.

14   Letter from Florence Nightingale to Sir Henry Acland, MS Acland, d.70, 20 July 1869 f.13.

15   Letter from Florence Nightingale to Sir Henry Acland, MS Acland d.70, 27 February 1872 f.1.

16   Ibid.

17   Anon., 'The Literature of Nursing', *Nursing Notes*, 1898, vol. ii, 28 August, p. 101.

18   Letter from Miss Nightingale to Sir Henry Acland, MS Acland d.70, 27 February 1872 f.16.

19   Ibid.

20   Ibid., f.3.

21   William Rathbone MP, Chairman of the Liverpool School and Home for Nurses, close associate of Miss Nightingale, is credited with being the originator of the first formalised scheme of district nursing. His text on the history of district nursing contained an anti-registrationist preface by Miss Nightingale. W. Rathbone, *Sketch of the History and Progress of District Nursing: From its Commencement in the Year 1859 to the Present Date, Including the Foundation by the 'Queen Victoria Jubilee Institute for Nursing the Poor in their Homes' with an Introduction by Florence Nightingale*, Edinburgh, R. and R. Clark, 1890. Rathbone gave oral evidence to the Select Committee of the House of Lords on the Metropolitan Hospitals: see *Select Committee of the House of Lords on the Metropolitan Hospitals, Providential and other Public Dispensaries and Charitable Institutions for the Sick Poor*, q. 531.

22   Ibid., f.16.

23   Burdett Papers, 1888, Letter on Nursing and Nurses by Florence Nightingale, 16 May 1888, Box 41 A1 f.1.

24   Ibid., f. 6.

25   Ibid., f. 3.

26 'History of the Movement in Favour of a Common Register', *Hospital*, 1889, vol. 2, p. 17.

27 A critical review of the use of the term and nomenclature on pressure groups in the political science literature is given in R. Klein, 'Policy-making in the British National Health Service', *Political Science*, 1974, vol. 22, pp. 1–14; C. Webster, 'Conflict and Consensus: Explaining the British Health Service', *Twentieth Century British History*, 1991, vol. 1, pp. 115–51.

28 For details of the origins of the Fund see C. Maggs, *Century of Change: The Story of the Royal National Pension Fund for Nurses*, London, Royal National Pension Fund for Nurses, 1988, pp. 15–40.

29 Maggs, *Origins*, p. 136.

30 Ibid.

31 Maggs, *Century of Change*, p. 14; G. Rivett, *The Development of the London Hospital System 1823–1982*, Oxford, Oxford University Press, 1986. The Hospitals Association later became the British Hospitals Association and strove to protect and promote the interests of the voluntary hospitals in England and Wales; a separate Association was established for Scotland.

32 Miss Luckes was matron at the London Hospital where early in her career Ethel Manson had been a sister. It is possible that it was as a sister at the London that Ethel Manson met her future husband, Dr Bedford Fenwick. Miss Luckes became an opponent of the BNA and registration and published a pamphlet discouraging nurses from joining the BNA as the Registration campaign was gaining momentum. The enmity and rivalry between Mrs Bedford Fenwick and Henry Burdett has been explored in a biographical comparison by C. Maggs, 'Ethel Manson and Henry Burdett: Two Great Minds Not Thinking Alike', *Bulletin of the History of Nursing Group*, 1989, vol. 2, pp. 1–6. For a biographical history of Miss Luckes and her role in nursing politics see McGann, *Battle of the Nurses*, pp. 9–34.

33 Maggs, *Century of Change*, pp. 33–4.

34 Abel-Smith maintains Miss Manson objected to nursing being subjected to interference from 'outsiders', such as Burdett: see Abel-Smith, *Nursing Profession*, p. 68.

35 Maggs, *Origins*, p. 136; Maggs, *Century of Change* pp. 33–5.

36 Bodleian Library, Oxford, Burdett Papers, Reports of the Hospital Association's Joint Sectional Committee on Registration, Box A1(2).

37 H. Bonham-Carter, *Is a General Register for Nurses Desirable?*, London, 1888; Burdett Papers, Box A1(2) f.34.

38 Letter from Miss Nightingale to Sir Henry Acland, MS Acland, d.70, 7 August 1889 f.127.

39 Letter from Miss Nightingale to Sir Henry Acland, MS Acland, d.70, 28 April 1893 f.170.

40 Burdett Papers, Box A1(2), 'Central Hospitals Council for London Statement on the State Registration of Nurses', 2 March 1909.

41 E. Luckes, *What Will Trained Nurses Gain by Joining the British Nurses Association?*, London, 1889, p. 2.

42   see Maggs, *Century of Change*, pp. 48–9, 54, 65, 88, 131 for details of the Bedford Fenwicks' campaign against Burdett waged in the *Lancet*.

43   Ibid., pp. 66–7. There are resonances of such arguments in the contemporary debate surrounding general and professional management in the National Health Service: see P. Strong and J. Robinson, *The NHS under New Management*, Milton Keynes, Open University Press, 1990.

44   British Nurses Association, *First Annual Report*, London, British Nurses Association, 1889, pp. 9–10.

45   *Select Committee on the Metropolitan Hospitals, Dispensaries and Charitable Institutions*, House of Lords, PP. 1890, vol. xvi.i, Minute of Evidence, Mrs Bedford Fenwick, pp. 9606.

46   For fuller details of these proposals see 'Editorial: Midwifery Legislation', *Nursing Record and Hospital World*, 1899, vol. 24, 11 November, p. 385; 'The Relative Position of Medical Practitioner and Midwife', *Nursing Record and Hospital World*, 1899, vol. 23, 29 September, p. 250; A.M. Rafferty, 'Mrs Bedford Fenwick and Project 2000', *Bulletin of the History of Nursing Group*, 1989, vol. 2, pp. 1–11.

47   For midwives' registration see B. Cowell and D. Wainwright, *Behind the Blue Door: The History of the Royal College of Midwives*, London, Cassell, 1981, pp. 11–36; R. Dingwall, A.M. Rafferty and C. Webster, *An Introduction to the Social History of Nursing*, London, Routledge, 1988, pp. 154–8; J. Donnison, *Midwives and Medical Men: A History of the Struggle for the Control of Childbirth*, 2nd edn, London, Heinemann, 1988, pp. 18–22, 236–7; A. Witz, *Professions and Patriarchy*, London, Routledge, 1992, pp. 104–27.

48   For details of the background to the establishment of the Select Committee see Rivett, *London Hospital System*, pp. 138–43. Its proceedings, evidence and appendices were published in three volumes between 1890 and 1892. See PP. 1890, vol. xvi.i, 1890–1, vol. xiii.i, and 1892, vol. xiii.i.

49   *Select Committee on the Metropolitan Hospitals, Dispensaries and Charitable Institutions*, House of Lords, PP. 1890, vol. xvi.i. Minute of Evidence, Miss Luckes, pp. 6604–92.

50   See the pamphlet by S. Holland, and E. Luckes, *State Registration of Nurses*, London, n.d., Royal College of Nursing; Parliamentary Papers, BAC 380; Maggs, *Origins*, p. 136.

51   Letter from Miss Nightingale to Sir Henry Acland, MS Acland d.70, 24 July 1889 f.152.

52   Letter from Florence Nightingale to Sir Henry Acland, MS Acland d.70, 24 July 1889 f.151. The memorial was published as an appendix to the *Report of the Select Committee on the Registration of Nurses, with Proceedings and Evidence, Appendix and Index*, London, PP. 1904 (281), vi. 701.

53   'History of the Movement'.

54   See extract from *Memorandum on the Registration of Nurses and the Royal British Nurses Association in Opposition to the Petition of Her Royal Highness Helena Princess Christian of Schleswig-Holstein, Princess of Great Britain and Ireland for the grant of a Charter for the*

Incorporation of the Royal British Nurses Association, London, 1892, p. 44; Burdett Papers, 1892, Box A1(2).

55 Letter from Miss Nightingale to Sir Henry Acland, MS Acland d.70, 24 July 1889 f.152; Ibid., 18 January 1894 f.176.

56 *Select Committee on the Metropolitan Hospitals, Dispensaries and Charitable Institutions*, House of Lords, PP. 1890, vol. xvi.i, Minute of Evidence, Mrs Bedford Fenwick, p. 9606.

57 Ibid., pp. 737.

58 Dr Bedford Fenwick was Senior Gynaecologist, Hospital for Women, Soho Square, London; Vice-president of the BNA; Fellow of the Royal Society of Medicine; Treasurer and Chairman of the Registered Nurses Society; editor of the *British Journal of Gynaecology*; and author of *The Nursing of Patients Suffering from Diseases of the Chest*, London, Nursing Record, 1901, and *Some Common Complaints of Women: Being a Series of Clinical Lectures delivered at the Hospital for Women, Soho Sq, London*, London, Medical Times, 1904. See *The Medical Directory*, London, Longmans, 1917, vol. 1.

59 *Select Committee on the Metropolitan Hospitals, Dispensaries and Charitable Institutions*, House of Lords, PP. 1892, vol. *xiii.i*, Minute of Evidence from Dr Bedford Fenwick, pp. 754.

60 British Nurses Association, *First Annual Report*, London, British Nurses Association, 1889, p. 28.

61 Dr James, later Sir James Crichton-Browne, President of the Medico-Psychological Association, Visitor in Lunacy and Director West Riding Asylum, was co-founding editor of *Brain*, see *The Medical Directory*, London, Longmans, 1890, p. 122. The British Nurses Association was established in 1887, the same year as the National Pension Fund for Nurses to secure registration for nurses. British Nurses Association, *First Annual Report*, London, British Nurses Association, 1888, p. 28.

62 *Select Committee on the Metropolitan Hospitals, Dispensaries and Charitable Institutions*, House of Lords, PP. 1892, vol. xiii.i, Minute of Evidence from Mrs Bedford Fenwick, p. 9606.

63 Ibid., p. 738.

64 Ibid., p. xc.

65 See Maggs, *Origins*, p. 196, for details of these issues in the representation of nurses in the Victorian novel.

66 N. Elias, *The Civilising Process: The History of Manners. vol. 1*, trans. E. Jephcott, New York, Urizen Books, 1978. For excellent discussions of the management of embarrassment, sexuality and 'closeness' involved in intimate contact between nurses and patients in contemporary nursing literature, see J. Lawler, *Behind the Screens: Nursing, Somology, and the Problem of the Body*, Edinburgh, Churchill Livingstone, 1991, pp. 117–227; J. Savage, *Nursing Intimacy: An Ethnographic Approach to Nurse–Patient Interaction*, London, Scutari Press, 1995, pp. 87–108.

67 W. Distant,'On the Mental Differences between the Sexes', *Journal of the Anthropological Institute*, 1875, vol. 4. pp. 78–85.

68 J. Burstyn, 'Education and Sex: The Medical and Religious Case against Higher Education for Women in England 1870–1900', *Proceedings of the American Philosophical Society*, 1974, vol. iii, pp.

79–89; O. Moscucci, *The Science of Woman: Gynaecology and Gender in England, 1800–1929*, Cambridge, Cambridge University Press, 1990.

69 C. Dyhouse, 'Social Darwinistic Ideas and the Development of Women's Education in England, 1880–1920', *History of Education*, 1976, vol. 5, pp. 41–50.

70 For a synoptic review of Crichton-Browne's career and significance in nineteenth-century psychiatry see J. Oppenheim, 'Sir James Crichton-Browne', in *'Shattered Nerves': Doctors, Patients, and Depression in Victorian England*, Oxford, Oxford University Press, 1991, pp. 54–78.

71 J. Crichton-Browne,'On the Weight of the Brain and its Component Parts in the Insane', *Journal of Mental Science*, 1879, vol. i, p. 515.

72 J. Burstyn, 'Brain and Intellect: Science Applied to a Social Issue 1876–1885', *Actes xiie Congres International D'Histoire des Sciences, Paris, Histoire Des Sciences Des Hommes*, 1971, vol. ix, pp. 13–16; E. Fee, 'Nineteenth Century Craniology: The Study of the Female skull', *Bulletin of the History of Medicine*, 1979, vol. 53, pp. 415–33.

73 For an incisive study of the 'politics' of observation see S. Shapin, 'Homo Phrenologicus: Anthropological Perspectives on an Historical Problem', in B. Barnes and S. Shapin (eds), *Natural Order: Historical Studies of Scientific Culture*, London, Sage, 1979, pp. 41–72.

74 S. Mosedale, 'Science Corrupted: Victorian Biologists Consider the Woman Question', *Journal of History Biology*, 1978, vol. ii, pp. 1–56.

75 R. Barnes, 'Women, Diseases of', in R. Quain (ed.), *A Dictionary of Medicine: Including General Pathology, General Therapeutics, Hygiene, and the Diseases Peculiar to Women and Children*, London, Longman, Green, 1882, vol. 2, p. 1789.

76 For the rise of public health and the beginnings of auxological epidemiology see J. Tanner, *A History of the Study of Human Growth*, Cambridge, Cambridge University Press, 1981. Tanner defines 'auxological epidemiology' as the use of growth data to research and define the correlates of health and ill-health. School surveys and surveillance as well as physical anthropology were important applications of this 'movement'.

77 For a discussion of the negative effects of sport and intellectual activity upon sexuality and childbirth see K. McCrone, *Sport and the Physical Emancipation of English Women 1870–1914*, London, Routledge, 1988, pp. 192–214; S. Vertinsky, *The Eternally Wounded Woman: Women, Exercise and the Doctors in the Late Nineteenth Century*, Cambridge, Cambridge University Press, 1990; A. Digby,'Women's Biological Straitjacket', in S. Mendus and J. Rendall (eds), *Sexuality and Subordination: Interdisciplinary Studies of Gender in the Nineteenth Century*, London, Routledge, 1989, pp. 192–220; C. Dyhouse, 'Social Darwinistic Ideas and the Development of Women's Education in England, 1880–1920', *History of Education*, 1976, vol. 5, pp. 41–50.

78 The most celebrated of these is E. Clark, *Sex in Education, or a Fair Chance to Girls*, Boston, J.R. Osgood & Co., 1875. Clark's observations on the deleterious effects of 'over-education' upon adolescent girls' reproductive functions provided the inspiration for Henry Maudsley to

publish his views: see H. Maudsley, 'Sex in Mind and in Education', *Fortnightly Review*, 1874, vol. 15, pp. 466–83. Thomas Clouston, the Edinburgh psychiatrist, publicised his anxieties in T. Clouston, *Female Education from a Medical Point of View: Being Two Lectures Delivered at the Philosophical Institution*, Edinburgh, MacNiven and Wallace, 1882.

79   For a review of the 'over-pressure' debate see A. Robertson, 'Children, Teachers and Society: The "Overpressure" Controversy, 1880–1886', *British Journal of Educational Studies*, 1972, vol. xx, pp. 315–23.

80   R. Brudenell Carter, *On the Influence of Education and Training in Preventing Diseases of the Nervous System*, London, Churchill, 1855.

81   In a sociological treatment of professionalism and bureaucracy, Novaks argues doctors looked to the state and state employment as a means of raising the status of the profession: S. Novaks, 'Professionalism and Bureaucracy: English Doctors and the Victorian Public Health Administration', *Journal of Social History*, 1973, vol. 6, pp. 440–62. For discussion of Crichton-Brown's contribution to the 'over-pressure' controversy see G. Sutherland, *Ability, Merit and Measurement: Mental Testing and English Education 1880–1940*, Oxford, Oxford University Press, 1984, pp. 6–8.

82   J. Langton Down, *On Some of the Mental Afflictions of Childhood and Youth: Being the Lettsonian Lectures Delivered for the Medical Society of London*, London, Churchill, 1887, p. 88. For a scholarly analysis of the responses of 'alienists' to psychiatric disorder in women see E. Showalter, *The Female Malady: Women, Madness and English Culture, 1830–1980*, London, Virago, 1985; M. Clark, 'The Data of Alienism: Evolutionary Neurology, Physiological Psychology and the Reconstruction of British Psychiatric Theory, 1850–1950', University of Oxford, DPhil thesis, 1982.

83   G. Bock and P. Thane (eds), *Maternity and Gender Policies: Women and the Rise of the European Welfare States, 1880s–1950s*, London, Routledge, 1991; D. Dwork, *War is Good for Babies and Other Young Children: A History of the Infant and Child Welfare Movement in England, 1898–1918*, London, Tavistock, 1989, pp. 124–66.

84   Clark, 'Data of Alienism', p. 240.

85   'Feckless' mothers arguably provided a scapegoat for medical inefficacy and political lethargy. For a case study of such 'victim blaming' see C. Dyhouse, 'Working Class Mothers and Infant Mortality in England, 1895–1914', in C. Webster (ed.), *Biology, Medicine, and Society 1840–1940*, Cambridge, Cambridge University Press, 1981, pp. 73–98; L. Duffin, 'Prisoners of Progress', in S. Delamont and L. Duffin (eds), *The Nineteenth Century Woman: Her Physical and Cultural World*, London, Croom Helm, 1978, pp. 57–91; J. Lewis, *The Politics of Motherhood: Child and Maternal Welfare in England, 1900–1939*, London, Croom Helm, 1980.

86   A. Davin, 'Imperialism and Motherhood', *History Workshop Journal*, 1978, vol. 5, pp. 9–66.

87   Dyce Duckworth, *Sick Nursing: Essentially A Woman's Mission*, London, Longmans Green, 1884, p. 24.

88   Ibid.
89   Dyce Duckworth, *Women: Their Probable Place and Prospects in the Twentieth Century. An Address Delivered in Glasgow before the Scottish Society of Literature and Art*, Glasgow, Maclehose and Sons, 1893, p. 9.
90   Ibid., pp. 18–19.
91   Ibid., p. 22.
92   Ibid., p. 26.
93   Ibid., p. 28. It was not just medical men who dubbed female dons as dowdy; the younger generation of students were apt to pass similar disparaging remarks: see C. Dyhouse, 'Storming the Citadel', p. 60.
94   B. Solomon, *In the Company of Educated Women: A History of Women and Higher Education in America*, New Haven, Yale University Press, 1985, p. 56.
95   See J. Bell, *Notes on Surgery for Nurses*, Edinburgh, Oliver and Boyd, 1887; Bedford Fenwick, *The Nursing of Patients* and *Some Common Complaints*; S. Benton, *Nurses and Nursing*, London, Henry Kimpton, 1877.
96   F. Gant, *Mock Nurses of the Latest Fashion: Professional Experiences in Short Stories and the Nursing Question*, London, Balliere, 1900. These amusing portraits included 'satan in petticoats' or nurse Lucretia, of Borgian blood; 'nurse gossip and scandal', 'the obscene nurse', 'the husband-huntress and trapper nurse', and 'the widow nurse and religious sisterhood nurses'.
97   Ibid., p. 154.
98   C. Dyhouse, *No Distinction of Sex?: Women in British Universities 1870–1939*, London, University College Press, 1995, pp. 191–2.
99   Frances Cobbe is reputed to have yelled enthusiastically to Charles Darwin on a walk in North Wales that J.S. Mill's essay *On the Subjection of Women*'s emancipationist ethos was 'perfect' for his study of human descent, especially the chapters on sexual selection: see J.S. Mill, *Three Essays*, London, Oxford University Press, 1975, first published 1868. Darwin, unimpressed, apparently responded that Mill 'could learn some things from biology' – men's superiority was the product of the 'struggle for existence'; their special 'vigour and courage' came with 'battling for possession for women'. See A. Desmond and J. Moore, *Darwin* London, Michael Joseph, 1991, p. 572; on the counter-arguments to the alleged negative biological impact of higher education for women see J. Burstyn, 'Educator's Response to Scientific and Medical Studies of Women in England 1860–1900', in S. Acker and D. Warren Piper (eds), *Is Higher Education Fair to Women?*, Guildford, Warren Piper, 1984, pp. 65–78.
100 *Select Committee on the Metropolitan Hospitals, Dispensaries and Charitable Institutions*, House of Lords, PP. 1892, vol. *xiii.i*, Minute of Evidence from Mrs Bedford Fenwick, pp. 9630.
101 H. Bonham-Carter, *Memorandum on the Registration of Nurses and the Royal British Nurses Association in Memorandum against the Petition*, London, 1892.
102 Central Hospitals Council for London, *State Registration of Nurses*, London, 1909; Burdett Papers, Box A1(2).

103   Miss Dock was also a suffragist, socialist and co-author of one of the first nursing history textbooks: see M. Nutting and L. Dock, *A History of Nursing*, New York, Putnam and Sons, 1907–12, vols 1–4. She was Honorary Secretary of the International Council of Nurses which Mrs Bedford Fenwick helped to found and contributed articles to the *British Journal of Nursing*, as well as a regular column in the *American Journal of Nursing* called the 'Foreign Department'. For a brief account of the early history of the Council and Anglo-American relations see A.M. Rafferty, 'Some Historical Aspects of the International Council of Nurses', in K. Robinson, A.M. Rafferty, G. Bergman, L. Quam and J. Quinlan, *Nursing in the World*, London, Polytechnic of the South Bank, 1989, pp. A11–12; M. Breay and E. Fenwick, 'History of the International Council of Nurses, 1899–1909', *International Council of Nurses Annual Reports*, London, 1928–9, pp. 215–75.

104   L. Dock, 'State Registration', *British Journal of Nursing*, 1905, vol. 34, 25 February, p. 149.

105   Ibid.

106   British Nurses Association, *First Annual Report*, London, British Nurses Association, 1889, p. 14.

107   *Select Committee on the Metropolitan Hospitals, Dispensaries and Charitable Institutions*, House of Lords, PP. 1892, vol. *xiii.i*, pp. 510.

108   British Nurses Association, *Annual Report*, p. 115.

109   Ibid., p. 117.

110   Letter from Miss Nightingale to Sir Henry Acland, MS Acland d.70, 19 July 1889, f.141.

111   Letter from Miss Nightingale to Sir Henry Acland, MS Acland d.70, 10 July 1889, f.1.

112   Ibid.

113   Letter from Henry Burdett to Sir Henry Acland, MS Acland d.70, 22 April 1991.

114   Abel-Smith, *Nursing Profession*, p. 72.

115   Letter from Miss Nightingale to Sir Henry Acland, MS Acland d.70, 14 December 1887 f.127.

116   For parallels with reformers of women's education see Dyhouse, 'Storming the Citadel', pp. 55–6.

117   Details of the constitution and committee structure of the BNA are given in British Nurses Association, *Annual Report*.

118   Nutting and Dock, *History*, vol. 1, pp. 51–2; S. Tooley, *The History of Nursing in the British Empire*, London, Blousfield, 1906, p. 375.

119   The chapter 'The Story of the Nurses of Great Britain and Ireland', in Nutting and Dock, *History*, vol. 1, p. 44, was written in collaboration with Mrs Bedford Fenwick. The tone of the chapter resembles Mrs Bedford Fenwick's intemperate language and appears to be the only surviving record of events. The 'arch anti-registrationist' in question was presumably Henry Burdett. It is not clear, but the authors of the chapter seem to be alluding to an alliance between Sir Henry Acland and Henry Burdett. Mrs Bedford Fenwick's authorship of the chapter might also be inferred further from the generous sprinkling of complimentary references to herself!

120 Nutting and Dock, *History*, vol. 1. p. 48.
121 Ibid., p. 43.
122 D. Bridges, *A History of the International Council of Nurses 1899–1964: The First Sixty Years*, Philadelphia, Lippincott, 1967; S. Quinn, *The ICN: Past and Present*, London, Scutari Press, 1989.
123 Nutting and Dock, *History*, vol. 3, p. 56.
124 The Hon. Sydney Holland, Lord Knutsford, Chairman of the London Hospital and co-author with Miss Luckes of *State Registration of Nurses*, London, n.d., referred to nursing as 'childishly simple': *Report of the Select Committee on the Registration of Nurses*, p. 830. Dr Norman Moore: ibid., p. 671.
125 Holland and Luckes, *State Registration*. For a review of Miss Luckes's writings see L. Parr, 'The Writings of Eva C.E. Luckes, Matron of the London Hospital 1880–1919', *History of Nursing Bulletin*, 1989, vol. 2, pp. 8–11; *Report of the Select Committee on the Registration of Nurses*, p. 830.
126 Ibid., p. 671.
127 See P. Bartrip, *Mirror of Medicine: A History of the British Medical Journal*, Oxford, British Medical Journal in Association with Oxford University Press, 1990, pp. 9–12, for an account of reactions to Wakely's diatribes.
128 E. Sherrington, 'Thomas Wakely and Reform 1823–1862', University of Oxford, DPhil thesis, 1973, p. 258–69.
129 Ibid., pp. 49–54.
130 Dingwall, Rafferty and Webster, *Introduction*, pp. 78–80.
131 Sherrington, 'Thomas Wakely', pp. 275–86. For a biography by the subsequent editor of the *Lancet* see S. Squire Sprigge, *The Life and Times of Thomas Wakely*, London, Longmans, 1897.
132 See Maggs, *Century of Change*, pp. 48–9, 54, 65, 88, 131, for details of the *Lancet's* pro-Bedford Fenwick stance.
133 For a recent evaluation of Cobbett's political journalism see M. Rustin, 'William Cobbett and the Invention of Popular Radical Journalism', *Soundings*, 1995, vol. 1, Autumn, pp. 139–56.
134 The Scottish Poor Law Nursing Service had a national system of credentials in operation from 1885: see C. Maggs, 'The Register of Nurses in the Scottish Poor Law Service 1885–1919', *Nursing Times*, 1981, vol. 77, pp. 129–32.
135 For an overview of early pro-suffragist campaigning by American nurses see T. Christy, 'Equal Rights for Women', *American Journal of Nursing*, 1971, vol. 71, pp. 288–93; S. Lewenson, *Taking Charge: Nursing, Suffrage and Feminism in America 1873–1920*, New York, Garland, 1993.
136 R. Cassell, 'Lessons in Medical Politics: Thomas Wakely and the Irish Medical Charities, 1827–39', *Medical History*, 1990, vol. 34, pp. 412–23; Sherrington, 'Thomas Wakely', p. 106.
137 I. Waddington, *The Medical Profession in the Industrial Revolution*, Dublin, Gill and Macmillan, 1984, p. 132.
138 'The Medical Practitioners Act', *Lancet*, 1858, vol. ii, p. 175.

4 THE NURSES' REGISTRATION ACT

1   C. Davies, 'Professionalising Strategies as Time and Culture-bound, Circa 1893', in E. Condliffe Lagemann (ed.), *Nursing History: New Perspectives, New Possibilities*, New York, Teachers College Press, 1983, p. 58.

2   D. Crane, *Invisible Colleges: Diffusion of Knowledge in Scientific Communications*, Chicago, University of Chicago Press, 1972; B. Shaw, 'The Diffusion of Innovation in Clinical Equipment', in R. Loveridge and K. Starkey (eds), *Continuity and Crisis in the NHS*, Milton Keynes, Open University Press, 1992, pp. 101–17.

3   Davies, 'Professionalising Strategies', p. 57.

4   N. Noel, 'Isabel Hampton Robb: Architect of American Nursing', Teachers' College, New York, EdD thesis, 1978, p. 97. Alumnae associations may have been intended as the analogue of the British nursing hospital leagues – or vice versa. For the importance of the leagues for career networking and for the creation of a sense of local corporate and more general occupational identity for early cohorts of trained nurses, see C. Maggs, *The Origins of General Nursing*, London, Croom Helm, p. 138. On the role of World Fairs and their influence upon the construction of ideas of 'empire', 'race', social and technological evolution and progress see R. Rydell, *All the World's a Fair: Visions of Empire at the American International Expositions, 1876–1916*, Chicago, University of Chicago Press, 1984.

5   D. Headrick, *The Tools of Empire: Technology and European Imperialism in the Nineteenth Century*, Oxford, Oxford University Press, 1982; R.W. Home and S.G. Kohlstedt (eds), *International Science and National Scientific Identity*, London, Kluwer Academic, 1991.

6   L. Dock, 'Editorial 1899–July 1929', *ICN*, 1929, vol. 9, pp. 14–151, cited by S. Lewenson, *Taking Charge: Nursing, Suffrage and Feminism, 1873–1929*, New York, Garland Press, 1993, p. 148.

7   M. Breay and E. Fenwick, 'History of the International Council of Nurses, 1899–1909: Compiled from Official Documents', *International Council of Nurses Reports*, London, 1928–9, pp. 218–19.

8   For a brief overview of the importance of feminism in the early professional organisation of American nurses see S. Poslusny, 'Feminist Friendship: Isabel Hampton Robb, Lavinia Dock and Mary Adelaide Nutting', *Image*, 1989, vol. xxi, pp. 64–8. Lewenson's excellent study is the first book-length treatment of the subject and the most comprehensive and detailed examination of the complex pressure group politics between nursing and women's organisations: see S. Lewenson, *Taking Charge: Nursing, Suffrage and Feminism 1873–1920*, New York, Garland, 1993.

9   Ibid., p. 66; B. Abel-Smith, *A History of the Nursing Profession*, London, Heinemann, 1960, p. 131.

10 B. Harrison, *Separate Spheres: The Opposition to Women's Suffrage in Britain*, London, Croom Helm, 1978, p. 51.

11 Ibid.

12 For a portrait of Edwardian feminism see B. Harrison, *Prudent Revolutionaries*, Oxford, Clarendon Press, 1991, pp. 1–16; Women's Social and Political Union, *Second Annual Report of the Women's Social and Political Union, 1908*, London, Women's Press, 1908, and *Sixth Annual Report of the Women's Social and Political Union, 1914*, London, Women's Press, 1914.

13 L. Dock, 'Foreign Department: The Cologne Congress', *American Journal of Nursing*, 1912, vol. 12, p. 814.

14 D. Bridges, *A History of the International Council of Nurses, 1899–1964: The First Sixty Years*, Philadelphia, Lippincott, 1967, pp. 45–6.

15 The settlement movement as a community ideal is discussed by M. Vicinus, *Independent Women: Work and Community for Single Women 1850–1920*, Chicago, University of Chicago Press, 1985, pp. 211–46; see also chapter on Jane Addams and Lilian Wald at the Henry St Settlement by B. Cook, 'A Utopian Female Support Network: The Case of the Henry St Settlement', in R. Rohrlich and E. Hoffman Baruch (eds), *Women in Search of Utopia*, New York, Schocken Books, 1984, pp. 109–116.

16 S. Tooley, *The History of Nursing in the British Empire*, London, Blousfield, 1906, p. i.

17 The establishment of the Select Committee on Registration was attributed to the activities of the State Society for the Registration of Nurses. See M. Nutting and L. Dock, *A History of Nursing*, vols 1–4, New York, Putnam, 1907-12; 1907, vol. 1, p. 56.

18 Miss Dock was deputy principal at the Johns Hopkins Training School for Nurses for part of the time when Miss Hampton was principal.

19 'Nursing at the World's Fair', *Nursing Record and Hospital World*, 1893, 26 January, p. 52. See also biographical tribute to Isabel Hampton Robb in Adelaide Nutting, 'Isabel Hampton Robb: Her Work in Organisation and Education', *American Journal of Nursing*, 1910, vol. 10, pp. 19–25.

20 International Council of Nurses Archives, Geneva (ICNA), ICN Records Book 2 1899–1904, excerpt from *British Journal of Nursing*, 1899.

21 Breay and Fenwick, 'History', p. 21. Miss McIssaac opened the 1901 Congress at Buffalo.

22 L. Dock, 'Foreign Department: Plans for the Cologne Congress', *American. Journal of Nursing*, 1911, vol. 11, pp. 719–20.

23 Breay and Fenwick, 'History', p. 20.

24 'Editorial: The Trained Nurse as a Factor in Civilization', *Nursing Record and Hospital World*, 1901, vol. xxvii.

25 C. Webster, *The Great Instauration: Science, Medicine and Reform 1626–1660*, London, Duckworth, 1975, pp. 57–66; G. Wersky, *The Visible College*, London, Allen Lane, 1978.

26 'Outside the Gates: Women', *Nursing Record and Hospital World*, 1896, 25 January, p. 82; 'Outside the Gates: Women, The International Congress', *Nursing Record and Hospital World* 1898, 3 December, p. 460; I. Merritt, 'The Brooklyn Associated Allumnae and the Organisation of its Registry', *Nursing Record and Hospital World*, 1897, 8 May, pp. 378–9; 'Superintendents' Convention, Baltimore, February, 1897',

Nursing Record and Hospital World, 1897, 29 May, pp. 437–8, 455–6, 476–7;'The American Society of Superintendents of Training Schools', *Nursing Record and Hospital World*, 1896, 7 March, p. 190; 'Women', *Nursing Record and Hospital World*, 1896, 23 May, p. 423; 'Matrons in Council: Their First Meeting in the United States', *Nursing Record and Hospital World*, 1894, 10 February, pp. 96–7. For a fuller discussion of Mrs Bedford Fenwick's pro-feminist journalism and politics more generally, see S. Hamer, 'Outside the Gates', University of York, MA thesis, 1994.

27   L. Dock, 'Nurses' Directories', *Nursing Record and Hospital World*, 1895, 20 April, p. 255; L. Dock, 'A National Association for Nurses and its Legal Organisation', *Nursing Record and Hospital World*, 1896, 14 March, pp. 208–9; S. Palmer, 'Alumnae Organisations', *Nursing Record and Hospital World*, 1895, 4 May, pp. 296–7; 'The Three Years Course of Training in Connection with the Eight-Hour Day', *Nursing Record and Hospital World*, 1895, 1 June, pp. 375–7, 395–6.

28   'Nursing at the World's Fair', *Nursing Record and Hospital World*, 1893, 26 January, p. 52.

29   'The International Council of Nurses: Ready for Affiliation in 1915', *Brit. Journal of Nursing*, 1914, 18 July, p. 51.

30   International Council of Nurses Archives, Geneva (ICNA), Mary Burr, 'The British Journal of Nursing and the British Nursing Press', *Rapports de la Conference Internationale du Nursing, Paris, 1907*, Bordeaux, International Council of Nurses, 1907, pp. 186–7.

31   For an analysis of dissemination patterns in scientific activity see Crane, *Invisible Colleges*, p. 76.

32   K. Blair, *The Torchbearers: Women and their Amateur Arts Associations in America, 1890–1930*, Bloomington, University of Indiana Press, 1994; A. Scot, *Making the Invisible Visible*, Urbana, University of Chicago Press; T. Martin, *The Sound of Our Own Voices: Women's Study Clubs 1860–1910*, Boston, Beacon Press, 1987. Lewenson notes that some state nursing organisations affiliated with the Federation of Women's Clubs as an additional platform of support: see Lewenson, *Taking Charge*, pp. 220–1.

33   Miss Wald, 'Nurses' Social Settlement', *Nursing Record and Hospital World*, 1901, 26 January, p. 69; Cook 'A Utopian Female Support Network'.

34   Marshall's biography of Adelaide Nutting is informative and lively but casts little light on the role of social networks in reform: see H. Marshall, *Mary Adelaide Nutting: Pioneer of Modern Nursing*, Baltimore, Johns Hopkins University Press, 1972. Winifred Hector's and Susan McGann's portraits of Bedford Fenwick (see below) are an excellent start, but we need more systematic research. For substantive accounts of Ethel Bedford Fenwick and Lavinia Dock see S. McGann, *The Battle of the Nurses: A Study of Eight Women who Influenced the Development of Professional Nursing, 1880–1930*, London, Scutari Press, 1992, pp. 35–57; W. Hector, *The Life of Mrs Bedford Fenwick*, London, Royal College of Nursing, 1973; Janet Wilson James (ed.), *A Lavinia Dock Reader*, New York, Garland Press, 1985, pp. vii–xix.

35   Useful reviews of social network studies in political, corporate and friendship circles are provided by S. Feld, 'The Focused Organisation of Social Ties', *American Journal of Sociology*, 1981, vol. 86, pp. 1015–34; R. Alba and C. Kadushin, 'The Intersection of Social Circles: A New Measure of Social Proximity on Networks', *Sociological Methods and Research*, 1976, vol. 5, pp. 77–103. For a rare study of collective biography in nursing see V. Bullough and B. Bullough, 'Achievements of Eminent American Nurses of the Past: A Prosopographical Study', *Nursing Research*, 1992, vol. 75, pp. 120–4.

36   The term 'Americanisation' refers to the policies and methods imported by British nurses from the USA in the attempt to raise the standard and quality of British nursing education and practice. This is an adaptation of the term 'Japanisation', used to denote the emulation of the methods and presumed success of methods of production used by large Japanese corporations. For further details see N. Oliver and B. Wilkinson, *The Japanisation of British Industry*, Oxford, Blackwell, 1988.

37   'Nursing at the World's Fair'.

38   See Lewenson, *Taking Charge*, pp. 23–7.

39   C. Davies, 'Professional Power and Sociological Analysis: Lessons from a Comparative Historical Study of Nursing in Britain and the USA', University of Warwick, PhD thesis, 1981.

40   Davies, 'Professionalising Strategies', pp. 47–64.

41   Miss Robb, for example, was well connected socially – the Astors attended her wedding at Westminster Abbey: see Noel, 'Isabel Hampton Robb', p. 96.

42   S. Armeny, 'Organised Nurses and Women Philanthropists, and the Intellectual Bases for Co-operation among Women', in E. Condliffe Lagemann (ed.), *Nursing History: New Perspectives, New Possibilities*, New York, Teachers College Press, 1983, pp. 13–45; K. Buhler-Wilkerson, 'Guarded by Standards and Directed by Strangers: Charleston, South Carolina's Response to a National Health Care Agenda, 1920–1930', *Nursing History Review*, 1993, 1, pp. 139–54.

43   D. Morgan, 'Woman Suffrage in Britain and America', in C. Emsley (ed.), *Essays in Comparative History: Economy, Politics and Society in Britain and America, 1850–1920*, Milton Keynes, Open University Press, 1984, p. 260; C. Bolt, *The Woman's Movements in the United States and Britain from the 1790s to the 1920s*, Amherst, University of Massachusetts Press, 1993.

44   Peretz considers the involvement of the local gentry over midwifery services in rural and urban areas: E. Peretz, 'A Maternity Service for England and Wales: Local Authority Maternity Care in the Inter-war Period in Oxfordshire and Tottenham', in J. Garcia, R. Kirkpatrick and M. Richards (eds), *The Politics of Maternity Care: Services for Childbearing Women in Twentieth Century Britain*, Oxford, Clarendon Press, 1990, pp. 16–29.

45   Lady Priestley's contribution to 'nursing' is mentioned in her son's obituary, Sir Joseph Priestley, first Chairman of the General Nursing Council for England and Wales: 'Sir Joseph Priestley K.C. Well-known

Probate and Divorce Counsel', *The Times*, 10 June 1941. His mother's reputation may well have been an important factor in his appointment to the chair of the Council. Lady Helen Munro Ferguson was the wife of Mr Munro Ferguson MP. See 'The Progress of State Registration', *British Journal of Nursing*, 1904, vol. 23, pp. 351–3; H. Ferguson, 'The State Registration of Nurses', *Nineteenth Century*, 1904, vol. 55, pp. 312–7.

46 C. Wood, 'Some Thoughts on the Recent Discussion on the Private Nurse', *Nursing Notes*, 1897, vol. 10, p. 59.

47 Ibid.

48 J. Paterson, 'A Nurses' Trade Union', *British Journal of Nursing*, 1919, vol. 66, pp. 267–8.

49 The social and intellectual connections between reformers of women's higher education and its sponsors are explored by G. Sutherland, 'The Movement for the Higher Education of Women: Its Social and Intellectual Context in England c.1840–80', in P. Waller (ed.), *Politics and Social Change in Modern Britain: Essays Presented to A.F. Thomson*, Brighton, Harvester, 1987, pp. 91–116.

50 See the brilliant study of nursing in South Africa by Shula Marks, *Divided Sisterhood: Race, Class and Gender in the South African Nursing Profession*, London, Macmillan, 1994, pp. 34, 40–1.

51 *Report from the Select Committee of the House of Commons on the Registration of Nurses with Proceedings of Evidence, Appendices and Index, 1905 (263)*, Minute of Evidence, Mrs E. G. Fenwick, q. 616–17.

52 Ibid., q. 617.

53 On the role of distance as a variable in colonial centre–periphery relations in scientific patronage see D. Chambers, 'Does Distance Tyrannize Science?', in R. Home and S. Kohlstedt (eds), *International Science and National Scientific Identity*, London, Kluwer Academic, 1991, pp. 19–38.

54 R. Dingwall, A.M. Rafferty and C. Webster, *An Introduction to the Social History of Nursing*, London, Routledge, 1988, pp. 77–89.

55 The origins and fate of VAD schemes are fully discussed by A. Summers, 'The Birth of the VAD: Nursing Reserve Schemes, 1906–14', in *Angels and Citizens: British Women as Military Nurses, 1854–1914*, London, Routledge, 1988, pp. 237–70.

56 'VAD's and the Nursing Profession', *British Journal of Nursing*, 1919, vol. 63, p. 35.

57 Ibid.

58 For the origins of the College of Nursing see G. Bowman, *The Lamp and the Book*, London, Queen Anne Press, 1967; Abel-Smith, *Nursing Profession*, pp. 87–8. For an account of Dame Sarah Swift's role see McGann, *Battle of the Nurses*, pp. 160–89.

59 The committee received representation from the RBNA, Matrons' Council for Great Britain and Ireland, the Society for the State Registration of Nurses, Fever Nurses Association, the Association for Promoting the Registration of Nurses in Scotland, the Scottish Nurses' Association, the Infirmary Nurses' Association, the British Medical Association and National Union of Trained Nurses.

60 Abel-Smith, *Nursing Profession*, p. 89.
61 Ibid., p. 91.
62 Ibid., p. 92.
63 After the end of World War I Parliament was favourably disposed towards women, and nurses in particular. Readings of the Nurses' Registration Bill followed that of the Representation of the People's Bill: see House of Commons Debates (1919), vol. 117, Friday 27 June, cols 557 and 558.
64 House of Commons Debates (1919), vol. 117, Major Nall, col. 1347.
65 Abel-Smith, *Nursing Profession*, pp. 94–5.
66 For details of the proposed constitution of the 'rival' councils, see Central Committee for the State Registration of Nurses, *State Registration of Nurses: A Statement issued by the Authority of the Central Committee of the State Registration of Nurses*, London, Royal College of Nursing, n.d., Parliamentary Papers file no. 380.
67 PRO Ministry of Health, MH55/462, 'Nurses' Registration' (No. 2) Bill, Standing Committee B, Arguments against Amendments to be proposed by Sir Watson Cheyne.
68 See 'Editorial: Midwifery Legislation', *Nursing Record and Hospital World*, 1899, vol. 23, pp. 385–6, for details of objections. For a discussion of the effect of the Midwives Act upon the Nurses' Registration Act see R. White, 'Some Political Influences Surrounding the Nurses' Registration Act 1919', *Journal of Advanced Nursing*, 1976, vol. 1, pp. 209–17.
69 Ibid., p. 386.
70 'The Relative Position of Medical Practitioner and Midwife', *Nursing Record and Hospital World*, 1899, vol. 23, p. 250.
71 'Editorial: Midwifery Legislation'.
72 'Editorial: The Midwives Bill', *Nursing Record and Hospital World*, 1902, vol. 28, p. 201.
73 For comment on the Nurses' Registration Bill of 1904 from a mental nursing point of view see D. Thomson, 'A Few Remarks on the Registration of Nurses and the Nurses' Registration Bill from the Mental Nursing Point of View', *Journal of Mental Science*, 1904, vol. 50, pp. 451–5. The author considered registration the 'one solid and reliable plank to paddle about on' in an otherwise 'troubled sea' of medico-politico 'flotsam and jetsam', p. 451.
74 T. Outterson Wood, 'Mental (or Asylum-trained) Nurses: Their Status and Registration', *Journal of Mental Science*, 1906, vol. 52, pp. 306–7.
75 Thomson, 'Mental Nursing', p. 453.
76 Ibid., p. 454.
77 A. Summers, 'Pride and Prejudice: Ladies and Nurses in the Crimean War', *History Workshop Journal*, 1983, vol. 16, pp. 33–56.
78 *Census of the Population for England and Wales* PP. 1911, vol. *lxxviii*, pp. 540–1, lists occupations of males and females at each of the four censuses, 1881–1911. Abel-Smith suggests that the census returns for males underestimate the numbers employed. Drawing on the Fifty-fifth Commission of Lunacy of 1905, he claims that the census excluded some 4,700 males employed as nurses by local authorities. For 1901,

therefore, one might suggest 5,792 as a more realistic estimate of male nurses, representing 9.1 per cent of the total female workforce: see Abel-Smith, *Nursing Profession*, p. 255.

79 M. Walsh, 'Male Nursing', in *Science and Art of Nursing*, London, Cassell, 1907, vol. 3, p. 168. Male nurses were excluded from membership of the Royal College of Nursing from 1916 to 1960: see J. Greene, 'Men in Nursing and the Royal College of Nursing', *History of Nursing Journal*, 1992/3, vol. 4, pp. 3–8.

80 P. Nolan, 'Psychiatric Nursing: Past and Present: The Nurses' Viewpoint', University of Bath, PhD thesis, 1989, p. 33.

81 Central Committee for the State Registration of Nurses, *State Registration of Nurses: A Statement*, London, 1919, p. 4; RCN archives Parliamentary Papers BAC 380; 'Nurses Fight for State Registration: The College of Nursing Bill Fully Discussed', *Hospital*, 1919, vol. lxv, p. 383.

82 Public Record Office, London, Kew, MH 55/462, 'Nurses' Registration', Sir Watson Cheyne, p. 2.

83 'Specialisation' as a sociological and political process has been studied by G. Rosen, 'Attitudes of the Medical Profession to Specialisation', *Bulletin of the History of Medicine*, 1942, vol. xi, pp. 342–54; G. Gritzer and A. Arluke, *The Making of Rehabilitation: A Political Economy of Medical Specialization, 1890–1980*, Berkeley, CA, University of California Press, 1985; L. Granshaw, *St Mark's Hospital: A Social History of a Specialist Hospital*, Oxford, Oxford University Press, 1987. A more detailed discussion of the politics of specialisation is provided in L. Granshaw, 'Fame and Fortune by Means of Bricks and Mortar: The Medical Profession and Specialisation in Britain 1800–1948', in L. Granshaw and R. Porter (eds), *The Hospital in History*, London, Routledge, 1989, pp. 199–220. For semantic shifts in the shades of meanings attached to the term see *Oxford English Dictionary*, 2nd edn, Oxford, Oxford University Press, vol. xvi, pp. 151–3.

84 C. Rosenberg, *The Care of Strangers: The Rise of America's Hospital System*, New York, Basis Books, 1987, p. 169; Granshaw, 'Bricks and Mortar', p. 199.

85 Each of these factors is identified although not evaluated by Rosen in relation to ophthalmology: see Rosen, *Specialisation*, pp. 342–54.

86 R. Stevens, *American Medicine and the Public Interest*, New Haven, Yale University Press, 1971, p. 49.

87 Granshaw, *St Mark's*, pp. 16–22.

88 Granshaw, 'Bricks and Mortar', pp. 200–4.

89 Rosen emphasises the role of instrumentation and technology in specialisation: see Rosen, *Specialisation*, pp. 342–54.

90 Granshaw, 'Bricks and Mortar', pp. 206–9.

91 Ibid., p. 207.

92 A. Flexner, *Medical Education in Europe: A Report to the Carneigie Foundation for the Advancement of Teaching*, New York, Bulletin/ Carneigie Foundation for the Advancement of Teaching, no. 6, 1912.

93 A. Flexner, *Medical Education in America and Canada: Carneigie Foundation for the Advancement of Teaching*, New York, 1910, no. 4, p. 67.

94 Stevens, *American Medicine*, p. 56.

95 C. Booth, 'Clinical Research', in J. Austoker and L. Bryder (eds), *Historical Perspectives on the Role of the MRC*, Oxford, Oxford University Press, 1989, pp. 205–6.

96 Ibid., p. 206.

97 C. Maggs, *Origins*; A. Simnet,'The Pursuit of Respectability: Women and the Nursing Profession, 1860–1900', in R. White (ed.), *Political Issues in Nursing: Past, Present and Future*, Chichester, John Wiley, 1986, pp. 1–24.

98 See M. Carpenter, *Working for Health: The History of the Confederation of Health Service Employees*, London, Lawrence and Wishart, 1988; C. Hart, *Behind the Mask: Nurses, their Unions and Nursing Policy*, London, Balliere Tindall, 1994.

99 Carpenter, 'Working for Health', p. 39.

100 See B. Drake, *Women in Trade Unions*, London, Virago, 1984 (first published 1921), p. 111. Overall trade union membership increased from 2,565,000 in 1920 to 8,347,000 in 1920. See R. McKibbin, *The Evolution of the Labour Party 1910–1924*, Oxford, Oxford University Press, 1974, p. 240.

101 Carpenter, *Working for Health*, p. 46.

102 Ibid., p. 71.

103 'The Trade Union Movement among Poor Law Nurses', *Nursing Times*, 1919, vol. xv, pp. 1081–2; 'Nurses and Trade Unions: Must they Be Driven to a Last Refuge?', *Hospital*, 1919, vol. lxv, p. 146. Miss MacCallum, President of the PUTN, referred to the bitter and malignant attacks on the union from the *Hospital*: see 'Nurses' Professional Union', *Nursing Times*, 1919, vol. xv, p. 1221. The ownership of the nursing press for commercial gain by men 'who know nothing about nursing' was condemned by Miss MacCallum. Presumably she was referring to Sir Henry Burdett: see 'A Nurses' Trade Union', *British Journal of Nursing*, 1919, vol. 63, p. 267.

104 Marsh and Ryan note that the PUTN was formed in 1920 with a membership of 268 but ceased to exist in 1930 when the membership fell to 14; A. Marsh and V. Ryan, *Historical Directory of Trade Unions: Non Manual Unions*, Aldershot, Gower, 1987, vol. 3, p. 184.

105 'Nurses' Trade Union', p. 266.

106 Ibid., p. 266.

107 'Editorial: Trade Union', *British Journal of Nursing*, 1919, vol. 62, 15 March. Mrs Bedford Fenwick approved of efforts by nurses to organise and combine to their advantage and published accounts of the meetings of the PUTN whose secretary was Maude MacCallum. Miss MaCallum was an important ally to Mrs Bedford Fenwick in the first nursing council. The objectives of the PUTN were consistent with Mrs Bedford Fenwick's: state registration, payment of a minimum wage and a proper regulation of working hours: see 'Nurses' Trade Union', p. 266.

108 K. Morgan, *Consensus and Disunity*, Oxford, Clarendon Press, 1979, p. 48.

109 W. Adams, 'Lloyd George and the Labour Movement', *Past and Present*, 1953, vol. 3, pp. 55–64.

110 'Editorial: Second Reading of our Nurses' Registration Bill', *British Journal of Nursing*, 1919, vol. 62, 29 March.

111 See Carpenter, *Working for Health*, p. 150. For details of the background to and operation of the Whitley machinery see J. Sheldrake, 'The Origin and Development of the Whitley System 1910–1939 with Particular Reference to Public Utilities', University of Kent, MPhil thesis, 1986.

112 *The Times*, 'A New Era for Nurses: Needs of Rural Areas', 9 January 1920, p. 7.

113 For details of the establishment of the Ministry of Health see P. Wilding, 'The Genesis of the Ministry of Health', *Public Administration*, 1967, vol. 45, pp. 149–68; S. Stacey, 'The Ministry of Health 1919–1929: Ideas and Practice in a Government Department', University of Oxford, DPhil thesis, 1984. Webster locates the origin of the idea of unifying health services in the 1869 Sanitary Commission, and traces the tortuous career of different interpretations of a unified comprehensive health service through the Minority Report on the Poor Law Commission to proposals to extend the health services by the Lloyd-George coalition government. For full details see C. Webster, *Problems of Health Care: The National Health Service before 1957*, London, HMSO, 1988, pp. 16–19.

114 Ministry of Reconstruction, *Machinery of Government Committee Report No. 1*, London, HMSO, Cmnd 9230, 1919, p. 4. Autobiographical reflections on the inception of the Ministry of Health are provided by its first Minister, Dr Christopher Addison, in C. Addison, *Politics from Within, 1911–1918, with Some Records of a Great National Effort*, London, Herbert Jenkins, 1924, vol. 2, pp. 221–32.

115 K. Morgan and J. Morgan, *Portrait of a Progressive: The Political Career of Viscount Addison*, Oxford, Oxford University Press, 1980, p. 95.

116 Ministry of Reconstruction, *Machinery of Government Committee Report No. 1*, p. 4.

117 PRO MH55/462, 'The Establishment of the General Nursing Council', memorandum by Dr Christopher Addison, Minister of Health to Cabinet on Nurses Registration, 1 October 1919, p. 1.

118 White, 'Political Influences', pp. 209–17.

119 Evidence of Mr Joseph Brown, President of Poor Law Unions Association for England and Wales, and Miss E.A. Wesley, certified midwife, Matron of the St George's in the East, to Departmental Committee on the Workings of the Midwives' Act, House of Commons, London, HMSO, 1909, Cmnd. 4822, pp. 39 and 373. Defensive attitudes to what was perceived of as 'voluntary snobbery' on the part of the CMB may well have coloured negative views of the it. See M. Crowther, *The Workhouse System 1834–1929: The History of An English Social Institution*, London, Batsford Academic and Educational, 1981, for a

discussion of the self-perception of Poor Law Officers and the conditions under which they worked.

120   White, 'Political Influences', pp. 209–17; R. White, *Social Change and the Development of the Nursing Profession: A Study of the Poor Law Nursing Service 1848–1948*, London, Henry Kimpton, 1978, pp. 117–18.

121   Association of Hospital Matrons, *Minutes of Meetings*, London, 1919, vol. 1, p. 3. The Association justified its initiation by the claim 'there is no Association which is representative of the nursing profession'.

122   L. Dock and I. Stewart, *A Short History of Nursing*, New York, Putnam and Sons, 1920, p. 244.

123   Mrs Bedford Fenwick's journal, *British Journal of Nursing*, provided a publicity outlet for the Council.

124   Association of Hospital Matrons, *Minutes of Meetings*, vol. 1, p. 13.

125   Ibid., p. 6.

126   'Nurses' Registration Debate', House of Commons Debates, 1919, vol. 117, 27 June, col. 557, Dr Christopher Addison.

127   PRO, MH55/462, Memorandum from Dr Christopher Addison, Minister of Health to Cabinet on Nurses' Registration', 1 October 1919, p. 1.

128   PRO, CAB 26/2, Minute Cabinet Committee of the Home Office, 25 September 1919.

129   PRO, MH55/462, Ministerial Conference on the Nurses' Registration Bill, 1 October 1919, p. 1.

130   Ibid., p. 3.

131   Ibid., p. 2.

132   Ibid., letter from Fisher-Harrison, Office of the Parliamentary Council, to Lawrence Brock, Ministry of Health, n.d.

133   Ibid., p. 3.

134   Ibid., memorandum from Lawrence Brock to Robert Morant, 31 October 1919.

135   For details of the breakdown of expenditure see Ibid., p. 3.

136   Ibid.

137   Mrs Bedford Fenwick described the introduction of the Bill for the State Registration of Nurses into the House of Commons as a 'splendid triumph' in 'Nurses' Trade Union', p. 302.

138   Bodleian Library, Oxford, Addison Papers, MS Addison, Box 61, Folder 223, 'Nurses' Registration'.

139   A. Beck, 'The British Medical Council and British Medical Education in the Nineteenth Century', *Bulletin of the History of Medicine*, 1956, vol. xx, pp. 150–3.

140   G. Webster, 'Medical Practitioners and Registration', *Lancet*, 1858, vol, ii, p. 175.

141   This could be justified initially on the grounds that the Ministry of Health lent the Council £5,000 to cover initial running costs of the first two years. A financial report was the only one the Council were required to submit to the Ministry. It was not until the advent of the National Health Service that the Council was obliged to produce a full annual report of all its activities.

142 See C. Maggs, 'Profit and Loss and the Hospital Nurse', in C. Maggs (ed.), *Nursing History: The State of the Art*, London, Croom Helm, 1987, pp. 154–76, for the calculus of nursing in teaching hospital economics. Administrators recognised the value of having the 'new' nurses on the wards, especially if their labour could be sold outside the institution. As Maggs comments, Burdett and others recognised the 'demand for private nurses for the middle classes was apparently insatiable': ibid., p. 187.

143 C. Maggs, 'The Register of Nurses in the Scottish Poor Law Service 1885–1919', *Nursing Times*, 1981, vol. 77, pp. 129–32.

144 British Nurses Association, *First Annual Report*, London, British Nurses Association, 1889, p. 28.

5 CRISIS AND CONFLICT IN THE CARETAKER COUNCIL (1919–23)

1 'Editorial', *Nursing Times*, 1919, vol. xv, 27 December, p. 355.

2 'Nurses and Trade Unions: Must they Be Driven to a Last Refuge?,' *Hospital*, 1919, vol. lxv, p. 146.

3 For an analysis of the 'career' of conflict theory in the sociology of the professions see C. Davies, 'Professionals in Bureaucracies: The Conflict Thesis Revisited', in R. Dingwall and P. Lewis (eds), *The Sociology of the Professions*, London, Macmillan, 1983, pp. 177–94.

4 Robert Morant had been Assistant Director of special enquiries and reports at the Education Department in 1895, Acting and then Secretary (1902–3) at the Board of Education, Vice-Chairman of the National Health Insurance Commission, where he identified Brock as one of his protégés. Morant was appointed First Secretary at the Ministry of Health in 1919. Laurence Brock was recruited from the Admiralty to the National Insurance Commission for England by Morant in 1912 and became Assistant Secretary of the Ministry of Health in 1919, Principal Assistant Secretary in 1925, and Chairman of the Board of Control in 1928. See biographical appendices in S. Stacey, 'The Ministry of Health: Ideas and Practice in a Government Department 1919–1929', University of Oxford, DPhil thesis, 1984; B. Allen, *Robert Morant*, London, Macmillan, 1934.

5 PRO, London, Kew, 'General Nursing Council for England and Wales, minutes of meetings, DT1/1, *Nurses' Registration Act*, 1919, 9 & 10 Geo. 5, p. 7.

6 PRO, MH55/469, draft list of members for the General Nursing Council for England and Wales, Morant's postscript to Brock in Brock's minute to Morant, 16 February 1920.

7 Ibid., p. 1.

8 PRO, MH55/462, 'Establishment of the General Nursing Council', list of Association of Hospital Matrons Executive members, p. 1.

9 PRO, MH55/469, 'Draft list,' p. 2.

10 Ibid., minute Brock to Morant 16 February 1920.

11 Ibid., 'Draft list', p. 4.

12   Ibid., p. 5.
13   Ibid.
14   See K. Robinson and A.M. Rafferty, *The Nursing Workforce*, London, Polytechnic of the South Bank, 1988, p. 52.
15   For details of union activity in the Poor Law sector, see M. Carpenter, *Working for Health: The History of the Confederation of Health Service Employees*, London, Lawrence and Wishart, 1988, pp. 137–243.
16   PRO, MH55/469, 'Draft list', minute Brock to Morant 16 February 1920.
17   PRO, DT2/2 'The Appointment of the Caretaker Council'.
18   Ibid. See also College of Nursing, 'The General Nursing Council', in *The Register of Nurses*, London, College of Nursing, 1922, p. vi.
19   Ibid., 'Caretaker Council'.
20   Full biographical details are provided in 'Who's Who on the General Nursing Council', *British Journal of Nursing*, 1920, vol. 64, 1 May, p. 256.
21   PRO, MH55/469, 'Draft list', notes on General Nursing Council members', p. 3.
22   B. Abel-Smith, *A History of the Nursing Profession*, London, Heinemann, 1960, p. 104.
23   *Report from the Select Committee of the House of Commons on the General Nursing Council with Minutes of Proceedings and Evidence,1924–5 (167)*, q. 33.
24   Ibid., q. 53.
25   Ibid., q. 62.
26   Ibid., q. 76.
27   Only two district nurses and two public health visitors were appointed to the Caretaker Council: Miss Annie Peterkin, General Superintendent, Queen Victoria's Jubilee Institute and Miss Ellinor Smith, Superintendent for Wales, Queen Victoria's Jubilee Institute for Nurses. Miss MacDonald and Miss Constance Smith, Health Visitor, were appointed under the section for public health. Two sick children's nurses, but only one mental nurse, were appointed to the Caretaker Council, Miss Agnes Coulton, Miss Constance Worsley and Tom Christian. For the fate of the representation of sick children's nursing interests in the Caretaker Council see M. Arton,'The Caretaker Council of the General Nursing Council and Sick Children's Nursing, 1920–23', *Bulletin of the History of Nursing Group*, 1987, vol. 2, p. 1.
28   E. Bendall and E. Raybould, *A History of the General Nursing Council for England and Wales 1919–1969*, London, Lewis, 1969.
29   PRO, MH55/469, Minute Brock to Addison, 3 March 1920, p. 1.
30   See 'Sir Joseph Priestley, K.C.', *The Times*, 10 June 1941, for biographical details; PRO, MH55/469, minute Brock to Addison, 3 March 1920.
31   Ibid., p. 3.
32   Ibid., minute Brock to Morant, 16 February 1920.
33   Ibid., letter Miss Maude MacCallum, secretary, Professional Union of Trained Nurses, to Dr Addison, 28 June 1920. It is likely that Mrs Bedford Fenwick had a hand in the letter.

34   Ibid., p. 2.
35   Ibid., minute Morant to Addison, 9 July 1920.
36   A. Flexner, *Medical Education in Europe: A Report to the Carnegie Foundation for the Advancement of Teaching*, New York, Bulletin/ Carnegie Foundation for the Advancement of Teaching, no. 6, 1912, p. 47.
37   Ibid.
38   Ibid., p. 66.
39   Bendall and Raybould, *History of the GNC*, pp. 38–9.
40   See Arton, 'Caretaker Council', pp. 1–2; PRO, DT2/3, 'Rules for Admission of Existing Nurses'.
41   PRO, MH55/463, 'Resignation of Members from the General Nursing Council: A Note on Some Outstanding Questions', p. 1.
42   Ibid.
43   PRO, DT48/1, 'Education and Examination Committee Minutes', 28 October 1921.
44   Arton, 'Caretaker Council', pp. 3–4.
45   PRO, MH55/463, 'Resignation of Members', minute Brock to Addison, 6 December 1921, p. 3.
46   Bendall and Raybould, *History of the GNC*, p. 40; Abel-Smith, *Nursing Profession*, p. 105.
47   Addison defended Mr Priestley with reference to the judicial functions performed by the Council; the removal of unfit persons from the register and the quasi-legal nature of the Council's work required a chairman with legal expertise: see 'General Nursing Council', *Nursing Times*, 1920, vol. xvi, 17 July, p. 839.
48   PRO, MH55/469, 'Resignation of Members', minute Brock to Addison, 10 July 1920.
49   Miss Tuke, Lady Hobhouse, Mrs Eustace Hills and the College Matrons were among those mentioned.
50   Sir Alfred Mond, industrialist, financier and politician, became managing director of his father's chemical business and amalgamated range of enterprises to form ICI Ltd in 1926. He was called to the Bar in 1894 and became First Commissioner of Works in 1916–1921, and Minister of Health, 1921–2: see *Dictionary of National Biography: The Concise Dictionary, Pt 2, 1901–70*, Oxford, Oxford University Press, 1982; Sir Alfred Mond, 'Nurses' Registration (Rules)', House of Commons, (1922), vol. 152, col. 626.
51   PRO, MH55/469, minute Brock to Addison 10 July 1920.
52   Ibid.
53   PRO, DT5/1,'Printed General Nursing Council Minutes', 16 July 1920,p. 1. These included Dr Goodall, Dr Bedford Pierce, Dr Bostock Hill, Mr Cronshaw, Lady Hobhouse, Mrs Eustace Hills, Miss Cox-Davies, Miss Lloyd Still, Miss Seymour Yapp, matron Birmingham, Miss Sparshott, Ashton-Under-Lyme, Miss Peterkin, Health Visitor, Miss Coulton, Miss Worseley, Miss Eleanor Smith and Miss Swiss.
54   PRO, MH55/463, notes of a meeting between resigning members of the Caretaker Council and Minister of Health, 21 December 1921, p. 1.

55 Ibid., Miss Villiers, Poor Law, Miss MacCallum, Miss MacDonald and Mr Christian.

56 Ibid., minute Brock to Addison 6 December 1921, p. 1.

57 'Editorial: The General Nursing Council and Resignations', *Nursing Times*, 1922, vol. xviii, 11 February, p. 119.

58 'Editorial: General Nursing Council Resignations', *Nursing Times*, xviii, 1922, 28 January, p. 69.

59 'Crisis in the General Nursing Council: A Striking Lesson', *British Journal of Nursing*, 1921, vol. 67, p. 380.

60 Mr Richardson, 'Nurses' Registration, (Rules)', House of Commons, 1922, vol. 152, 22 March, col. 628.

61 PRO, MH55/463, list of reasons given by Council members for their resignation.

62 Ibid., letter from GNC Members to Minister of Health, 6 December 1921.

63 Ibid., minute Brock to Addison, 6 December 1921, p. 1.

64 PRO, DT20/231, 'Correspondence of Members', Miss Riddell to Mr Priestley, letter of 16 September 1921; DT20/72 Part 1, correspondence with Mrs Bedford Fenwick.

65 PRO, MH55/463, minute Brock to Minister, 6 December 1921.

66 Ibid., minute Brock to Robinson, 16 December 1921, p. 2.

67 Ibid., p. 3.

68 Ibid., p. 2.

69 Ibid., pp. 2–3.

70 Sir Arthur Robinson 1874–1950; Queen's College, Oxford, 1897 Second and First Clerk, Colonial Office. 1912 appointed Assistant Secretary, Office of Works. 1917, Secretary, Ministry of Air. 1920 First Secretary, Ministry of Health: see S. Stacey, 'Ministry of Health', Appendix 1.

71 PRO, MH55/463, notes of a meeting between the Minister of Health and deputation of resigning members of the General Nursing Council, 21 December 1921, p. 2.

72 Ibid.

73 Ibid., pp. 2–3.

74 Ibid., p. 3.

75 Bendall and Raybould, *History of the GNC*, p. 56.

76 Other suggestions included Lord Buckmaster, who helped the College Bill in the House of Lords, Lord Cave, governor of St Bartholomew's, and Mr Charles Lyle MP, Chairman of East Ham Hospital. See PRO, MH55/463, letters Cooper Perry to Robinson, 24 January 1922, 26 January 1922.

77 Ibid., letter Cooper Perry to Robinson, 26 January 1922.

78 Ibid., notes of a meeting between the Minister of Health and deputation of resigning members of the General Nursing Council, 21 December 1921, pp. 3–4.

79 Ibid.

80 Ibid., p. 5.

81 This line of questioning clearly bears the hallmark of Mrs Bedford Fenwick.

82 'Nurses' Registration (Rules)', Mr Kenny, House of Commons (1922), 22 February, vol. 152, col. 483.
83 'Nurses' Registration (Rules)', Captain Elliott, House of Commons (1922), vol. 152, col. 634.
84 'Nurses' Registration (Rules)', Sir Alfred Mond, House of Commons, 22 March (1922), col. 624.
85 Abel-Smith, *Nursing Profession* pp. 106–9.
86 Bendall and Raybould, *History of the GNC*, pp. 72–4.
87 See M. Arton, 'The Chapple Amendment: Parliamentary Intervention and the General Nursing Council', *History of Nursing Journal*, 1992/3, vol. 4, pp. 178–83.
88 PRO, DT 2/5, 'General Nursing Council, Rules', Dr Chapple's Amendment, Rule 9(1) (g).
89 Ibid.
90 Ibid.
91 Bendall and Raybould, *History of the GNC* p. 64; Abel-Smith, *Nursing Profession*, p. 106.
92 Men were not admitted as full members of the Royal College of Nursing until 1960: see R. Dingwall, 'Men in Nursing', in M. College and D. Jones (eds), *Readings in Nursing*, Edinburgh, Churchill Livingstone, 1979, pp. 199–209.
93 'Registers Official and Otherwise', *Nursing Times*, 1920, vol. xvi, 14 August, p. 946.

6 THE EDUCATION POLICY OF THE GENERAL NURSING COUNCIL (1919–32)

1 Members volunteered for membership of various committees and the following were appointed to the Education and Examinations Standing Committee: Miss Dowbiggin, Mrs Bedford Fenwick, Miss Lloyd Still, Miss Sparshott, Miss Swiss, Miss Tuke or Mrs Hills, Miss Villiers, Miss Worsley and the chairman. The chairman was Alicia Lloyd Still. See E. Bendall and E. Raybould, *A History of the General Nursing Council for England and Wales 1919–1969*, London, Lewis, 1969, p. 39.
2 A. Flexner, 'Medical Education in Europe: A Report to the Carnegie Foundation for the Advancement of Teaching', New York, Bulletin/ Carnegie Foundation for the Advancement of teaching, no. 6, 1912: Henry Burdett produced a number of volumes containing details of hospitals and training schools but these excluded material on training content and organisation; they also predated the councils' needs: see H. Burdett, *Hospitals and Asylums of the World*, London, Scientific Press, 1893.
3 PRO, DT48/101 microfilm reel no 4830, 'General Nursing Council, Education and Examinations Committee Minutes'.
4 The length of the working week was the subject of heated debate in nursing and trade union circles: see R. Lowe, 'Hours of Labour: Negotiating Industrial Legislation in Britain 1919–1939', *Economic History Review*, 1982, vol. 35, pp. 254–71.

5   PRO, DT16/246, memorandum respecting the Poor Law Nursing Service.

6   *Report from the Select Committee of the House of Commons on the General Nursing Council, with Proceedings and Evidence, 1924–5 (167)*, q.3.

7   Other members of the Education and Examinations Committee between May 1920 and November 1921 were Miss Dowbiggin, Mrs Bedford Fenwick, Miss Sparshott, Miss Swiss, Miss Tuke or Miss Hills, Miss Villiers, Miss Worsley: Bendall and Raybould, *History of the GNC*, p. 39; L. Seymer, *Dame Alicia Lloyd Still 1869–1944*, London, Nightingale Fund, 1953. Miss Lloyd Still was born in Ceylon, daughter of a Henry Lloyd Still, member of the Ceylon Civil Service. Miss Lloyd Still was also a founder member of the College of Nursing, a member of College Council, founder and President of the Association of Hospital Matrons (1919–1937), and prominent in the International Council of Nurses from 1919.

8   Seymer, *Alicia Lloyd Still*, p. 17.

9   Ibid., p. 4.

10   Ibid.

11   PRO, DT5/1,'Education and Examinations Committee Minutes'.

12   PRO, DT20/231, correspondence of Mr Priestley, letter Mrs Bedford Fenwick to Mr Priestley on the education and examination syllabus, 9 August 1921.

13   PRO, DT 5/1, p. 6.

14   Ibid., p. 7.

15   Ibid. See comments by Miss Cox-Davies, p. 503.

16   PRO, DT5/1, meeting with delegation from the conference of Poor Law training schools, p. 9.

17   Ibid., p. 9.

18   Ibid.

19   Ibid.

20   Ibid.

21   Ibid.

22   PRO, DT5/2, letter from County Medical Officers of Health for England and Wales containing extract from the Annual Report of the Medical Officers of Health for the County of Salop n.d.

23   Ibid.

24   Ibid., p. 2.

25   Ibid., p. 3.

26   PRO, DT5/1, p. 499.

27   Ibid.

28   'Making the Future Nurse: Great Conference on the Syllabus of Training and Affiliation Schemes', *Nursing Times*, 1921, vol. xvii, 7 May, p. 498.

29   Ibid., p. 498.

30   Ibid., p. 498.

31   Ibid.

32   Ibid., p. 501.

33   Ibid., p. 503.

34   Ibid.
35   Miss Musson was subsequently to be elected as the first nurse Chairman of Council between 1928 and 1938.
36   'Making the Future Nurse', p. 501.
37   Ibid.
38   Ibid.
39   Ibid.
40   Ibid. See also comments of Miss Scovell, Swansea General Hospital, Ibid., p. 502.
41   'Making the Future Nurse', p. 498.
42   Ibid., p. 512.
43   Lancet, *The Final Report of the Lancet Commission on Nursing*, London, 1932, pp. 125–6.
44   Ibid.
45   'Making the Future Nurse', p. 504.
46   Ibid.
47   R. Dingwall, A.M. Rafferty and C. Webster, *An Introduction to the Social History of Nursing*, London, Routledge, 1988, p. 90.
48   This was the central advisory machinery established for professional advice in matters of health policy. Nurses were denied representation on the grounds that their interests could be represented by a hospital administrator. This provoked a hostile response from certain quarters of nursing opinion: see A.M. Rafferty, 'Nursing Policy and Nationalization of Nursing: The Representation of "Crisis" and "Crisis" of Representation', in J. Robinson, A.M. Gray and R. Elkan (eds), *Policy Issues in Nursing*, Buckingham, Open University Press, 1992, pp. 67–83.
49   Ministry of Health, *Consultative Council on Medical and Allied Services, Interim Report on the Future Provision of Medical and Allied Services*, Chairman Lord Dawson, London, HMSO, Cmnd 693, 1920.
50   *Final Report of the Voluntary Hospitals Commission*, Chairman Lord Cave, London, HMSO, Cmnd 1335, 1921.
51   R. Spann, 'The Use of Advisory Bodies by the Ministry of Health', in R. Vernon and N. Mansreigh (eds), *Advisory Bodies: A Study in their Use in Relation to Central Government 1919–1939*, London, Allen and Unwin, 1940, p. 239.
52   Addison Papers, Box 453: Lord Sandford, Lord Knutsford, Sir Arthur Stanley and Earl of Athlone attended the meeting.
53   Ibid.
54   C. Webster, *Problems of Health Care: The National Health Service before 1957*, London, HMSO, 1988, pp. 20–1.
55   C. Webster, 'Conflict and Consensus: Explaining the British Health Service', *Twentieth Century British History*, 1991, vol. 1, pp. 115–51.
56   N. MacKenzie and J. MacKenzie, *The First Fabians*, London, Weidenfeld and Nicolson, 1977, p. 356. For a less flattering if not embittered portrait of Morant's character and work see W. Braithwaite in H. Bunbury and R. Titmuss (eds), *Lloyd-George's Ambulance Wagon: Being the Memoirs of William J. Braithwaite, 1911–12*, London, Methuen, 1957. Braithwaite accused Morant of underhand dealings and claimed 'it was

always said of Morant that if you invited him into your house and left the front door open he would prefer to climb in by the pantry window', p. 304.

57   F. Watson, *Dawson of Penn*, London, Chatto and Windus, 1950, p. 58.
58   Bodleian Library, Addison Papers, Box 53, Morant to Addison, n.d.
59   L. Selby-Bigge, *The Board of Education*, London, Putnam and Sons, 1927, p. 20.
60   College of Nursing Council, *Minutes*, August 1919, p. 486.
61   PRO, ED50/56, 'Grants for Nurse Training, Board of Education'.
62   PRO, ED50/56, minute Pelham to Dr Janet Campbell, 27 September 1921.
63   Ibid., marginalia of Morant in Pelham's minute to Newman, 20 November 1919.
64   PRO, ED50/58, 'Representatives of the Board of Education on the General Nursing Council', minute Pelham to Newman, 20 November 1919.
65   *Final Report of the Voluntary Hospitals Commission*, p. 48.
66   PRO, ED50/56, minute Brock to Dr Janet Campbell, 12 October 1921.
67   Ibid., minute Dr Janet Campbell to Pelham, 16 December 1920.
68   Ibid., minute Brock to Dr Janet Campbell, 12 October 1921.
69   Ibid.
70   Ibid., minute Pelham to Dr Janet Campbell, 27 September 1921.
71   PRO, ED50/58, marginalia of Morant and comments upon minute from Pelham to Newman, 20 November 1919.
72   K. Morgan, 'Dr Christopher Addison and Social Reform', *Society for the Social History of Medicine Bulletin*, 1981, December, p. 23.
73   P. Musgrave, 'The Definition of Technical Education', in P. Musgrave (ed.), *Sociology, History and Education*, London, Methuen, 1970, p. 70.
74   'Making the Future Nurse', p. 501.
75   *National Insurance Commission, Scotland Report Hospital and Nursing Services*, Edinburgh, HMSO, Cmnd 699, 1920.
76   For a fuller discussion of the origins and fate of the Dawson report see Webster,'Conflicts and Consensus', pp. 121–5.
77   S. Glynn and J. Oxborrow, *Inter-war Britain: A Social and Economic History*, London, Allen and Unwin, 1976, p. 127.
78   'Making the Future Nurse', p. 498.
79   The eugenic language may have been merely a rhetorical device rather than signifying any deeper ideological commitment.
80   Ibid., pp. 498–9.
81   Ibid., p. 499.
82   Ibid.
83   Ibid.
84   Ibid.
85   Ibid.
86   Ibid., p. 501.
87   Ibid., p. 502.
88   Miss Todd, St James's Infirmary, Balham, Miss McIntosh, St Bartholomew's Hospital, Miss Pearse, NUTN. See evidence of Miss Rodgers, St Luke's Municipal Hospital Bradford, Miss Finch, University College

Hospital, for reports of sister-tutors already installed in such hospitals to good effect: ibid., p. 502.

89   PRO, DT6/5, Dr Goodall, meeting of the Education and Examination Committee, 25 May 1921, p. 3.
90   Ibid., Mrs Bedford Fenwick, p. 1.
91   Ibid., p. 3.
92   Ibid., Dr Goodall, p. 2.
93   Ibid., p. 2.
94   Miss Tuke, ibid., p. 3.
95   Ibid., p. 3.
96   Ibid., p. 4.
97   Ibid., p. 5.
98   Ibid., Miss Cox-Davies, p. 5.
99   PRO, DT38/141, Education and Examinations Committee, letter Brock to Priestley, 4 August 1921.
100   Ibid.
101   Ibid., p. 3.
102   Ibid., letter Brock to Priestley, 28 July 1921.
103   Ibid., p. 4.
104   Ibid., p. 2.
105   *Report from the Select Committee of the House of Commons on the General Nursing Council, with the Proceedings and Evidence, 1924–5 (167)*, q. 449–55.
106   PRO, DT38/141, letter Brock to Registrar of the General Nursing Council, 15 November 1922, p. 2.
107   Ibid.
108   PRO, DT38/141, letter Brock to Registrar, 7 February 1923.
109   Ibid., letter Brock to Herringham, 1 March 1923.
110   Ibid., letter Brock to Herringham, 6 March 1923.
111   *Report from the Select Committee of the House of Commons on the General Nursing Council, with the Proceedings and Evidence, 1924–5 (167)*, pp. iv–v.
112   Ibid., evidence of Mrs Bedford Fenwick, q. 194; Mr Herbert Paterson, q. 678–84; Miss MacCallum, q. 841; Miss Beatrice Kent, q. 1028; Miss Pearse, q. 1174, q. 1181, who argued that raising the standard of training would raise the calibre of probationers attracted to the occupation.
113   Ibid., evidence of Miss MacCallum, q. 829–913.
114   Ibid., q. 841.
115   Ibid., Miss Beatrice Kent, q. 1028.
116   Ibid., Brock q. 45.
117   Ibid., p. ix.
118   Ibid., Mrs Bedford Fenwick, q. 307.
119   Ibid., q. 918, q. 922.
120   Ibid., Miss MacCallum, q. 915.
121   Ibid., Brock, q. 20.
122   Ibid., Haywood q. 44.
123   Ibid., p. xix.
124   'Making the Future Nurse', p. 504.

125 P. Nolan, 'Mental Nurse Training in the 1920's', *Bulletin of the History of Nursing Group*, 1986, spring, pp. 15–23; see also P. Nolan, 'Psychiatric Nursing Past and Present: The Nurses' Viewpoint', University of Bath, PhD thesis, 1989.

126 For a general discussion of exclusionary strategies present in men's unions post-World War I see S. Rose, 'Gender Antagonism and Class Conflict: Exclusionary Strategies of Male Trade Unionists in Nineteenth Century Britain', *Social History*, 1988, vol. 13, pp. 192–208.

127 Dingwall, Rafferty and Webster, *Introduction*, p. 93.

128 A.M. Rafferty, 'The Education Policy of the General Nursing Council for England and Wales', *Society for the Social History of Medicine Bulletin*, 1987, 41, December, pp. 56–9.

129 PRO, DT6/50, Education and Examination Committee Shorthand Notes, 23 March 1922.

130 Ibid., 30 March 1922.

131 Ibid., p. 4.

132 PRO, MH55/465, 'Inspection of Rate-paid Hospitals by the General Nursing Council', report of deputation from the General Nursing Council to Ministry of Health, n.d., *c.* July 1931.

133 Ibid., minute Dr Janet Campbell to Dr MacEwan, 23 September 1931.

134 Ibid., chronology of General Nursing Council for England and Wales Scheme of Inspection of Hospitals, 3 November 1932.

135 Ibid., deputation from the General Nursing Council, 18 October 1933, pp. 1–4.

136 Ibid.

137 Dingwall, Rafferty and Webster, *Introduction*, p. 94.

138 Webster, *Problems of Health Care*, p. 19.

139 Watson, *Dawson of Penn*, p. 311.

140 D. Fox, 'The National Health Service and the Second World War: The Elaboration of Consensus', in H. Smith (ed.), *War and Social Change: British Society in the Second World War*, Manchester, University of Manchester Press, 1986, pp. 32–57.

141 Ibid., p. 34; Webster, 'Conflict and Consensus', pp. 123–42.

142 Ibid., p. 126.

7 COMMISSION AND COMMITTEE IN NURSE EDUCATION POLICY (1930-9)

1 PRO, DT5/1. The Bill was debated at the Council meeting of 15 October 1920. Ten members voted for, compared with thirteen against, inclusion in the legislation.

2 Lancet, *The Final Report of the Lancet Commission on Nursing*, London, 1932.

3 R. Lowe, 'Hours of Labour: Negotiating Industrial Legislation in Britain 1919–1939', *Economic History Review*, 1982, vol. 35, pp. 254–71. For a fuller discussion of the work of the Ministry of Labour in inter-war Britain see R. Lowe, *Adjusting to Democracy: The Role of the Ministry of Labour in British Politics 1916–1939*, Oxford, Clarendon

Press, 1986. Lowe's study represents an attempt to salvage the reputation of the Ministry from unflattering views of its influence as a 'second-rate' 'Ministry... occupied by a stodgy, uninspiring people': A. Bullock, *The Life and Times of Ernest Bevin: Minister of Labour*, London, Heinemann, 1967, vol. 2, p. 119.

4 College of Nursing Council, *Minutes*, 1920–1, letter from the Deputy Medical Secretary of the British Medical Association G.C. Anderson, 23 March 1920, p. 5.

5 College of Nursing, *Report of the Salaries Committee on Salaries and Conditions of Service and Conditions of Service and Employment of Nurses*, London, 1919, p. 5.

6 College of Nursing Council, *Minutes*, 1920–1, p. 170. The response rate to the College's questionnaire was low; out of 20,000 questionnaires only 3,000 replies were received, 80 per cent voting against inclusion in the Bill.

7 College of Nursing Council, *Minutes*, 1920–1, report of Minister of Labour's enquiry, 5 January 1921, p. 171.

8 College of Nursing Council, *Minutes*, 1922, p. 97, letter from Ministry of Labour Employment and Insurance Department to College of Nursing, 17 October 1922.

9 College of Nursing, *Minutes*, 1920–1, p. 80; ibid., *Report of Parliamentary Committee No. 2, Interim Report*, p. 35.

10 College of Nursing Council, *Minutes*, letter from College secretary to Clerk of West Ham Board of Guardians, 29 May 1924.

11 The College claimed about one third of its membership was drawn from the Poor Law sector – 7,302 out of 22,771 on 30 September 1923: College of Nursing Council, *Minutes*, 1923, p. 70.

12 College of Nursing Council, *Minutes*, 1923, p. 16.

13 College of Nursing Council, *Minutes*, 1925, p. 97. Letter J.C. Muir, Whipps Cross Infirmary, to Miss Rundle, College of Nursing Secretary, 3 October 1924. The College responded promptly to the situation and instituted a student nurses' association in January 1925.

14 Labour Party, *The Nursing Profession: A Statement of Policy with Regard to Nursing*, London, Labour Party, 1927, p. 29.

15 A draft report was prepared by a subcommittee of the Standing Joint Committee of Industrial Women's Organisations and the Labour Party's Advisory Committee on Public Health: Labour Party, *Nursing Profession*, pp. 24, 25.

16 Ibid., p. 6.

17 Ibid.

18 Ibid.

19 Ibid., p. 20.

20 Ibid., p. 23.

21 Ibid.

22 Ibid., pp. 20–1.

23 F. Brockway, *Towards Tomorrow: The Autobiography of Fenner Brockway*, London, Hart-Davis with Macgibbon, 1977, plate facing p. 224.

24 Fenner Brockway wrote extensively on social issues in his capacity as a political journalist: see his autobiography, n. 23, for details.

25   The College of Nursing was incorporated by royal charter in 1930.
26   Royal College of Nursing Council, *Minutes*, 1931, p. 39.
27   Royal College of Council, *Minutes*, report of meeting between Mr Fenner Brockway and the Parliamentary Committee, 29 May 1931, pp. 72–3.
28   Royal College of Nursing Council, *Minutes*, 1930, p. 141, Education Committee Report, November 1930.
29   Royal College of Nursing Council, *Minutes*, 1930, p. 170.
30   Royal College of Nursing Council, *Minutes*, 1930, p. 142.
31   E. Carling, 'Recruitment for Nursing', the *Lancet*, 1930, vol. ii, 11 October, p. 826.
32   L. Bryder, *Below the Magic Mountain*, Oxford, Clarendon Press, 1988, p. 213.
33   Ibid., pp. 241–2.
34   'Incidence of Tuberculosis amongst Hospital Nurses', *Lancet*, 1930, vol. i, pp. 874–5.
35   J. Walker, *The Modern Nursing of Consumption*, London, Scientific Press, 1924.
36   Lancet, *Final Report*, pp. 142–8.
37   'Editorial: Where are we Drifting?', *Nursing Times*, 1930, vol. 26, 18 October, p. 1233. G. Carter,'Recruitment for Nursing', *Lancet*, 1930, vol. ii, 25 October, p. 937.
38   Carter, 'Recruitment', p. 938.
39   'The Position of Nursing: Past and Present', *Lancet*, 1930, vol, ii, 15 November, pp. 1090–2.
40   'The Position of Nursing – The Public Health', *Lancet*, 1930, vol. ii, 25 November, p. 1025.
41   Throughout 1930, approximately 53 articles were published in the *Lancet* on various aspects of TB diagnosis and treatment. This total was roughly equivalent to the space devoted to university issues: Lancet, *Final Report*, pp. 142–8.
42   Bryder, *Magic Mountain*, p. 171.
43   Lancet, *Final Report*, preface.
44   Of the ten members who were not staff of the *Lancet*, six had voluntary hospital or academic connections mainly in London. They were Miss Dorothy Brock, headmistress of Mary Datchelor Girl's School; Miss Edith Thompson, member of Council Bedford College, University of London; Miss R.E. Derbyshire, matron of University College Hospital; Professor Henry Clay, late Professor of Social Economics, University of Manchester; Professor F.R. Fraser, Professor of Medicine in the University of London, Physician to St Bartholomew's Hospital; Dr Robert Huchinson, Physician to the London Hospital and to the Hospital for Sick Children, Great Ormond Street.
45   Dr Dorothy Brock was the sister of Lawrence Brock: see PRO, MH71/31, letter Brock to Chrystal, 4 October 1937.
46   Correspondence between Mr Kettle, secretary to the Lancet Commission, and Miss Rundle, Secretary Royal College of Nursing, on requests for information on preliminary training schools, Royal College of

Nursing Council, *Minutes,* 19 November 1931; ibid., 'Salary Scales', 25 September 1931.

47 T. Mellor, *Report of the Salaries Committee on Salaries and Conditions of Employment of Nurses as Submitted to the College Council in April 1919,* London, 1919; Royal College of Nursing, *Report on the Questionnaire on the Supply of Suitable Candidates for the Nursing Profession and Unemployment amongst Nurses,* London, Royal College of Nursing, 1931.

48 For a review of the work of Professor Austin Bradford Hill at the Medical Research Council see J. Austoker and L. Bryder, *Historical Perspectives on the Role of the MRC: Essays in the History of the MRC of the United Kingdom and its Predecessor, the Medical Research Committee, 1913–1953,* Oxford, Oxford University Press, 1988, pp. 46–7; A. Landsborough Thomson, *Half a Century of Medical Research. vol. 2: The Programme of the Medical Research Council,* London, HMSO, 1975, p. 136; 'The Lancet Commission on Nursing: First Interim Report', *Lancet,* 1931, vol. 1, pp. 451–6; 'Second Interim Report: The Lancet Commission on Nursing', *Lancet,* 1932, vol. i, pp. i–xxii.

49 A. Bradford Hill, 'Statistical Analysis of the Questionnaire issued to Hospitals by the "Lancet" Commission on Nursing. Final Report submitted to the Commission by Bradford Hill', *Lancet,* 1932, supplement, p. i.

50 'Lancet Commission', pp. 454–5.

51 'Second Interim Report', p. vii.

52 Ibid., p. xi.

53 Ibid.

54 'Lancet Commission', p. 456.

55 Association of Hospital Matrons, *Memorandum of the Association of Hospital Matrons to the Lancet Commission on Nursing,* London, 1930, p. 1. Both the AHM and the College of Nursing recommended a fifty-six-hour week when other workers were demanding a forty-four-hour week. Much of the concern expressed in their memorandum revolved around the difficulties some matrons had in asserting their authority as heads of nursing staffs in their hospitals: ibid., p. 2.

56 Royal College of Nursing, *Memorandum of Evidence submitted to the Lancet Commission on Nursing: Suggested Improvements for the Nursing Profession,* London, 1931, p. 1.

57 Royal College of Nursing, *Memorandum of the Salaries and Superannuation Committee of the Royal College of Nursing to the Lancet Commission,* London, 1931, p. 1.

58 Royal College of Nursing, *Memorandum to the Lancet Commission on Nursing submitted by the Royal College of Nursing,* 1931, pp. 1–3.

59 Sister from Glasgow, letter to the Honorary Secretary of the *Lancet,* n.d., Royal College of Nursing, correspondence on Lancet Commission.

60 Maggs examined recruitment to two large voluntary hospitals and two large Poor Law infirmaries between 1881 and 1921. At various times, all had difficulty in attracting recruits for training and responded partly by

lowering educational requirements. Immigrants from Ireland, Wales and Scotland made up 15 per cent of the recruits. More than 70 per cent of recruits had some previous work experience in domestic service, clerical and commercial posts, clothing and textiles, shopwork, war work and 'education'. Less than 10 per cent of these were secondary schoolteachers, the majority being uncertificated pupil teachers, and a few private teachers: see C. Maggs, *The Origins of General Nursing*, London, Croom Helm, 1983, pp. 73–101.

61 M. Viney, 'The Nursing Service of Great Britain: A Career for Girls', *Journal of Education*, 1930, February, pp. 88–90.

62 H. Balme, *The Reform of Nurse Education*, Oxford, Oxford University Press, 1930. Many of the criticisms related to the restricted lifestyles of nurses. Compulsory attendance at meals, regulated bedtimes, and the rigid hierarchical form of social relationships were all features of the earlier report by Mellor, *Report of the Salaries Committee.*

63 This was a recapitulation of an earlier recommendation of the *Report from the Select Committee of the House of Commons on the Registration of Nurses with Proceedings, Evidence, Appendices and Index, 1905 (263)*, p. v.

64 Lancet, *Final Report*, p. 47.

65 Ibid., p. 50.

66 Royal College of Nursing, *First Draft: The Royal College of Nursing Committee on the Lancet Commission Report*, London, 1931, p. 3.

67 'Correspondence between the College of Nursing and the General Nursing Council', *British Journal of Nursing*, 1932, vol. 80, August, p. 224.

68 Royal College of Nursing Council, *Minutes*, 20 October 1932, p. 92.

69 'Editorial: The One Portal to the State Register', *British Journal of Nursing*, 1932, vol. 80, March.

70 'Nursing as a Profession', *The Times*, 4 March 1932.

71 Ibid.

72 'The Nurses' Calling', *The Times*, 14 August 1931. The *Church Times* also condemned poor salaries but emphasised the importance of the fostering of the vocational element in nursing and advocated thorough improvements in education, tuition, salaries, leisure and freedom: 'Lancet Commission', *Church Times*, 26 February 1932; 'The Nurses' Night Out', *Birmingham Post*, 20 January 1932; 'Hospital Nursing', *The Spectator*, 27 February 1932.

73 'The Nurse's Life', *The Times*, 19 February 1932.

74 'The Final Report of the Lancet Commission on Nursing', *Nursing Times*, 1932, vol. 27, February, pp. 207–8.

75 Ibid., p. 203.

76 'Editorial: The One Portal'.

77 M. Hitch, 'The Education of the Nurse as a Problem of the Future', *Nursing Times*, 1932, vol. 30, 12 November, p. 1163.

78 'The Hospital Nursing Service', *British Medical Journal*, 1932, 20 February, vol. 1, p. 344.

79 'Entry to the Nursing Profession', *Lancet*, 1933, vol. ii, 28 October, p. 1020.

80   Lancet, *Final Report*, pp. 162–4.
81   Ibid., p. 163.
82   Ibid.
83   Ibid.
84   PRO, DT5/4, Education and Examinations Committee, *Minutes*, 24 November 1933.
85   C. Wood, 'Sick Nursing', *Englishwoman's Yearbook*, 1899, p. 61.
86   PRO, DT20/231, letter Brock to Priestley, 22 July 1920.
87   Royal College of Nursing, *Memorandum of Evidence*, p. 3.
88   PRO, DT5/4. The Matrons' Council and British Council of Nurses, an organisation established by Mrs Bedford Fenwick as a competitor to the Royal College of Nursing, opposed the division of the preliminary examination until 1938.
89   'The Lancet Commission on Nursing', *Lancet*, 1933, vol. i, 18 February, pp. 369–70.
90   Ibid.
91   PRO, MH55/1447, 'Admission of Foreigners as Probationers in English Hospitals', letter Director of Education, Royal College of Nursing, to Minister of Health, 2 November 1933.
92   J. Austoker, 'Biological Education and Social Reform: The British Social Hygiene Movement', University of London, MA dissertation, 1981; N. Blakestad, 'The Place of Domestic Subjects in the Curriculum of Girls' Secondary Education in late Victorian and Edwardian England', University of Oxford, MPhil thesis, 1988, and 'King's College of Household and Social Science and the Household Science Movement in English Higher Education, 1908–1939', University of Oxford, DPhil thesis, 1995; C. Manthorpe, 'Science or Domestic Science?: The Struggle to Define an Appropriate Science Education for Girls in the Early Twentieth Century', *History of Education*, 1986, vol. 15, pp. 195–213.
93   PRO, ED50/51, 'Representations of Board of Education on General Nursing Council', letter Brock to Secretary of Board of Education, 5 February 1920.
94   PRO, ED50/58, minute Cleary to Dame Janet Campbell, 30 January 1930.
95   PRO ED 50/56, 'Grants for Nurse Training Board of Education', Brock to Wood, 17 May 1920.
96   For an analysis of the debate in the USA see S.J. Gould, *The Mismeasure of Man*, Harmondsworth, Penguin, 1981. For the UK see A. Wooldridge, 'Child Study and Educational Psychology in England 1918–1950', University of Oxford, DPhil thesis, 1985; G. Sutherland, *Ability, Merit and Measurement: Mental Testing and English Education 1880–1940*, Oxford, Oxford University Press, 1986; A. Wooldridge, *Measuring the Mind: Education and Psychology, c.1860–1990*, Cambridge, Cambridge University Press, 1994.
97   K. Robinson and A.M. Rafferty, *The Nursing Workforce*, London, Polytechnic of the South Bank, 1988, pp. 55–6.
98   PRO DT34/97, 'Test Educational Examination', report of meeting at Board of Education, 6 May 1937, to discuss the suggestion that the Board of Education should act as assessors for the test.

99 Ibid., Miss Musson's introductory remarks during conference with Minister of Health, 30 November 1936.
100 Ibid., conference at Ministry of Health, 30 November 1936, on test for probationers. The BHA had five representatives at the conference compared with four from the GNC and two from the AHM.
101 PRO, ED50/203, 'Draft Rule regarding Educational Test for Probationer Nurses'.
102 PRO, DT34/97, conference at Ministry of Health, 30 November 1936, note on test for probationers.
103 Ibid., comments of Miss Musson at Conference at Ministry of Health, 30 November 1936, on test for probationers.
104 PRO, DT50/203, 'Draft Rule regarding Educational Test for Probationer Nurses'.
105 Ibid.
106 Ibid., letter Eustace Hill, Ministry of Health, to Cecil Maudsley, Board of Education, 20 March 1937.

8 NATIONALISING NURSING EDUCATION (1939-48)

1 Ministry of Health, Department of Health for Scotland, Ministry of Labour and National Service, *Working Party on the Recruitment and Training of Nurses*, London, HMSO, 1947; Ministry of Health, Department of Health for Scotland, Ministry of Labour and National Service, *Working Party on the Recruitment and Training of Nurses, Minority Report*, London, HMSO, 1948.
2 PRO, MH71/31, minute Eustace Hill to Neville, 10 May 1937.
3 Ibid., letter Sir Fredrick Menzies to Sir Kingsley Wood, March 1937; ibid., minute Eustace Hill to Neville, 10 May 1937.
4 Ibid., letter Women's Medical Federation to Sir Kingsley Wood, Minister of Health, 23 June 1937. Dame Janet Campbell (1877–1954) graduated BM, 1901, from the London School of Medicine for Women, and qualified MD and MS, 1904–5. Following house and senior medical officer jobs at the Royal Free and Belgrave Hospital for Children respectively, she was appointed assistant school medical officer in the London School Medical Service in 1904. In 1907 she joined the Board of Education as their first full-time medical officer, and moved to the Ministry of Health in 1919 under George Newman, Chief Medical Officer. She was appointed Senior Medical officer for Maternal and Child Welfare in 1919, retaining her connection with the Board of Education as Chief Woman Adviser. She published extensively on the recruitment and training of midwives, maternal and child welfare. In 1934 she married Michael Hesletine, registrar of the GMC and under civil service rules was obliged to renounce her office: see E. Williams and H. Palmer (eds), *Dictionary of National Biography 1951–60*, Oxford, Oxford University Press, 1971, pp. 181–2.
5 Ibid., letter Dame Janet Campbell to Minister of Health, 7 November 1936.

6 Ibid.
7 Trades Union Congress, *Report of the Proceedings of the 69th Annual Trade Union Congress 1937*, London, Trades Union Council, 1937, p. 96.
8 Ibid., p. 97.
9 Ibid., Mr Ben Smith, Distributive and Allied Trades, pp. 96–7.
10 'A Charter for Nurses', *Star*, 9 September 1937; 'Nurses' Charter Campaign', *Nottingham Journal and Express*, 25 October 1937; 'A Charter for Nurses', *Spectator*, 20 August 1937.
11 'Support for New Union', *Nottingham Journal and Express*, 3 November 1937; 'Nurses' Fight to End "Anarchy"', *Daily Mirror*, 9 November.
12 See J. Fyrth and S. Alexander (eds), *Women's Voices from the Spanish Civil War*, London, Lawrence and Wishart, 1991, pp. 55–7.
13 'The National Association of Local Government Officer's Charter for Nurses', *Daily Independent*, 12 December 1937; 'Why T.U.C. Charter is a Vital Necessity', *Reynolds News*, 22 August 1937; 'Charter for Nurses, Disapproval of T.U.C. Plan', *Western Morning News*, 21 August 1937; 'Nursing Profession and Trade Union Protection', *Evening Herald*, 2 September 1937.
14 Royal College of Nursing Council, *Minutes*, letter Royal College of Nursing Secretary to Branch Secretaries, September 1937.
15 M. Carpenter, *Working for Health: The History of the Confederation of Health Services Employees*, London, Lawrence and Wishart, 1988, pp. 211–18.
16 Ibid., p. 216.
17 'Nursing Profession Problem', *Scotsman*, 9 November 1937; 'Dragooned by Petty Rules', *Daily Sketch*, 9 November 1937; 'Nurses' Conditions', *Daily Worker*, 18 September 1937; 'The Shortage of Nurses', *Nottingham Evening News*, 15 December 1937; 'Ministering Angels Minus', *Tribune*, 27 August 1937; 'What the "Life" of the Probationer and Training for the Nurse in the Average Hospital is Like', *Public Opinion*, 10 December 1937.
18 'Supply of Nurses: School and Hospital', *The Times*, 27 February 1937.
19 'What Is There to Attract Nurses?', *Lincoln and Stamford Mercury*, 22 October 1937; 'Nurses' Hours: Profession Above Trade Unionism', *Nottingham Evening News*, 30 October 1937; 'Welcome News for Bradford Nurses', *Yorkshire Observer*, 29 December 1937; 'Nurses' Pay and Conditions', *Daily Telegraph*, 28 September 1937.
20 'The Nurse's Training II: The Path of Reform by a Medical Correspondent', *Spectator*, 16 July 1937; G.B. Carter, 'The Nurse's Training: Letter to the Editor', *Spectator*, 23 July 1937.
21 'Nurse's Training II'.
22 Carter, 'Nurse's Training'.
23 'Nursing is Hard Work but it is Well Worth It', *Leeds Mercury*, 10 September 1937; 'Hospital Nurse's Lot: Some of the Advantages', *Daily Telegraph*, 22 September 1937; 'The Nurse's Training – Another Side', *Spectator*, 6 August 1937.
24 'Nurses of Britain Plan their Case', *Daily Sketch*, 2 November 1937; A.J. Cronin, 'The Worst Job in the World', *Daily Mirror*, 3 November 1937.

A.J. Cronin was medically qualified and critical of his own profession. His novel *The Citadel*, London, Victor Gollancz, 1932, was an attack upon the Harley Street mentality in medicine, and was subsequently made into a successful feature film: see M. Shortland, *Medicine and Film: A Checklist, Survey and Research Resource*, Oxford, Wellcome Unit for the History of Medicine, 1988.

25 ' "Scares" Responsible for Shortage of Candidates', *Birmingham Post*, 10 November 1937; Hart hints that the mask is symbolic of the muted militancy within nursing. See C. Hart, *Behind the Mask: Nurses' Unions and Nursing Policy*, London, Balliere Tindall, 1995.

26 PRO, MH71/31, handwritten note Sir Arthur MacNalty to Secretary, Ministry of Health, 13 May 1937.

27 Ibid.

28 Royal College of Nursing, *Professional Association Committee Report to Council*, London, 1936, p. 1.

29 'Nursing Inquiry to be Instituted', *Daily Worker*, 24 September 1937; 'Ladies with the Lamp', *Evening Standard*, 23 September 1937; 'More Nurses Wanted', *Birmingham Daily*, 23 September 1937.

30 PRO, MH71/31, minute Minister of Health to Secretary, 8 June 1937.

31 Ibid., minute Eustace Hill to Chief Medical Officer, 11 May 1937.

32 In 1934 the Secretary of State for Scotland appointed a Scottish Departmental Committee on the Training of Nurses, which published an interim report in 1936: Department of Health for Scotland, *Training of Nurses*, London, HMSO, 1935–6. The report recommended the harmonisation of general and specialists training. This committee was reconstituted with Lord Alness as chairman: Department of Health for Scotland, *Scottish Departmental Report*, London, HMSO, Chairman Lord Alness, Cmnd 5866, 1937–8.

33 The ideal balance of interests was considered to include one chairman, two matrons, two local authority representatives, one 'mental' services representative, one medical officer of health, one voluntary hospital representative, one representative of the teaching profession, one consultant, one sister-tutor, one private medical practitioner, one representative of the GNC, one representative of district nursing: PRO, MH71/31, minute Hill to Neville, 11 August 1937, p. 6.

34 Ibid., minute Eustace Hill to Neville, 11 August 1937.

35 Ibid., note on constitution of Inter-departmental Committee, 15 May 1937.

36 'Inquiry into Nursing Services, Committee's Constitution Explained', *The Times*, 17 January 1938.

37 PRO, MH71/31, terms of reference and personnel of nursing committee, 9 November 1937.

38 Dr Rees-Thomas was the representative of mental nursing, a Medical Senior Commissioner at the Board of Control. Only details supplementary to those contained in the interim report of the committee are included here: Ministry of Health, Board of Education and Department of Health for Scotland, *Interim Report of the Inter-departmental Committee on Nursing Services*, London, HMSO, 1939. Sir Arthur Hall, formerly Professor of Medicine at Sheffield Uni-

versity, was consultant physician at Sheffield Royal Hospital. Dr Gilbert Orme was a doctor in private practice, 'actively interested in nursing questions': PRO MH71/31, notes on members, 9 November 1937.

39 Ibid., letter Brock to Chrystal, 4 October 1937.

40 Alexander Augustus Fredrick William Alfred George Athlone, third son of Princess Mary Adelaide and Duke of Teck and brother of the future Queen Mary. In 1914 he was nominated Governor General of Canada, but did not take up the appointment due to the war. After the army and the war he took an active interest in social work, and was nominated as chairman of the Middlesex Hospital in 1910. In 1921 he was appointed chairman of a committee to investigate the needs of medical practitioners. His comprehensive report recommended public funds for postgraduate education to promote postgraduate instruction and research. This led to the establishment of the postgraduate medical school at the Hammersmith Hospital. He was also Chairman of Senate at the University of London, 1932–55. See Williams and Palmer, *Dictionary of National Biography*, pp. 176–7.

41 PRO, MH71/31, letter Brock to Chrystal, 4 October 1937.

42 'Nursing Services Committee Objects Explained', *Manchester Guardian*, 17 January 1938.

43 PRO, DT20/201, pp. 9–10.

44 Ibid., p. 10.

45 PRO, DT20/201, Mrs Keynes, Board of Education, p. 23.

46 Ibid., p. 14.

47 Ibid., p. 4. Evidence submitted by the Women's Employment Federation to the Inter-departmental Committee on Nursing Services.

48 Ibid.

49 Ibid., p. 5.

50 'Special Meeting to Present Reasons for Opposition to Division of Preliminary Examination of Nurses', *British Journal of Nursing*, 1934, vol. 84, p. 94.

51 Ibid.

52 Ibid.

53 Ibid.

54 PRO, DT20/201, British Medical Association, *Memorandum of Evidence to the Inter-departmental Committee on Nursing Services*, London, 1938, p. 2; Royal College of Nursing, *Memorandum of Evidence Relating to Conditions in the Nursing Profession Submitted to the Inter-departmental Committee on Nursing Services*, London, 1938; Royal College of Nursing Student Nurses' Association, 'Memorandum of Evidence Relating to Conditions in the Nursing Profession Submitted to the Inter-departmental Committee on Nursing Services'; National Council of Women of Great Britain, *Memorandum of Evidence Relating to Conditions in the Nursing Profession Submitted to the Inter-departmental Committee on Nursing Services*, London, 1938.

55 PRO, DT20/199, Association of Headmistresses, *Memorandum of Evidence to the Inter-departmental Committee on Nursing Services by the Association of Headmistresses*, London, 1938, p. 1.

56 PRO, DT20/201, p. 17.
57 PRO, DT20/201, British Medical Association (1938), *Memorandum of Evidence*, p. 3.
58 Ibid., evidence of Tuberculosis Association, Royal College of Nursing, Association of Headmistresses, TUC and BMA.
59 H. Balme, 'A Criticism of Nursing Education with Suggestions for Constructive Reform', *Nosokomeion*, 1938, vol. ix, p. 54.
60 PRO, DT20/201, Voluntary Hospitals Committee County of London, *Statement of Evidence for Submission to the Inter-departmental Committee on Nursing*, London, HMSO, 1938, p. 4.
61 PRO, MH71/31, minute Sir Arthur MacNalty, Minister of Health, to Neville, Secretary, 31 July 1937.
62 PRO, DT20/201, British Medical Association, *Memorandum of Evidence*, p. 2.
63 PRO, MH77/33, note on nurses, n.d., pp. 2–3.
64 Ibid., p. 3.
65 'The Interim Report', *Nursing Times*, 1939, vol. 35, 4 February, p. 120.
66 'Ways and Means', *Nursing Times*, 1938, vol. 34, 28 May, p. 1726.
67 'The Nurse and the Nation', *Time and Tide*, 1939, vol. 50, pp. 129–30. It is not clear whether Mrs Bedford Fenwick was behind this charge or not. The tone of the article, Mrs Bedford Fenwick's journalist connections and feminist sympathies suggest it may be a strong possibility.
68 PRO, MH71/33, *Interim report of the Inter-departmental Committee on Nursing Services*, note of a discussion on 23 March 1939, p. 4.
69 Ibid.
70 Ibid., p. 5.
71 Ibid., letter Tribe to Hughes, 12 May 1939, p. 2.
72 Ibid.
73 Letter Earl of Athlone to Frances Goodall, General Secretary of the Royal College of Nursing, 27 April 1940.
74 C. Webster, 'Conflict and Consensus: Explaining the British Health Service', *Twentieth Century British History*, 1991, vol. 1, pp. 115–51; D. Fox, 'The National Health Service and the Second World War: The Elaboration of Consensus', in H. Smith, *War and Social Change: British Society in the Second World War*, Manchester, Manchester University Press, 1986, pp. 32–57.
75 C. Webster, *Problems of Health Care: The National Health Service before 1957*, London, HMSO, p. 393.
76 'Trained Nurses: The Steel Framework', *Time and Tide*, 1939, vol. 50, p. 1461.
77 R. Titmuss, *Problems of Social Policy: History of the Second World War*, London, HMSO, 1950, p. 56.
78 Ibid.; K. Watt, 'The Civil Nursing Services in War-time', in C. Dunn (ed.), *The Emergency Medical Services*, London, 1952, p. 438. Dame Katherine Watt was Chief Nursing Officer and Principal Matron, Ministry of Health. Her qualifications are listed as Royal Red Cross (RRC), not SRN, which possibly reflects the marginal status of registration.

79 Ibid., p. 438.

80 The committee contained representatives from the General Nursing Council (GNC), RCN, Matrons-in-Chief of the Army, Navy and Air Force and representatives from County Councils Associations, Municipal Corporations and the LCC. Miss Puxley from the Ministry of Health was appointed secretary: see ibid.

81 Ibid., p. 439.

82 Details of the fate and fortunes of the Civil Nursing reserve and the workforce distribution are provided by S. Ferguson and H. Fitzgerald, *Studies in the Social Services*, London, HMSO, 1954, pp. 305–9.

83 Titmuss, *Problems of Social Policy*, p. 64.

84 Ibid., p. 67.

85 C. Dunn, *The Emergency Medical Service. vol. 1: England and Wales*, London, HMSO, 1952, p. 67.

86 Ibid., p. 446.

87 Ibid., p. 188.

88 A. MacNalty (ed.), *The Civilian Health and Medical Services*, London, HMSO, 1953, vol. 1, p. 188.

89 Watt, 'Civil Nursing Services', p. 444.

90 Interview with Sir George Godber, former Chief Medical Officer at the Ministry of Health, 15 March 1988.

91 C. Webster, 'Nursing and the Crisis of the Early Health Service', *Bulletin of the History of Nursing Group*, 1985, vol. 2, pp. 4–12.

92 Ibid., p. 6.

93 PRO, MH55/886, letter Ernest Bevin to Rushcliffe, 25 August 1941.

94 B. Abel-Smith, *A History of the Nursing Profession*, London, Heinemann, 1960, pp. 172–80.

95 PRO, MH55/886, notes of discussion of nurses' salaries committee with the Royal College of Nursing, 24 July 1941. For an analysis of the development of the Whitley Council system see J. Sheldrake, 'The Origins and Development of the Whitley System 1910–1939 with Particular Reference to Public Utilities', University of Kent, MPhil thesis, 1986.

96 R. Dingwall, A.M. Rafferty and C. Webster, *An Introduction to the Social History of Nursing*, London, Routledge, 1988, pp. 104–5.

97 PRO, MH55/1994, 'Grants in Respect of Increases in Nurses Salaries'.

98 Webster, 'Nursing and Crisis', p. 6.

99 Letter from Frances Goodall, Royal College of Nursing Secretary, to Earl of Athlone, 22 April 1940.

100 For details of the reconstruction and planning movements prior to and during World War II, see J. Stevenson, 'Planner's Moon?: The Second World War and the Planning Movement', in H. Smith (ed.), *War and Social Change*, Manchester, Manchester University Press, 1986, pp. 58–77.

101 Thomas Jeeves Horder (1871–1955), physician, appointed senior physician to St Bartholomew's Hospital in 1921, honorary consultant physician to the Ministry of Pensions in 1939, and medical adviser to London Transport, 1940–55. He is described as an outstanding physi-

cian and committed to the application of laboratory science to clinical medicine. His patients included King George V, King George VI, Bonar Law and Ramsay MacDonald. He was antagonistic to many aspects of the NHS. See Williams and Palmer, *Dictionary of National Biography 1951–60*, pp. 501–3.

102   Details of the report its findings and effects are discussed by Abel-Smith, *Nursing Profession*, pp. 170–3; R. White, *The Effect of the National Health Service upon the Nursing Profession 1948–1960*, Oxford, Oxford University Press, 1988, pp. 14–20.

103   Abel-Smith *Nursing Profession*, p. 169.

104   Ibid., p. 170.

105   Royal College of Nursing, *Nursing Reconstruction Committee, Section i: The Assistant Nurse*, London, Royal College of Nursing, 1942, p. 5.

106   PRO, MH55/887, letter Brock, Board of Control, to Wrigley, Ministry of Health, 21 November 1941.

107   Letter from Miss Lavinia Dock cited in 'Editorial: A Demand for Justice for the State Registered Nurse', *British Journal of Nursing*, 1943, vol. 91, p. 209.

108   'Editorial: The Rise and Decline of Nursing in England and Wales', *British Journal of Nursing*, 1943, vol. 91, pp. 37–8.

109   Certificated status was to be offered to uncertificated teachers of 'long and meritorious' service, but after an appointed day their absorption was to be curtailed: National Union of Teachers, *A Report of Proposals by the Executive of the National Union of Teachers*, Gloucester, National Union of Teachers, 1943, p. 31.

110   Ferguson and Fitzgerald, *Studies in the Social Services*, p. 322, fn. 1.

111   Royal College of Nursing, *Nursing Reconstruction Commmittee Report, Section ii: Education and Training*, London, Royal College of Nursing, 1943, p. 5.

112   Ibid., p. 5.

113   Lord Horder, 'Eugenics as I See It', *Eugenics Review*, 1936, vol. 38, p. 267.

114   Royal College of Nursing, 'Nursing Reconstruction Commmittee, Education and Training Sub-committee', *Minutes*, 20 January 1942, p. 59.

115   G. Hardy, 'A Quest for Qualification', *British Journal of Nursing*, 1943, vol. 90, May, p. 50.

116   Royal College of Nursing 'Nursing Reconstruction Committee', *Minutes*, 20 January 1942, p. 57.

117   Ibid., p. 60.

118   Royal College of Nursing, *Nursing Reconstruction Commmittee Report, Section ii*, p. 9.

119   Ibid., pp. 15–7.

120   Ibid., pp. 32–3.

121   Ministry of Health, *First Report of Nurses' Salaries Committee*, London, HMSO, Chairman Lord Rushcliffe, 1943, pp. 7–8.

122   Ferguson and Fitzgerald, *Studies in the Social Services*, pp. 320–2.

123   Watt,'Civil Nursing Services', p. 442.

124   Ferguson and Fitzgerald, *Studies in the Social Services*, pp. 323–6.

125 PRO, LAB 8/1632, 'Registration for Employment, National Service Order Special Registration of Nurses and Midwives, 1952'.

126 A. MacNalty and W. Mellor, *Medical Services in War: The Principal Medical Lessons of the Second World War: Based on the Official Histories of the United Kingdom, Canada, Australia, New Zealand and India*, London, HMSO, 1968, p. 309.

127 *Lancet*, 1945, vol. ii, p. 413.

128 Ministry of Health, Ministry of Labour and National Service and Department of Health for Scotland, *Staffing the Hospitals: An Urgent National Need*, London, HMSO, 1945.

129 See Ferguson and Fitzgerald, *Studies in the Social Services*, p. 325, for the details of the target audience and timing of campaigns.

130 Ministry of Health, *Nursing in a National Health Service*, London, HMSO, 1945.

131 'Mr Bevan at the Royal College of Nursing – The Minister of Health Speaks at the Fourth Nation's Nurses Conference', *Nursing Times*, 1948, vol. 44, 12 June, p. 426.

132 Webster, *Problems of Health Care*, pp. 107–20; C. Webster, *Aneurin Bevan on the National Health Service*, Oxford, Wellcome Unit for the History of Medicine, 1991, p. 10; A.M. Rafferty, 'Nursing Policy and Nationalization of Nursing: The Representation of "Crisis" and "Crisis" of Representation', in J. Robinson, A.M. Gray and R. Elkan (eds), *Policy Issues in Nursing*, Buckingham, Open University Press, 1992, pp. 68–83.

133 'Lord Horder's Speech in the USA', *Lancet*, 1948, vol. ii, 25 June, p. 1124.

134 Socialist Medical Association, *Nursing in the Post-War World: A Memorandum on the Shortage of Nurses with Constructive Proposals*, London, Socialist Medical Association, 1945.

135 Sir Robert Wood (1886–1963), educationist, entered the Board of Education in 1911 as inspector of schools. Subsequently he held a number of positions: private secretary to the President of the Board of Education, Lord Eustace Percy, 1926–8; Director of Establishments, 1928–36, and Principal Assistant Secretary for technical education, 1936–40. It was during this period that he first made contact with the University College of Southampton, of which he eventually became Vice-chancellor. In 1938 he was seconded for special service with Sir John Anderson, then Lord Privy Seal, later Home Secretary. The arrival of R.A. Butler at the Presidency of the Board of Education opened up a range of opportunities in technical education policy-making, in which Wood became actively involved. He was largely responsible for promoting a variety of schemes, including the section on higher education in the government's White Paper of 1943. After the Act, the Board became the Ministry of Education, and it was widely believed that Wood would become Permanent Secretary. A change of government prevented this, much to Wood's disappointment. It was shortly after this he took up an appointment as Principal of University College Southampton. He was a strong advocate of rational planning and Labour's ideal of extending equality of opportunity. Biographical details derived from Williams and

Nicholls, *Dictionary of National Biography 1961–70*, pp. 1101–2. For a review of his role in shaping the 1944 Education Act see D. Thom, 'The 1944 Education Act: The "Art of the Possible" ', in H. Smith (ed.), *War and Social Change*, Manchester, Manchester University Press, 1986, pp. 101–28; P. Gosden, *Education in the Second World War: A Study in Policy and Administration*, London, Methuen, 1976, pp. 237–331.

136   See PRO, MH55/2959, 'Provisional Scheme of Work for the Working Party', letter to Miss Katherine Watt from National League of Nursing, 9 April 1946. Ten of the thirty-six reports collated as evidence by the committee were international in origin: Ministry of Health, Department of Health for Scotland, Ministry of Labour and National Service, *Working Party on Recruitment and Training*. Miss Cockayne was also secretary to the AHM. Miss Bridges was recommended in preference to Miss Russell, head of the Toronto School of Nursing. Miss Russell, like Miss Cockayne, had been awarded a Rockefeller fellowship and study tour of nurse education in London: see A.M. Rafferty, 'Internationalising Nursing Education', in P. Weindling (ed.), *International Health Organisations and Movements 1870–1939*, Cambridge, Cambridge University Press, 1995, pp. 275–6.

137   There was some cross-membership between the Working Party and Steering Committee; Dr Inch and Sir Robert Wood were members of both.

138   Ministry of Health, Department of Health for Scotland, Ministry of Labour and National Service, *Working Party on Recruitment and Training*, p. iii.

139   PRO, MH55/2959, 'Provisional Scheme of Work for the Working Party', pp. 1–5.

140   Ibid., p. 6.

141   PRO, MH55/2060, 'Statistics of Nursing: Nursing Working Party', 22 February 1946.

142   Ministry of Health, Department of Health for Scotland, Ministry of Labour and National Service, *Working Party on Recruitment and Training*, pp. 17–21.

143   Webster, 'Conflict and Consensus', pp. 138–9.

144   PRO, MH55/2061, note of a meeting held 4 March 1947 to discuss action on the first instalment of the Working Party Report; Socialist Medical Association, 'Nursing in the Post-war World'.

145   Ministry of Health, Department of Health for Scotland, Ministry of Labour and National Service, *Working Party on the Recruitment and Training of Nurses*, p. 80.

146   Ibid., p. 81.

147   PRO, MH55/2061, 'Nursing policy consequent on Working Party's Report'.

148   Ibid., note from T.J. Hotton to Miss Enid Smith, n.d.

149   Ibid., note of a meeting to discuss the first instalment of the Working Party Report, 4 March 1947.

150   Ibid., note on the trend of observations submitted by organisations on the report of the Working Party on the Recruitment and Training of Nurses.

151 'Reconstruction: The New Utilitarianism', *Lancet*, 1949, vol. i, 7 May, pp. 792–3.
152 General Nursing Council, *Memorandum submitted to the Working Party on Nurse Recruitment and Training*, London, 1948, p. 6.
153 Ministry of Health, Department of Health for Scotland, Ministry of Labour and National Service, *Working Party on Recruitment and Training*, p. 68.
154 'Correspondence', *Nursing Times*, 1948, vol. 44, 20 November, p. 852; R. White, 'The Nurses Act 1949', *Nursing Times*, Occasional Papers, 1982, vol. 78, no. 3, 27 January, and no. 4, 3 February; Royal College of Nursing, Council, minutes, September 1948.
155 White, 'The Nurses Act 1949: 2', pp. 13–15.
156 PRO, MH77/160, 'NHS Nurses and Nursing Associations' Representations 1943–5'; MH77/161, 'NHS Nurses and Nursing Associations' Representations 1946'.
157 'Missing Nurses' Report Mystifies Councils', *Daily Worker*, 7 June 1947.
158 'Recruits for Nursing', *The Times*, 16 September 1948.
159 Ministry of Health, Department of Health for Scotland, Ministry of Labour and National Service, *Working Party on the Recruitment and Training of Nurses, Minority Report*, London, HMSO, 1948, p. 16.
160 Ibid., p. v.
161 Ibid., pp. iv–v.
162 Ibid., p. 9.
163 R. Thomson, *The Pelican History of Psychology*, Harmondsworth, Pelican, 1968, p. 328.
164 J. Cohen, 'The Analysis of Physique', *Eugenics Review*, 1940–1, vol. 32, pp. 81–4; A. Wooldridge, 'Child Study and Educational Psychology in England 1918–1950', University of Oxford, DPhil thesis, 1985; B. Norton, 'Psychologists and Class', in C. Webster (ed.), *Biology, Medicine and Society 1840–1940*, Cambridge, Cambridge University Press, 1981, pp. 289–314.
165 Ministry of Health, Department of Health for Scotland, Ministry of Labour and National Service, *Minority Report*, p. 3.
166 Interview with Dame Elizabeth Cockayne, 24 August 1987.
167 'Nursing Problems and Dr Cohen', *Nursing Mirror*, 1948, 2 October, p. 2.
168 Ministry of Health, Department of Health for Scotland, Ministry of Labour and National Service, *Minority Report*, p. 6.
169 Ibid., p. 13.
170 Ibid., p. 17.
171 Ibid., pp. 20–1.
172 J. Cohen, 'The Nurse as Citizen', *Nursing Times*, 1948, vol. 44, 20 November, p. 850.
173 Ministry of Health, Department of Health for Scotland, Ministry of Labour and National Service, *Minority Report*, p. 19.
174 Ibid., p. 49.
175 'Nursing Problems and Dr Cohen', pp. 1–2.

176   Ministry of Health, Department of Health for Scotland, Ministry of Labour and National Service, *Minority Report*, pp. 39–41; Thomson, *Pelican History of Psychology*, pp. 345–7.
177   Ibid., p. 52.
178   Reverby provides a review of the impact of early operational research upon changing perceptions of nursing work in the USA: see S. Reverby, *Ordered to Care: The Dilemma of American Nursing*, Cambridge, Cambridge University Press, 1987, pp. 143–58.
179   'Nursing Problems and Dr Cohen', pp. 1–2.
180   'Working Party Minority Report: Summary of Conclusions and Recommendations', *Nursing Mirror*, vol. 87, 1948, 25 September, pp. 405, 409; 'The Working Party on the Recruitment and Training of Nurses – Minority Report: Summary of Comments made by John Cohen', *Nursing Times*, vol. 44, 1948, 25 September, pp. 700–1.
181   Ibid., p. 1.
182   Ibid.
183   Ibid., p. 2.
184   'Ward Sisters Meet Dr Cohen', *Nursing Times*, 1948, vol. 44, 19 March, p. 231; Cohen, 'Nurse as Citizen', pp. 850–1.
185   'Recruitment of Nurses, Minority Report of Working Party', *The Times*, 16 September 1948.
186   Ibid.
187   Ibid., 'Student Nurses Tell Why They Left Training, "Bullied, Can't Do Anything Right" ', *Daily Worker*, 16 September 1948; 'No Time to be Sergeant-Majors, Dear Dr Cohen, It Just Isn't True', *Daily Record*, 16 September 1948.
188   W. McAllister, 'Thoughts upon Dr Cohen's Report', *Nursing Times*, 1948, vol. 44, 20 November, p. 852.
189   'How Many Nurses?', *Lancet*, 1948, vol. ii, p. 498.
190   Ibid.
191   Ibid.
192   Webster, 'Nursing and Crisis', pp. 4–12.
193   *Royal Commission on the Poor Laws and Relief of Distress*, London, HMSO, Cmnd 4499, Minority Report, 1909, reissued separately as S. Webb and B. Webb, *The Break-up of the Poor Law: Being Part of the Minority Report of the Poor Law Commission*, London, Longmans and Green, 1909.

CONCLUSION

1   H. Perkin, *The Rise of Professional Society: England Since 1800*, London, Routledge, 1988, p. 130.
2   Ibid., pp. 131–2.
3   G. Sutherland, 'Recent Trends in Administrative History', *Victorian Studies*, 1970, vol. xiii, p. 410.
4   S. Stacey, 'The Ministry of Health 1919–1929: Ideas and Practice in a Government Department', University of Oxford, DPhil thesis, 1984, p. 35.

5   R. MacLeod (ed.), *Government and Expertise: Specialists, Administrators and Professionals, 1860–1919*, Cambridge, Cambridge University Press, 1986.

6   See M. Bartlett, 'Education for Industry: Attitudes and Policies affecting the Provision of Technical Education in Britain 1916–1929', University of Oxford, DPhil thesis, 1995.

7   M. Carpenter, *Working for Health: The History of the Confederation of Health Service Employees*, London, Lawrence and Wishart, 1988; C. Davies, 'Experience of Dependency and Control in Work: The Case of Nurses', *Journal of Advanced Nursing*, vol. 1, pp. 273–83; M. Carpenter, *Gender and the Professional Predicament in Nursing*, Buckingham, Open University Press, 1995; C. Maggs, *The Origins of General Nursing*, London, Croom Helm, 1983; P. Nolan, *A History of Mental Health Nursing*, London, Chapman Hall, 1993; A. Summers, *Angels and Citizens: British Women as Military Nurses, 1854–1914*, London, Routledge, 1988; A. Simnet, 'The Pursuit of Respectability, Women and the Nursing Profession, 1860–1900', in R. White (ed), *Political Issues in Nursing: Past, Present and Future*, London, John Wiley, vol. 2, 1986, pp. 1–24.

8   B. Turner, *Medical Power and Social Knowledge*, London, Sage, 1987, pp. 146–156.

9   A. Witz, *Professions and Patriarchy*, London, Routledge, 1992; Davies, *Gender and the Professional Predicament*.

10   Witz, *Professions and Patriarchy*.

11   Davies, *Gender and the Professional Predicament*.

12   See C. Emden, 'Ways of Knowing in Nursing', in G. Gray and R. Pratt (eds), *Towards a Discipline of Nursing*, Edinburgh, Churchill Livingstone, 1991, p. 22.

13   Useful contributions to the sociology of medical knowledge are beginning to emerge but the focus for these tends to be intra- rather than inter-disciplinary analysis: see L. Jordonova, 'The Social Construction of Medical Knowledge', *Social History of Medicine*, 1995, vol. 8, pp. 361–82; A. Treacher and P. Wright (eds), *The Problem of Medical Knowledge: Examining the Social Construction of Medicine*, Edinburgh, Edinburgh University Press, 1982.

14   D. Ross, 'American Social Science and the Idea of Progress', in T.L. Haskell (ed.), *The Authority of Experts: Essays in History and Theory*, Bloomington, Indiana University Press, 1978, p. 157.

15   See especially the critical analysis of science that emerged from the Science Studies Unit at the University of Edinburgh: B. Barnes, *Scientific Knowledge and Sociological Theory*, London, Routledge, Kegan Paul, 1974; B. Barnes, *Interests and the Growth of Knowledge*, London, Routledge, Kegan Paul, 1977; D. Bloor, *Knowledge and Social Imagery*, 2nd edn, Chicago, University of Chicago Press, 1991.

16   Ross, 'American Social Science', p. 160.

17   Ibid., pp. 160–1.

18   For a review of the sources of nursing knowledge see K. Robinson and B. Vaughan (eds), *Knowledge for Nursing Practice*, London, Heinemann, 1992.

19 See C. Rosenberg, 'Towards an Ecology of Knowledge: On Discipline, Context, and History', in A. Olesen and J. Voss (eds), *The Organization of Knowledge in Modern America, 1860–1920*, Baltimore, Johns Hopkins University Press, 1979, pp. 440–55, for a particularly prescient discussion of these factors, and a review of relevant literature and case examples.

20 J. Guy and I. Small, *Politics and Value in English Literature*, Cambridge, Cambridge University Press, 1994; H. Kaye, *The Powers of the Past: Reflections on the Crisis and Promise of History*, Minneapolis, University of Minnesota Press, 1991; J. Lewis, *What Price Community Medicine?: The Philosophy, Practice and Politics of Public Health since 1919*, Brighton, Harvester, 1983.

21 The tentative nature of any claims to being a discipline is encapsulated in the title of G. Gray and R. Pratt (eds), *Towards a Discipline of Nursing*, Edinburgh, Churchill Livingstone, 1991.

22 Guy and Small, *Politics and Value*.

23 For a rare synthesis and overview of the professionalisation of disciplines such as English studies, history and economics, see Guy and Small, *Politics and Value*, pp. 29–67, 156–182. For an analysis of different disciplinary traditions in the USA in the humanities, social science and science, see L. Veysey, 'The Plural Organized Worlds of the Humanities', D. Ross, 'The Development of the Social Sciences', M. Rossiter, 'The Organization of the Agricultural Sciences', G. Allen, 'The Transformation of a Science: T.H. Morgan and the Emergence of the a New American Biology', and Rosenberg, 'Towards an Ecology of Knowledge', all in A. Oleson and J. Voss (eds), *The Organization of Knowledge in Modern America, 1860–1920*, Baltimore, Johns Hopkins University Press, 1979, pp. 51–269, 440–455. For a full-length work on American social science, see D. Ross, *The Origins of American Social Science*, Cambridge, Cambridge University Press, 1991. For the UK, see P. Abrams, *The Origins of British Sociology 1834–1914*, Chicago, University of Chicago Press, 1968. For anthropology, see George Stocking Jnr, *Race, Culture and Evolution: Essays in the History of Anthropology*, New York, Free Press, 1968. For psychology in the UK, see R. Thomson, *The Pelican History of Psychology*, Harmondsworth, Pelican, 1968; A. Wooldrige, *Measuring the Mind: Education and Psychology in England c.1860–1990*, Cambridge, Cambridge University Press, 1994.

24 G. Lemaine, R. MacLeod, M. Mulkay and P Weingart (eds), *Perspectives on the Emergence of New Disciplines*, Chicago, Aldine, 1976, p. 14.

25 Commonalities do exist in terms of the purposes to which the writing of disciplinary histories are put. See L. Graham, W. Lepeneis and P. Weingart (eds), *Functions and Uses of Disciplinary Histories*, Lancaster, D. Reidel, 1983. I am grateful to Paul Weindling for this reference.

26 E. Freidson, *Professional Powers: A Study in the Institutionalization of Formal Knowledge*, Chicago, University of Chicago Press, 1986.

27 See P. Atkinson and S. Delamont, 'Professions and Powerlessness', *Sociological Review*, 1990, vol. 38, pp. 90–110; M. Larson, *The Rise of Professionalism*, Berkeley, CA, University of California Press, 1977.

28   See M. Carpenter, 'The Subordination of Nurses in Health Care', in E. Riska and K. Wegar, (eds), *Gender, Work and Medicine: Women and the Medical Division of Labour*, London, Sage, 1992, p. 98.

29   Ibid., p. 98. On the new nursing see J. Salvage, 'The New Nursing: Empowering Patients or Empowering Nurses?', in J. Robinson, A. Gray and R. Elkan (eds), *Policy Issues in Nursing*, Milton Keynes, Open University Press, 1992, pp. 9–23.

30   Rosenberg, 'Towards An Ecology of Knowledge', p. 442.

31   Ibid., p, 447.

32   S. Beishon, S. Virdee and A. Hagell, *Nursing in a Multi-ethnic National Health Service*, London, Policy Studies Institute, 1995; S. Marks, *Divided Sisterhood: Race, Class and Gender in the South African Nursing Profession*, London, Macmillan, 1994.

Bibliography

PRIMARY SOURCES

Archives

London, Public Record Office

CAB 26	Cabinet Committee for the Home Office Meetings.
DT 1	General Nursing Council: Rules.
DT 2	Rules for training.
DT 3	Rules for training.
DT 4	Temporary rules.
DT 5	General Nursing Council minutes, amendments to rules.
DT 6	Council and Committee minutes.
DT 7	Schemes of election, nominations to Council.
DT 16	Training hospitals.
DT 20	Correspondence of members.
DT 27	Examination results.
DT 28	Examination results.
DT 34	Test examination.
DT 38	Syllabus and schemes for training, approved institutions.
DT 48	Education and Examination Committee minutes, microfilm.
ED 50	Nurse training.
LAB 8	Nurses and midwives recruitment.
MH 55	Hospital nursing: miscellaneous.
MH 71	Nursing organisations and NHS.
MH 77	National Health Service and nursing policy.
MH 78	Nursing establishments.
MH 80	Nurses' Bill.
MH 87	Nurses' and midwives' conditions of service.
MH 123	Nurses and domestic staff.
MH 133	Standing Nursing Advisory Committee, appointments.
T 161	Miscellaneous files on hospitals.

London/Edinburgh, Royal College of Nursing

Council Minutes 1916–48.
Association of Hospital Matrons: Minutes of Executive Committee, 1919–39.
Education and Examination Committee Minutes, 1925–39.
Special Committees: correspondence and evidence to the Lancet Commission, 1930–2.
Correspondence and evidence to the Inter-departmental Committee on Nursing Services, 1938–9.
Minutes of Sub-committee on Nurses' Reconstruction Committee, 1942–6.
General files relating to the work of the Nurses' Reconstruction Committee, 1942–9.
Parliamentary files on nurses' registration.
Correspondence and evidence to the Working Party on the Recruitment and Training of Nurses.

Oxford University, Bodleian Library

Acland Papers.
Addison Papers.
Burdett Papers.

Oxford, Radcliffe Infirmary

Recruitment records of probationers entering training, 1891–1939.

International Council of Nurses, Geneva

Files related to Congresses and foundation of Council.

London, Trades Union Congress

Reports of the Proceedings of the Annual Trades Union Congresses, London, 1919–39.

Parliamentary papers

Report of the Schools Inquiry Commission, PP 1867–8 Vol. XXVIII, London, HMSO, Cmnd 3966.
Select Committee of the House of Lords on the Metropolitan Hospitals, Provident and other Public Dispensaries and Charitable Institutions PP. 1890 (392), Vol. XVI.I.
Select Committee on the Metropolitan Hospitals, Dispensaries and Charitable Institutions, House of Lords, PP. 1890, vol. xvi.i.
Report of the Select Committee on the Registration of Nurses, with Proceedings and Evidence, Appendix and Index, London, PP 1904 (281), vi. 701.

Report from the Select Committee of the House of Commons on the Registration of Nurses, with Proceedings and Evidence, Appendix and Index, 1904–5 (281).

Report from the Select Committee of the House of Commons on the Registration of Nurses with Proceedings of Evidence, Appendices and Index, 1905 (263).

Royal Commission on the Poor Laws and Relief of Distress London, HMSO, Cmnd 4499, Minority Report, 1909.

Report from the Select Committee of the House of Commons on the General Nursing Council with Minutes of Proceedings and Evidence, 1924–5 (167).

Select Committee of the House of Lords on the Metropolitan Hospitals, Providential and other Public Dispensaries and Charitable Institutions for the Sick Poor.

Other official publications

Hansard's Parliamentary Debates, 1919–48.
Ministry of Health Annual Reports, 1919–48.

Official reports related to hospitals and nursing

House of Commons *Departmental Committee on the Workings of the Mid-wives' Act*, London, HMSO, Cmnd 4822, 1909.

Ministry of Reconstruction *Machinery of Government Committee Report No. 1*, London, HMSO, Cmnd 9230, 1919.

Ministry of Health *Consultative Council on Medical and Allied Services, Interim Report on the Future Provision of Medical and Allied Services*, London, HMSO, Chairman Lord Dawson, Cmnd 693, 1920.

National Insurance Commission, Scotland Report Hospital and Nursing Services, Edinburgh, HMSO, Cmnd 699, 1920.

Final Report of the Voluntary Hospitals Commission, London, HMSO, Chairman Lord Cave, Cmnd 1335, 1921.

Department of Health for Scotland, *Training of Nurses*, London, HMSO, 1935–6.

Department of Health for Scotland *Scottish Departmental Report*, London, HMSO, Chairman Lord Alness, Cmnd 5866, 1937–8.

Ministry of Health, Board of Education and Department of Health for Scotland *Interim Report of the Inter-departmental Committee on Nursing Services*, London, HMSO, 1939.

Ministry of Health *First Report of Nurses' Salaries Committee*, London, HMSO, Chairman Lord Rushcliffe, 1943.

Ministry of Health, *Nursing in a National Health Service*, London, HMSO, 1945.

Ministry of Health, Department of Health for Scotland, Ministry of Labour and National Service *Working Party on the Recruitment and Training of Nurses*, London, HMSO, 1947.

Ministry of Health, Department of Health for Scotland, Ministry of Labour and National Service *Working Party on the Recruitment and Training of Nurses, Minority Report*, London, HMSO, 1948.

Special reports and memoranda

Acland, H. *Memorandum concerning Medical Education of Women in reply to communication through Lord President, from Earl Granville and the Russian Ambassador at the Court of St James by the President of the Medical Council*, London, 1884.

Association of Headmistresses *Memorandum of Evidence to the Inter-departmental Committee on Nursing Services*, London, 1938.

Association of Hospital Matrons *Memorandum of the Association of Hospital Matrons to the Lancet Commission on Nursing*, London, 1930.

Bonham-Carter, H. *Memorandum on the Registration of Nurses and the Royal British Nurses Association in Memorandum against the Petition*, London, 1892.

British Medical Association *Memorandum of Evidence to the Inter-depart-mental Committee on Nursing Services*, London, 1938.

British Nurses Association *First Annual Report*, London, British Nurses Association, 1889.

Central Committee for the State Registration of Nurses *State Registration of Nurses: A Statement issued by the Authority of the Central Committee of the State Registration of Nurses*, London, n.d.

College of Nursing *Report of the Salaries Committee on Salaries and Conditions of Employment of Nurses*, London, 1919.

General Nursing Council *Memorandum submitted to the Working Party on Nurse Recruitment and Training*, London, 1948.

International Council of Nurses Archives, Geneva (ICNA), Mary Burr 'The British Journal of Nursing and the British Nursing Press', *Rapports de la Conference Internationale du Nursing, Paris, 1907*, Bordeaux, International Council of Nurses, 1907, pp. 186–7.

Labour Party *The Nursing Profession: A Statement of Policy*, London, Labour Party, 1927.

Lancet *The Final Report of the Lancet Commission on Nursing*, London, 1932.

Mellor, T. *Report of the Salaries Committee on Salaries and Conditions of Employment of Nurses as Submitted to the College Council in April 1919*, London, 1919.

Memorandum on the Registration of Nurses and the Royal British Nurses Association in Opposition to the Petition of Her Royal Highness Helena Princess Christian of Schleswig-Holstein, Princess of Great Britain and Ireland for the Grant of a Charter for the Incorporation of the Royal British Nurses Association, London, 1892.

Ministry of Health, Ministry of Labour and National Service and Department of Health for Scotland *Staffing the Hospitals: An Urgent National Need*, London, HMSO, 1945.

National Council of Women of Great Britain *Memorandum of Evidence Relating to Conditions in the Nursing Profession submitted to the Inter-departmental Committee on Nursing Services*, London, 1938.

National Union of Teachers *A Report of Proposals by the Executive of the National Union of Teachers*, Gloucester, National Union of Teachers, 1943.

Royal College of Nursing *First Draft: The Royal College of Nursing Committee on the Lancet Commission Report*, London, 1931.

Royal College of Nursing *Memorandum of Evidence submitted to the Lancet Commission on Nursing: Suggested Improvements for the Nursing Profession*, London, 1931.

Royal College of Nursing *Memorandum of the Salaries and Superannuation Committee of the Royal College of Nursing to the Lancet Commission*, London, 1931.

Royal College of Nursing, *Memorandum to the Lancet Commission on Nursing submitted by the Royal College of Nursing*, 1931.

Royal College of Nursing *Salaries and Superannuation Committee: Report on the Questionnaire on the Supply of suitable candidates for the Nursing Profession and Unemployment amongst Nurses*, London, 1931.

Royal College of Nursing *Professional Association Committee Report to Council*, London, 1936.

Royal College of Nursing *Memorandum of Evidence Relating to Conditions in the Nursing Profession Submitted to the Inter-departmental Committee on Nursing Services*, London, 1938.

Royal College of Nursing *Nursing Reconstruction Committee Report, Section i: The Assistant Nurse*, London, Royal College of Nursing, 1942.

Royal College of Nursing *Nursing Reconstruction Committee Report, Section ii: Education and Training*, London, Royal College of Nursing, 1943.

Royal College of Nursing *Nursing Reconstruction Committee Report, Section iii: Recruitment*, London, Royal College of Nursing, 1943.

Royal College of Nursing *Nursing Reconstruction Committee Report, Supplement A: Minimum Standards for Nurse Training Schools, Supplement B: Post-registration Training for Nurses*, London, Royal College of Nursing, 1945.

Royal College of Nursing *Nursing Reconstruction Committee, Section iv: The Social and Economic Condition of the Nurse*, London, Royal College of Nursing, 1949.

Royal College of Nursing Student Nurses' Association *Memorandum of Evidence relating to Conditions in the Nursing Profession submitted to the Inter-departmental Committee on Nursing Services,* London, 1938.

Socialist Medical Association *Nursing in the Post-War World: A Memorandum on the Shortage of Nurses with Constructive Proposals*, London, Socialist Medical Association, 1945.

Voluntary Hospitals Committee County of London *Statement of Evidence for Submission to the Inter-Departmental Committee on Nursing*, London, HMSO, 1938.

Webb, S. and Webb, B. *The Break-up of the Poor Law: Being Part of the Minority Report of the Poor Law Commission*, London, Longmans and Green, 1909.

Contemporary journals and newspapers

American Journal of Nursing
Birmingham Daily
Birmingham Post
British Journal of Nursing
British Medical Journal
Church Times
Daily Independent
Daily Mirror
Daily Record
Daily Sketch
Daily Telegraph
Daily Worker
Englishwoman's Magazine
Englishwoman's Yearbook
Eugenics Review
Evening Herald
Evening Standard
Fortnightly Review
Hospital
Journal of the Anthropological Institute
Journal of Medical Psychology
Journal of Mental Science
Lancet
Leeds Mercury
Lincoln and Stamford Mercury
Manchester Guardian
Nineteenth Century
North Evening News
Nosokomeion
Nottingham Evening News
Nottingham Journal and Express
Nursing Mirror
Nursing Notes
Nursing Record and Hospital World
Nursing Times
Public Opinion
Reynolds News
Scotsman
Spectator
Star
Time and Tide
The Times
Transactions of the National Association for the Promotion of Social Science
Tribune
Western Morning News
Yorkshire Observer

Contemporary books and pamphlets

Addison, C. *Politics from Within, 1911–1918, with Some Records of a Great National Effort*, vol. 2, London, Herbert Jenkins, 1924.

Anon. *The Nurse and the Nursery: Being a Digest of Important Information by a Physician*, London, Hope, 1854.

Anon. 'Hospital Nursing without Alcoholic Drinks', *Pamphlets on Temperance*, 1882, vol. 24, pp. 2–16.

Balme, H. *The Reform of Nurse Education*, Oxford, Oxford University Press, 1930.

Barnes, J. *Notes on Surgical Nursing: Being a Short Course of Lectures on Surgical Nursing delivered at the School for Nurses in Connection with the Liverpool Workhouse*, London, Churchill, 1865.

Barwell, R. *The Care of the Sick: A Course of Practical Lectures Delivered at the Working Women's College, London*, London, Chapman and Hall, 1857.

Bedford Fenwick, S. *The Nursing of Patients Suffering from Diseases of the Chest*, London, Nursing Record, 1901.

Bedford Fenwick, S. *Some Common Complaints of Women: Being a Series of Clinical Lectures delivered at the Hospital for Women, Soho Square, London*, London, Medical Times, 1904.

Bell, J. *Notes on Surgery for Nurses*, Edinburgh, Oliver and Boyd, 1887.

Benton, S. *Nurses and Nursing*, London, Henry Kimpton, 1887.

Bonham-Carter, H. *Is a General Register for Nurses Desirable?*, London, 1888.

Brudenell Carter, R. *On the Influence of Education and Training in Preventing Diseases of the Nervous System*, London, Churchill, 1855.

Burdett, H. *Hospitals and Asylums of the World*, London, Scientific Press, 1893.

Childe, C. *Operative Nursing and Technique: A Book for Nurses, Dressers, House Surgeons*, London, Balliere, 1916.

Clark, E. *Sex in Education, or a Fair Chance to Girls*, Boston, J.R. Osgood Co ., 1875.

Clouston, T. *Female Education from a Medical Point of View: Being Two Lectures Delivered at the Philosophical Institution*, Edinburgh, MacNiven and Wallace, 1882.

College of Nursing, 'The General Nursing Council', in *The Register of Nurses*, London, 1922.

Croft, J. *Notes of Lectures: St Thomas's Hospital*, London, Blades Co ., 1863.

Cronin, A.J. *The Citadel*, London, Victor Gollancz, 1932.

Dickens, C. *Martin Chuzzlewit*, Oxford, Oxford University Press, 1984 (first published 1844).

Dock, L. and Stewart, I. *A Short History of Nursing*, New York, Putnam and Sons, 1920.

Drake, B. *Women in Trade Unions*, London, Virago, 1984 (first published 1921).

Duckworth, Dyce, *Women: Their Probable Place and Prospects in the Twentieth Century. An Address Delivered in Glasgow before the Scottish Society of Literature and Art*, Glasgow, Maclehose and Sons, 1893.

Duckworth, Dyce *Sick Nursing: Essentially a Woman's Mission*, London, Longmans Green, 1894.

Flexner, A. *Medical Education in America and Canada: Carnegie Foundation for the Advancement of Teaching*, New York, no. 4, 1910.

Flexner, A. *Medical Education in Europe: A Report to the Carnegie Foundation for the Advancement of Teaching*, New York, Bulletin/Carnegie Foundation for the Advancement of Teaching, no. 6, 1912.

Gairdner, W. *On Medicine and Medical Education: Three Lectures with Notes and an Appendix*, Edinburgh, Sutherland and Knox, 1858.

Gant, F. *Mock Nurses of the Latest Fashion: Professional Experiences in Short Stories and the Nursing Question*, London, Ballière, 1900.

Gordon, M.M. 'The Double Cure or What is a Medical Mission?', *Theological Pamphlets*, 1869, vol. 27, pp. 68–9.

Higgins, J. 'The Improvement of Nurses in County Districts', *Transactions of the National Association for the Promotion of Social Science*, London, Parker, 1861, pp. 574–77.

Holland, S. and Luckes, E. *State Registration of Nurses*, London, n.d.

Jex-Blake, S. *Medical Women: A Thesis and a History*, Edinburgh, Oliphant, Anderson and Ferrier, 1872.

Langton Down, J. *On Some of the Mental Afflictions of Childhood and Youth: Being the Lettsonian Lectures Delivered for the Medical Society of London*, London, Churchill, 1887.

Lankester, E. *Sanitary Defects and Medical Shortcomings: A Lecture by E. Lankester before the Ladies' Sanitary Association*, London, Jarrold and Sons, 1883.

Lees, F. *A Handbook for Hospital Sisters*, London, Isbister, 1874.

Luckes, E. *What Will Trained Nurses Gain by Joining the British Nurses Association?*, London, 1889.

Marshall Humphrey, L. *A Manual of Nursing: Medical and Surgical*, London, 1889.

Martineau, H. *Life in the Sickroom: Essays by an Invalid*, London, Moxon, 1844.

Medical Directory, vol. 1, London, Longmans, 1917.

Mill, J.S. *Three Essays*, London, Oxford University Press, 1975 (first published 1868).

National Temperance League, *Alcohol in Hospital Practice*, London, National Temperance League, 1934.

Nightingale, F. *Suggestions for Thought for the Searchers after Truth of the Artizans of England*, 3 vols, London, Eyre and Spottiswoode, 1860.

Nightingale, F. *Cassandra as an Appendix to Suggestions for Thought for the Searchers after Truth of the Artizans of England*, 3 vols, London, Eyre and Spottiswoode, 1860.

Nightingale, F. *Notes on Nursing: What it Is and What it Is Not*, London, Harrison, 1860.

Nightingale, F. *Notes on Hospitals*, London, Longmans, Green, Longman, Roberts and Green, 1883.

Nutting, M. and Dock, L. *A History of Nursing*, vols 1–4, New York, Putnam, 1907–12.

Quain, R. (ed.), *A Dictionary of Medicine: Including General Pathology, General Therapeutics, Hygiene, and the Diseases Peculiar to Women and Children*, London, Longman, Green, 1882.

Quinlan, M. *Victorian Prelude: A History of English Manners 1700–1830*, London, Cassell, 1941.

The Old Statutes and Rules for the Government of the General Hospital near Nottingham open to the Sick and Lame Poor of any County, Nottingham, 1783.

Ranyard, Mrs *The Missing Link, or Bible Women in the Homes of the London Poor*, London, James Nisbet & Co., 1859.

Rathbone, W. *Sketch of the History and Progress of District Nursing: From its Commencement in the Year 1859 to the Present Date, Including the Foundation by the 'Queen Victoria Jubilee Institute for Nursing' the Poor in their Homes with an Introduction by Florence Nightingale*, Edinburgh, R and R. Clark, 1890.

Selby-Bigge, L. *The Board of Education*, London, Putnam and Sons, 1927.

Sprigge, S. Squire *The Life and Times of Thomas Wakely*, London, Longmans, 1897.

Strachey, R. *The Cause: A Short History of the Women's Movement in Great Britain*, London, Bell and Sons, 1928.

Thompson, A.T. *The Domestic Management of the Sick Room: Necessary, in Aid of Medical Treatment for the Cure of Disease*, London, Orme, Brown, Green, Longman, 1841.

Tooley, S. *The History of Nursing in the British Empire*, London, Blousfield, 1906.

Trimmer, Mrs *The Oeconomy of Charity, or an Address to Ladies, Adapted to the Present State of Charitable Institutions in England with a Particular View to the Cultivation of Religious Principles among the Lower Orders of Society*, London, J. Johnson and F.C. Rivington with G.G. and J. Robinson and Longman and Rees, 1801.

Twining, L. *Nurses for the Sick: With a Letter to Young Women*, London, Longman Green, Longman Roberts, 1863.

Veitch, Z. *Handbook for Nurses of the Sick*, London, Churchill, 1870.

Walker, J. *The Modern Nursing of Consumption*, London, Scientific Press, 1924

Contemporary articles

'The American Society of Superintendents of Training Schools', *Nursing Record and Hospital World*, 1896, March 7, p. 190.

Anon., 'The Literature of Nursing', *Nursing Notes*, 1898, vol. ii, 28 August, p. 101.

Balme, H. 'A Criticism of Nursing Education with Suggestions for Constructive Reform', *Nosokomeion*, 1938, vol. ix, p. 54.

Bradford Hill, A. 'Statistical Analysis of the Questionnaire Issued to Hospitals by the "Lancet" Commission on Nursing. Final Report submitted to the Commission by Bradford Hill, *Lancet*, 1932, supplement, pp. i–iii.

Breay, M. and Fenwick, E. 'History of the International Council of Nurses, 1899–1909: Compiled from Official Documents', *International Council of Nurses Reports*, London, 1928–9, pp. 218–91.

Carling, E. 'Recruitment for Nursing', *Lancet*, 1930, vol. ii, 11 October, p. 826.

Carter, G. 'Recruitment for Nursing', *Lancet*, 1930, vol. ii, 25 October, p. 937.

Cohen, J. 'The Analysis of Physique', *Eugenics Review*, 1940–1, vol. 32, pp. 81–4.

Cohen, J. 'The Nurse as Citizen', *Nursing Times*, 1948, vol. 44, 20 November, pp. 850–1.

College of Nursing, 'The General Nursing Council', in *The Register of Nurses*, London, College of Nursing, 1922, p. vi.

'Correspondence', *Nursing Times*, 1948, vol. 44, 20 November, p. 852.

'Correspondence between the College of Nursing and the General Nursing Council', *British Journal of Nursing*, 1932, vol. 80, August, p. 224.

Crichton-Browne, J. 'On the Weight of the Brain and its Component Parts in the Insane', *Journal of Mental Science*, 1879, vol. 1, p. 515.

'Crisis in the General Nursing Council: A Striking Lesson', *British Journal of Nursing*, 1921, vol. 67, p. 380.

Distant, W. 'On the Mental Differences between the Sexes', *Journal of the Anthropological Institute*, 1875, vol. 4. pp. 78–85.

Dock, L. 'Nurses' Directories', *Nursing Record and Hospital World*, 1895, 20 April, p. 255

Dock, L. 'A National Association for Nurses and its Legal Organisation', *Nursing Record and Hospital World*, 1896, 14 March, pp. 208–9

Dock, L. 'State Registration', *British Journal of Nursing*, 1905, vol. 34, 25 February, p. 149.

Dock, L. 'Foreign Department: Plans for the Cologne Congress', *American Journal of Nursing*, 1911, vol. 11, pp. 719–20.

Dock, L. 'Foreign Department: The Cologne Congress', *American Journal of Nursing*, 1912, vol. 12, p. 814.

Dock, L. 'Editorial 1899–July 1929', *ICN*, 1929, vol. 9, pp. 14–151, cited by S. Lewenson, *Taking Charge: Nursing, Suffrage and Feminism, 1873–1929*, New York, Garland Press, 1993, p. 148.

'Editorial: Midwifery Legislation', *Nursing Record and Hospital World*, 1899, vol. 23, pp. 385–6.

'Editorial: Midwifery Legislation', *Nursing Record and Hospital World*, 1899, vol. 24, 11 November, p. 385.

'Editorial: The Trained Nurse as a Factor in Civilization', *Nursing Record and Hospital World*, 1901, vol. xxvii.

'Editorial: The Midwives Bill', *Nursing Record and Hospital World*, 1902, vol. 28, p. 201.

'Editorial', *Nursing Times*, 1919, vol. xv, 27.

'Editorial: Second Reading of our Nurses' Registration Bill', *British Journal of Nursing*, 1919, vol. 62, 29 March.

'Editorial: Trade Union', *British Journal of Nursing*, 1919, vol. 62, 15 March.

'Editorial: General Nursing Council Resignations', *Nursing Times*, xviii, 1922, 28 January, p. 69.

'Editorial: The General Nursing Council and Resignations', *Nursing Times*, 1922, vol. xviii, 11 February, p. 119.

'Editorial: Where are We Drifting?' *Nursing Times*, 1930, vol. 26, 18 October, p. 1233. December, p. 355.

'Editorial: The One Portal to the State Register', *British Journal of Nursing*, 1932, vol. 80, March.

'Editorial: A Demand for Justice for the State Registered Nurse', *British Journal of Nursing*, 1943, vol. 91, p. 209.

'Editorial: The Rise and Decline of Nursing in England and Wales', *British Journal of Nursing*, 1943, vol. 91, pp. 37–8.

'Entry to the Nursing Profession', *Lancet*, 1933, vol. ii, 28 October, p. 1020.

Ferguson, H. 'The State Registration of Nurses', *Nineteenth Century*, 1904, vol. 55, pp. 312–17.

'General Nursing Council', *Nursing Times*, 1920, vol. xvi, 17 July, p. 839.

Hampton, I. 'Educational Standards for Nurses', in L. Petry (ed.), *Congress of Charities, Correction and Philanthropy, Chicago*, New York, 1893, pp. 1–12.

Hardy, G. 'A Quest for Qualification', *British Journal of Nursing*, 1943, vol. 91, May, p. 50.

'History of the Movement in favour of a Common Register', *Hospital*, 1889, vol. 2, p. 17.

Hitch, M. 'The Education of the Nurse as a Problem of the Future', *Nursing Times*, 1932, vol. 30, 12 November, p. 1163.

Horder, Lord, 'Eugenics as I see it', *Eugenics Review*, 1936, vol. 38, p. 267.

'The Hospital Nursing Service', *British Medical Journal*, 1932, 20 February, vol. 1, p. 344.

'Incidence of Tuberculosis amongst Hospital Nurses', *Lancet*, 1930, vol. i, pp. 874–5.

'The Interim Report', *Nursing Times*, 1939, vol. 35, 4 February, p. 120.

'The International Council of Nurses: Ready for Affiliation in 1915', *British Journal of Nursing*, 1914, 18 July, p. 51.

Kris, E. and Gombrich, E. 'The Principles of Caricature', *Journal of Medical Psychology*, 1937, vol. xvii, pp. 319–42.

'The Lancet Commission on Nursing', *Lancet*, 1933, vol. i, 18 February, pp. 369–70.

'The Lancet Commission on Nursing: First Interim Report', *Lancet*, 1931, vol. i, pp. 451–6.

'Lord Horder's Speech in the USA', *Lancet*, 1948, vol. ii, 25 June, p. 1124.

'Making the Future Nurse: Great Conference on the Syllabus of Training and Affiliation Schemes', *Nursing Times*, 1921, vol. xvii, 7 May, p. 501.

'Matrons in Council: Their First Meeting in the United States', *Nursing Record and Hospital World*, 1894, 10 February, pp. 96–7.

Maudsley, H. 'Sex in Mind and in Education', *Fortnightly Review*, 1874, vol. 15, pp. 466–83.

McAllister, W. 'Thoughts upon Dr Cohen's Report', *Nursing Times*, 1948, vol. 44, 20 November, p. 852.

'The Medical Practitioners Act', *Lancet*, 1858, vol. ii, p. 175.

Merritt, I. 'The Brooklyn Associated Allumnae and the Organisation of its Registry', *Nursing Record and Hospital World*, 1897, 8 May, pp. 378–9.

'Mr Bevan at the Royal College of Nursing – the Minister of Health Speaks at the Fourth Nation's Nurses Conference', *Nursing Times*, 1948, vol. 44, 12 June, p. 426.

'The Nurse and the Nation', *Time and Tide*, 1939, vol. 50, pp. 129–30.

'Nurses and Trade Unions: Must they be Driven to a Last Refuge?', *Hospital*, 1919, vol. lxv, p. 146.

'Nurses Fight for State Registration: The College of Nursing Bill Fully Discussed', *Hospital*, 1919, vol. lxv, p. 383.

'Nurses' Professional Union', *Nursing Times*, 1919, vol. xv, p. 1221.

'A Nurses' Trade Union', *British Journal of Nursing*, 1919, vol. 63, p. 266.

'Nursing at the World's Fair', *Nursing Record and Hospital World*, 1893, 26 January, p. 52.

Nutting, A. 'Isabel Hampton Robb: Her Work in Organisation and Education', *American Journal of Nursing*, 1910, vol. 10, pp. 19–25.

'Outside the Gates: Women', *Nursing Record and Hospital World*, 1896, 25 January, p. 82.

'Outside the Gates: Women, the International Congress', *Nursing Record and Hospital World* 1898, 3 December, p. 460.

Outterson Wood, T. 'Mental (or Asylum-trained) Nurses: Their Status and Registration', *Journal of Mental Science*, 1906, vol. 52, pp. 306–7.

Palmer, S. 'Alumnae Organisations', *Nursing Record and Hospital World*, 1895, 4 May, pp. 296–7

Paterson, J. 'A Nurses' Trade Union', *British Journal of Nursing*, 1919, vol. 66, pp. 267–8.

'The Position of Nursing: Past and Present', *Lancet*, 1930, vol. ii, 15 November, pp. 1090–2.

'The Position of Nursing – the Public Health', *Lancet*, 1930, vol. ii, 25 November, p. 1025.

'The Progress of State Registration', *British Journal of Nursing*, 1904, vol. 23, pp. 351–3.

'Reconstruction: The New Utilitarianism', *Lancet*, 1949, vol. i, 7 May, pp. 792–3.

'Registers Official and Otherwise', *Nursing Times*, 1920, vol. xvi, 14 August, p. 946.

'The Relative Position of Medical Practitioner and Midwife' *Nursing Record and Hospital World*, 1899, vol. 23, p. 250.

'Second Interim Report: The Lancet Commission on Nursing', *Lancet*, 1932, vol. i, pp. i–xxii.

Sieveking, E. 'Training Institutions for Nurses', *Englishwoman's Magazine*, 1852, vol. 7, p. 294.

Spann, R. 'The Use of Advisory Bodies by the Ministry of Health', in R. Vernon and N. Mansreigh, *Advisory Bodies: A Study in their Use in Relation to Central Government 1919–1939*, London, Allen and Unwin, 1940, 227–81.

'Special Meeting to Present Reasons for Opposition to Division of Preliminary Examination of Nurses', *British Journal of Nursing*, 1934, vol. 84, p. 94.

'Superintendents' Convention, Baltimore, February, 1897', *Nursing Record and Hospital World*, 1897, 29 May, pp. 437–8, 455–6, 476–7.

Thomson, D. 'A Few Remarks on the Registration of Nurses and the Nurses Registration Bill from the Mental Nursing Point of View', *Journal of Mental Science*, 1904, vol. 50, pp. 451–5.

'The Three Years Course of Training in Connection with the Eight-Hour Day', *Nursing Record and Hospital World*, 1895, 1 June, pp. 375–7, 395–6.

'The Trade Union Movement among Poor Law Nurses', *Nursing Times*, 1919, vol. xv, pp. 1081–2.

'Trained Nurses: The Steel Framework', *Time and Tide*, 1939, vol. 50, p. 1461.

Tufts, M. 'Hospital Discipline and Ethics', *Nursing Times*, 1917, vol. 17, 20 October, pp. 1231–2.

Tufts, M. 'Hospital Discipline and Ethics', *Nursing Times*, 1917, vol. 17, 24 November, pp. 1338–9.

Tufts, M. 'Hospital Discipline and Ethics', *Nursing Times*, 1917, vol. 17, 1 December, pp. 1422–5.

'VAD's and the Nursing Profession', *British Journal of Nursing*, 1919, vol. 63, p. 35.

Viney, M. 'The Nursing Service of Great Britain: A Career for Girls', *Journal of Education*, 1930, February, pp. 88–90.

Wald, Miss 'Nurses' Social Settlement', *Nursing Record and Hospital World*, 1901, 26 January, p. 69

Walsh, M. 'Male Nursing', in *Science and Art of Nursing* vol. 3, London, Cassell, 1907, p. 168.

Way, H. 'Authority and Discipline', *Nursing Times*, 1960, 29 April, pp. 545–6.

'Ways and Means', *Nursing Times*, 1938, vol. 34, 28 May, p. 1726.

Webster, G. 'Medical Practitioners and Registration', *Lancet*, 1858, vol, ii, p. 175.

'Who's Who on the General Nursing Council', *British Journal of Nursing*, 1920, vol. 64, 1 May, p. 256.

'Women', *Nursing Record and Hospital World*, 1896, 23 May, p. 423.

Women's Social and Political Union *Second Annual Report of the Women's Social and Political Union, 1908*, London, Women's Press, 1908.

Women's Social and Political Union *Sixth Annual Report of the Women's Social and Political Union, 1914*, London, Women's Press, 1914.

Wood, C. 'Some Thoughts on the Recent Discussion on the Private Nurse', *Nursing Notes*, 1897, vol. x, p. 59.

Wood, C. 'Sick Nursing', *Englishwoman's Yearbook*, 1899, p. 61.

Oral interviews

Dame Elizabeth Cockagne, 24 August 1987.

Sir George Godber, 15 March 1988.

SECONDARY SOURCES

Journals and newspapers

American Anthropologist
British Journal of Educational Studies
Bulletin of the History of Medicine
Bulletin of the History of Nursing Group, also published as *History of Nursing Society Journal/Journal of History of Nursing*
Historical Research
History Today
History Workshop Journal
Human Organisation
Image
Journal of Advanced Nursing
Journal of the History of Ideas
Journal of the History of Biology
Journal of Social History
Medical History
Nursing Inquiry
Nursing Research
Nursing Times
Political Science
Proceedings of the American Philosophical Society
Public Administration
Signs
Social History
Social History of Medicine
Society for the Social History of Medicine Bulletin
Sociological Methods and Research
Sociological Review
Soundings
Twentieth Century British History
Victorian Studies
Women's Studies Quarterly

Unpublished theses

Austoker, J. 'Biological Education and Social Reform: The British Social Hygiene Movement'. University of London, MA Dissertation, 1981.

Baly, M. 'The Influence of the Nightingale Fund from 1855 to 1914 on the Development of Nursing'. University of London, PhD thesis, 1984.

Bartlett, M. 'Education for Industry: Attitudes and Policies affecting the Provision of Technical Education in Britain 1916–1929'. University of Oxford, DPhil thesis, 1995.

Blakestad, N. 'The Place of Domestic Subjects in the Curriculum of Girls' Secondary Education in late Victorian and Edwardian England'. University of Oxford, MPhil thesis, 1988.

Blakestad, N. 'King's College of Household and Social Science and the Household Science Movement in English Higher Education, 1908–1939'. University of Oxford, DPhil thesis, 1995.

Clark, M. 'The Data of Alienism: Evolutionary Neurology, Physiological Psychology and the Reconstruction of British Psychiatric Theory, 1850–1950'. University of Oxford, DPhil thesis, 1982.

Davies, C. 'Professional Power and Sociological Analysis: Lessons from a Comparative Historical Study of Nursing in Britain and the USA'. University of Warwick, PhD thesis, 1981.

Gamarnikov, E. 'Women's Employment and the Sexual Division of Labour: The Case of Nursing 1860–1923'. University of London, PhD thesis, 1985.

Hamer, S. 'Outside the Gates'. University of York, MA thesis, 1994.

Hogg, S. 'The Employment of Women in Great Britain 1891–1921'. University of Oxford, DPhil thesis, 1967.

Lawrence, S. 'Science and Medicine at the London Hospitals: The Development of Teaching and Research, 1750–1815'. University of Toronto, PhD thesis, 1985.

Martin, R. 'The Pan-Evangelical Impulse in Britain 1795–1830 with Special Reference to Four London Societies'. University of Oxford, DPhil thesis, 1974.

Noel, N. 'Isabel Hampton Robb: Architect of American Nursing'. Teachers' College, New York, EdD thesis, 1978.

Nolan, P. 'Psychiatric Nursing Past and Present: The Nurses' Viewpoint'. University of Bath, PhD thesis, 1989.

Pedersen, J.B.S. 'The Reform of Women's Secondary and Higher Education: A Study in Elite Groups'. University of California, PhD thesis, 1974.

Prince, J. 'Florence Nightingale's Reform of Nursing 1860–1887'. London School of Economics, PhD thesis, 1982.

Sheldrake, J. 'The Origins and Development of the Whitley System 1910–1939 with Particular Reference to Public Utilities'. University of Kent, MPhil thesis, 1986.

Sherrington, E. 'Thomas Wakely and Reform 1823–1862'. University of Oxford, DPhil thesis, 1973.

Stacey, S. 'The Ministry of Health 1919–1929: Ideas and Practice in a Government Department'. University of Oxford, DPhil thesis, 1984.

Underhill, P. 'Science, Professionalism and the Development of Medical Education in England: An Historical Sociology'. University of Edinburgh, PhD thesis, 1987.

Wooldridge, A. 'Child Study and Educational Psychology in England 1918–1950'. University of Oxford, DPhil thesis, 1985.

Yeo, E. 'Social Science and Social Change: A Social History of Some Aspects of Social Science and Social Investigation in Britain 1830–1890'. University of Sussex, PhD thesis, 1972.

Later books

Abel-Smith, B. *A History of the Nursing Profession*, London, Heinemann, 1960.

Abel-Smith, B. *The Hospitals 1848–1948*, London, Heinemann, 1964.

Abrams, P. *The Origins of British Sociology 1834–1914*, Chicago, University of Chicago Press, 1968.

Allen, B. *Robert Morant*, London, Macmillan, 1934.

Armstrong, D. *Political Anatomy of the Body: Medical Knowledge in Britain in the Twentieth Century*, Cambridge, Cambridge University Press, 1983.

Austoker, J. and Bryder, L. *Historical Perspectives on the Role of the MRC: Essays in the History of the MRC of the United Kingdom and its Predecessor, the Medical Research Committee, 1913–1953*, Oxford, Oxford University Press, 1988.

Baly, M. *Florence Nightingale and the Nursing Legacy*, London, Croom Helm, 1986.

Baly, M. *As Miss Nightingale Said...*, London, Scutari Press, 1991.

Barfoot, M. ' " To Do Violence to the Best Feelings of their Nature": The Controversy Over the Clinical Teaching of Women Medical Students at the Royal Infirmary of Edinburgh', Edinburgh, Lothian Health Board Medical Archives Centre, 1992.

Barnes, B. *Scientific Knowledge and Sociological Theory*, London, Routledge and Kegan Paul, 1974.

Barnes, B. *Interests and the Growth of Knowledge*, London, Routledge and Kegan Paul, 1977.

Bartrip, P. *Mirror of Medicine: A History of the British Medical Journal*, Oxford, British Medical Journal in Association with Oxford University Press, 1990.

Beishon, B., Virdee, S. and Hagell, A. *Nursing in a Multi-ethnic National Health Service*, London, Policy Studies Institute, 1995.

Bendall, E. and Raybould, E. *A History of the General Nursing Council for England and Wales 1919–1969*, London, Lewis, 1969.

Bennett, D. *Emily Davies and the Liberation of Women*, London, Andre Deutsch, 1990.

Berlant, J. *Profession and Monopoly: A Study of Medicine in the United States and Britain*, Berkeley, CA, University of California Press, 1975.

Bishop, W.J. and Goldie, S. *A Bio-bibliography of Florence Nightingale*, London, Dawsons of Pall Mall for the International Council of Nurses and Florence Nightingale International, 1962.

Blair, K. *The Torchbearers: Women and their Amateur Arts Associations in America, 1890–1930*, Bloomington, University of Indiana Press, 1994.

Blake, C. *The Charge of the Parasols: Women's Entry to the Medical Profession*, London, Women's Press, 1990.

Bloor, D. *Knowledge and Social Imagery*, 2nd edn, Chicago, University of Chicago Press, 1991.

Bock, G. and Thane, P. (eds), *Maternity and Gender Policies: Women and the Rise of the European Welfare States, 1880s-1950s*, London, Routledge, 1991.

Bolt, C. *The Woman's Movements in the United States and Britain from the 1790s to the 1920s*, Amherst, University of Massachusetts Press, 1993.

Bowman, G. *The Lamp and the Book*, London, Queen Anne Press, 1967.

Braverman, H. *Labour and Monopoly Capital: The Degradation of Work in the Twentieth Century*, New York, Monthly Review Press, 1974.

Bridges, D. *A History of the International Council of Nurses, 1899–1964: The First Sixty Years*, Philadelphia, Lippincott, 1967.

Brockway, F. *Towards Tomorrow: The Autobiography of Fenner Brockway*, London, Hart-Davis, Macgibbon, 1977.

Bryder, L. *Below the Magic Mountain*, Oxford, Clarendon Press, 1988, p. 213.

Bullock, A. *The Life and Times of Ernest Bevin: Minister of Labour*, London, Heinemann, 1967.

Bunbury, H. and Titmuss, R. (eds) *Lloyd-George's Ambulance Wagon: Being the Memoirs of William J. Braithwaite, 1911–12*, London, Methuen, 1957.

Burstyn, J. *Victorian Education and the Ideal of Womanhood*, London, Croom Helm, 1980.

Bynum, B. and Porter, R. (eds) *Medical Fringe and Medical Orthodoxy*, London, Croom Helm, 1987.

Carpenter, M. *Working for Health: The History of the Confederation of Health Service Employees*, London, Lawrence and Wishart, 1988.

Carr-Saunders, A.M. and Wilson, P. *The Professions*, Oxford, Clarendon Press, 1933.

Chevalier, L. *Labouring Classes and Dangerous Classes in Paris during the First Half of the Nineteenth Century*, London, Routledge and Kegan Paul, 1973.

Cope, Z. *Florence Nightingale and the Doctors*, London, Museum Press, 1958.

Cowell, B. and Wainwright, D. *Behind the Blue Door: The History of the Royal College of Midwives*, London, Cassell, 1981.

Crane, D. *Invisible Colleges: Diffusion of Knowledge in Scientific Communications*, Chicago, University of Chicago Press, 1972.

Crowther, M. *The Workhouse System 1834–1929: The History of An English Social Institution*, London, Batsford Academic and Educational, 1981.

Davidoff, L. *The Best Circles: Society, Etiquette and the Season*, London, Croom Helm, 1974.

Davidoff, L. and Hall, C. *Family Fortunes: Men and Women of the English Middle Class 1780–1850*, London, Hutchinson, 1987.

Davies, C. *Gender and the Professional Predicament in Nursing*, Buckingham, Open University Press, 1995.

Desmond, A. and Moore, J. *Darwin*, London, Michael Joseph, 1991.

Dictionary of National Biography: The Concise Dictionary, Pt 2, 1901–70, Oxford, Oxford University Press, 1982.

Digby, A. *Pauper Palaces: Studies in Economic History*, London, Routledge and Kegan Paul, 1978.

Dingwall, R., Rafferty, A.M. and Webster, C. *An Introduction to the Social History of Nursing*, London, Routledge, 1988.

Donnison, J. *Midwives and Medical Men: A History of the Struggle for the Control of Childbirth*, 2nd edn, London, Heinemann, 1988.

Dunn, C. *The Emergency Medical Service: vol. 1. England and Wales*, London, HMSO, 1952.

Dwork, D. *War is Good for Babies and Other Young Children: A History of the Infant and Child Welfare Movement in England, 1898–1918*, London, Tavistock, 1989.

Dyhouse, C. *Girls Growing Up in Late Victorian and Edwardian England*, Routledge and Kegan Paul, 1981.

Dyhouse, C. *No Distinction of Sex?: Women in British Universities 1870–1939*, London, University College Press, 1995.

Elias, N. *The Civilising Process: The History of Manners: vol. 1.*, trans. E. Jephcott, New York, Urizen Books, 1978.

Ellsworth, E. *Liberators of the Female Mind: The Shireff Sisters, Educational Reform and the Women's Movement*, Westport, CT, Greenwood Press, 1979.

Euler, J. *Victorian Social Medicine: The Ideas and Methods of William Farr*, Baltimore, Johns Hopkins University Press, 1979.

Ferguson, S. and Fitzgerald, H. *Studies in the Social Services*, London, HMSO, 1954.

Finch, F. *Education as Social Policy*, London, Longman, 1984.

Finch, F. and Groves, D. (eds) *A Labour of Love: Women, Work and Caring*, London, Routledge, 1983.

Fletcher, S. *Feminists and Bureaucrats: A Study of Girls' Education in the Nineteenth Century*, Cambridge, Cambridge University Press, 1980.

Foucault, M. *Discipline and Punish: The Birth of the Prison*, New York, Pantheon, 1971.

Freidson, E. *Professional Powers: A Study in the Institutionalization of Formal Knowledge*, Chicago, University of Chicago Press, 1986.

Freidson, E. *Professionalism Reborn: Theory, Prophecy and Practice*, Chicago, University of Chicago Press, 1994.

Fyrth, J. and Alexander, S. (eds) *Women's Voices from the Spanish Civil War*, London, Lawrence and Wishart, 1991.

Gelfand, T. *Professionalising Modern Medicine: Paris Surgeons and Medical Science and Institutions in the Eighteenth Century*, Westport, CT, Greenwood Press, 1980.

Glynn, S. and Oxborrow, J. *Inter-war Britain: A Social and Economic History*, London, Allen and Unwin, 1976.

Gosden, P. *Education in the Second World War: A Study in Policy and Administration*, London, Methuen, 1976.

Gould, S.J. *The Mismeasure of Man*, Harmondsworth, Penguin, 1981.

Graham, L., Lepeneis, W. and Weingart, P. (eds) *Functions and Uses of Disciplinary Histories*, Lancaster, D. Reidel, 1983.

Granshaw, L. *St Mark's Hospital: A Social History of a Specialist Hospital*, Oxford, Oxford University Press, 1987.

Granshaw, L. and Porter, R. (eds) *The Hospital in History*, London, Routledge, 1989.

Gray, G. and Pratt, R. (eds) *Towards a Discipline of Nursing*, Edinburgh, Churchill Livingstone, 1991.

Gritzer, G. and Arluke, A. *The Making of Rehabilitation: A Political Economy of Medical Specialization, 1890–1980*, Berkeley, CA, University of California Press, 1985.

Guy, J. and Small, I. *Politics and Value in English Literature*, Cambridge, Cambridge University Press, 1994.

Harrison, B. *Separate Spheres: The Opposition to Women's Suffrage in Britain*, London, Croom Helm, 1978.

Harrison, B. *Drink and the Victorians: The Temperance Question in England, 1815–1872*, London, Faber and Faber, 1983.

Harrison, B. *Prudent Revolutionaries*, Oxford, Clarendon Press, 1991,

Hart, C. *Behind the Mask: Nurses' Unions and Nursing Policy*, London, Ballière Tindall, 1995.

Headrick, D. *The Tools of Empire: Technology and European Imperialism in the Nineteenth Century*, Oxford, Oxford University Press, 1982.

Hector, W. *The Life of Mrs Bedford Fenwick*, London, Royal College of Nursing, 1973.

Heyck, T. *The Transformation of Intellectual Life in Victorian England*, London, Croom Helm, 1982.

Holcombe, L. *Wives and Property: Reform of the Married Women's Property Law in Nineteenth Century England*, Newton Abbott, David and Charles, 1983.

Home, R.W. and Kohlstedt, S.G. (eds) *International Science and National Scientific Identity*, London, Kluwer Academic, 1991.

Hugman, R. *Power in Caring Professions*, London, Macmillan, 1991.

Hunt, F. (ed.) *Lessons for Life: The Schooling of Girls and Women 1850–1950*, Oxford, Blackwell, 1989.

Hurt, J.S. *Elementary Schooling and the Working Classes 1786–1918*, London, Routledge and Kegan Paul, 1979.

James, Janet Wilson (ed.) *A Lavinia Dock Reader*, New York, Garland Press, 1985.

John, A. *Unequal Opportunities: Women's Employment in England 1800–1918*, Oxford, Blackwell, 1986.

Johnson, T., Larkin, G. and Saks, M. (eds), *Health Professions and the State in Europe*, London, Routledge, 1995.

Jordonova, L. *Sexual Visions: Images of Gender in Science and Medicine between the Eighteenth and Twentieth Centuries*, Hemel Hempstead, Harvester Wheatsheaf, 1989.

Kamm, J. *Hope Deferred: Girls' Education in English History*, London, Methuen, 1965.

Kaye, H. *The Powers of the Past: Reflections on the Crisis and Promise of History*, Minneapolis, University of Minnesota Press, 1991.

Larkin, G. *Occupational Monopoly and Modern Medicine*, London, Tavistock, 1983.

Larson, M. *The Rise of Professionalism*, Berkeley, CA, University of California Press, 1977.

Lawler, J. *Behind the Screens: Nursing, Somology, and the Problem of the Body*, Edinburgh, Churchill Livingstone, 1991.

Lemaine, G. et al. (eds) *Perspectives on the Emergence of New Disciplines*, Chicago, Aldine, 1976.

Lewenson, S. *Taking Charge: Nursing, Suffrage and Feminism in America 1873–1920*, New York, Garland, 1993.

Lewis, J. *The Politics of Motherhood: Child and Maternal Welfare in England, 1900–1939*, London, Croom Helm, 1980.

Lewis, J. *What Price Community Medicine?: The Philosophy, Practice and Politics of Public Health Since 1919*, Brighton, Harvester, 1983.

Lewis, J. *Women in England 1870–1950: Sexual Divisions and Social Class*, Brighton, Wheatsheaf, 1984.

Lewis, J. (ed.) *Labour of Love: Women's Experience of Work and the Family*, Oxford, Blackwell, 1986.

Loudon, I.S.L. *Medical Care and the General Practitioner 1750–1850*, Oxford, Clarendon Press, 1986.

Lowe, R. *Adjusting to Democracy: The Role of the Ministry of Labour in British Politics 1916–1939*, Oxford, Clarendon Press, 1986.

MacKenzie, N. and MacKenzie, J. *The First Fabians*, London, Wedenfield and Nicolson, 1977.

MacLeod, R. (ed.) *Government and Expertise: Specialists, Administrators and Professionals, 1860–1919*, Cambridge, Cambridge University Press, 1986.

MacNalty, A. (ed.) *The Civilian Health and Medical Services*, vol. 1, London, HMSO, 1953.

MacNalty, A. and Mellor, W. *Medical Services in War: The Principal Medical Lessons of the Second World War: Based on the Official Medical Histories of the United Kingdom, Canada, Australia, New Zealand and India*, London, HMSO, 1968.

Maggs, C. *The Origins of General Nursing*, London, Croom Helm, 1983.

Maggs, C. *Century of Change: The Story of the Royal National Pension Fund for Nurses*, London, Royal National Pension Fund for Nurses, 1988.

Maggs, C. and Newby, M. (eds) *Sources for the History of Nursing in Great Britain*, London, King's Fund Centre, 1984.

Manton, J. *Elizabeth Blackwell: England's First Female Physician*, London, Methuen, 1987.

Marks, S. *Divided Sisterhood: Race, Class and Gender in the South African Nursing Profession*, London, Macmillan, 1994.

Marsh, A. and Ryan, V. *Historical Directory of Trade Unions: Non Manual Unions*, vol. 3, Aldershot, Gower, 1987.

Marshall, H. *Mary Adelaide Nutting: Pioneer of Modern Nursing*, Baltimore, Johns Hopkins University Press, 1972.

Martin, T. *The Sound of Our Own Voices: Women's Study Clubs 1860–1910*, Boston, Beacon Press, 1987.

McCrone, K. *Sport and the Physical Emancipation of English Women 1870–1914*, London, Routledge, 1988.

McGann, S. *The Battle of the Nurses: A Study of Eight Women who Influenced the Nursing Profession 1880–1930*, London, Scutari Press, 1992.

McKibbin, R. *The Evolution of the Labour Party 1910–1924*, Oxford, Oxford University Press, 1974.

Melosh, B. *The Physician's Hand: Work, Culture and Conflict in American Nursing*, Philadelphia, Temple University Press, 1982.

Monod, S. *Martin Chuzzlewit*, London, Allen and Unwin, 1985.

Morantz Sanchez, R. *Sympathy and Science*, Oxford, Oxford University Press, 1985.

Morgan, K. *Consensus and Disunity*, Oxford, Clarendon Press, 1979.

Morgan, K. and Morgan, J. *Portrait of a Progressive: The Political Career of Viscount Addison*, Oxford, Oxford University Press, 1980.

Morrell, J. and Thrackray, A. *Gentlemen of Science: Early Years of the British*

Association for the Advancement of Science, Oxford, Clarendon Press, 1981.

Moscucci, O. *The Science of Woman: Gynaecology and Gender in England, 1800–1929*, Cambridge, Cambridge University Press, 1990.

Newman, C. *The Evolution of Medical Education in the Nineteenth Century*, Oxford, Oxford University Press, 1957.

Nicholson, L. *Gender and Society: The Limits of Social Theory in the Age of the Family*, New York, Columbia University Press, 1986.

Nolan, P. *A History of Mental Health Nursing*, London, Chapman Hall, 1993.

Nutton, V and Porter, R. (eds) *The History of Medical Education in Britain*, Clio Medica vol. 30, Amsterdam, Rodopi, 1995.

Oleson, A. and Voss, J. (eds) *The Organization of Knowledge in Modern America, 1860–1920*, Baltimore, Johns Hopkins University Press, 1979.

Oliver, N. and Wilkinson, B. *The Japanisation of British Industry*, Oxford, Blackwell, 1988.

Parry, N. and Parry, J. *The Rise of the Medical Profession*, London, Croom Helm, 1980.

Pearson, C. and Pope, K. *The Female Hero in American and British Literature*, New York, Bowker, 1983.

Pennington, S. and Westover, B. *A Hidden Workforce: Homeworkers in England 1850–1939*, Basingstoke, Macmillan, 1989.

Perkin, H. *The Rise of Professional Society: England Since 1800*, London, Routledge, 1988.

Peterson, M.J. *The Medical Profession in Mid-Victorian England*, London, Croom Helm, 1978, pp. 14–15.

Pinchbeck, I. *Women Workers and the Industrial Revolution 1750–1850*, London, Virago, 1985.

Pinker, R. *English Hospital Statistics 1861–1938*, London, Heinemann, 1966.

Pollard, S. *The Genesis of Modern Management*, London, Edward Arnold, 1965.

Purvis, J. *Hard Lessons: The Schooling of Working Class Girls*, Cambridge, Polity Press, 1989.

Pyke-Lees, W. *Centenary of the General Medical Council 1858–1958*, London, General Medical Council, 1958.

Quinn, E. and Prest, J. *Dear Miss Nightingale: A Selection of Benjamin Jowett's Letters 1860–1893*, Oxford, Clarendon Press, 1987.

Quinn, S. *The ICN: Past and Present*, London, Scutari Press, 1989.

Reverby, S. *Ordered to Care: The Dilemma of American Nursing 1850–1945*, Cambridge, Cambridge University Press, 1987.

Risse, G. *Hospital Life in Enlightenment Scotland*, Cambridge, Cambridge University Press, 1986.

Rivett, G. *The Development of the London Hospital System 1823–1982*, Oxford, Oxford University Press, 1986.

Robinson, K. and Rafferty, A.M. *The Nursing Workforce*, London, Polytechnic of the South Bank, 1988.

Robinson, K. and Vaughan, B. (eds) *Knowledge for Nursing Practice*, London, Heinemann, 1992.

Rosenberg, C. *The Care of Strangers: The Rise of America's Hospital System*, New York, Basic Books, 1987.

Rosner, L. *Medical Education in the Age of Improvement*, Edinburgh, Edinburgh University Press, 1991.

Ross, D. *The Origins of American Social Science*, Cambridge, Cambridge University Press, 1991.

Rothblatt, S. *The Revolution of the Dons: Cambridge and Society in Victorian England*, London, Faber and Faber, 1968.

Rydell, R. *All the World's a Fair: Visions of Empire at the American International Expositions, 1876–1916*, Chicago, University of Chicago Press, 1984.

Savage, J. *Nursing Intimacy: An Ethnographic Approach to Nurse–Patient Interaction*, London, Scutari Press, 1995.

Scot, A. *Making the Invisible Visible*, Urbana, University of Chicago Press.

Selby-Bigge, L. *The Board of Education*, London, Putnam and Sons, 1927.

Seymer, L. *Dame Alicia Lloyd Still 1869–1944*, London, Nightingale Fund, 1953.

Shanley, M. *Feminism, Marriage and the Law in Victorian England*, London, Tauris, 1989.

Shortland, M. *Medicine and Film: A Checklist, Survey and Research Resource*, Oxford, Wellcome Unit for the History of Medicine, 1988.

Showalter, E. *The Female Malady: Women, Madness and English Culture, 1830–1980*, London, Virago, 1987.

Silver, H. *The Concept of Popular Education: A Study of Ideas in the Social Movements of the Nineteenth Century*, London, Methuen, 1977.

Simon, B. *Education and the Labour Movement 1870–1920*, London, Lawrence and Wishart, 1965.

Smith, F.B. *Florence Nightingale: Reputation and Power*, London, Croom Helm, 1982.

Solomon, B. *In the Company of Educated Women: A History of Women and Higher Education in America*, New Haven, Yale University Press, 1985.

Stedman Jones, G. *Outcast London: A Study of the Relationship between Classes in Victorian Society*, Oxford, Oxford University Press, 1971.

Stevens, R. *American Medicine and the Public Interest*, New Haven, Yale University Press, 1971.

Stevens, R. *In Sickness and in Wealth: American Hospitals in the Twentieth Century*, New York, Basic Books, 1989.

Stocking, George, Jnr *Race, Culture and Evolution: Essays in the History of Anthropology*, New York, Free Press, 1968.

Strong, P. and Robinson, J. *The NHS Under New Management*, Milton Keynes, Open University Press, 1990.

Summers, A. *Angels and Citizens: British Women as Military Nurses, 1854–1914*, London, Routledge, 1988.

Sutherland, G. *Ability, Merit and Measurement: Mental Testing and English Education 1880–1940*, Oxford, Oxford University Press, 1984.

Tanner, J. *A History of the Study of Human Growth*, Cambridge, Cambridge University Press, 1981.

Thompson, J. and Goldin, G. *The Hospital: A Social and Architectural History*, New Haven, Yale University Press, 1975.

Thomson, A. Landsborough *Half a Century of Medical Research: vol. 2. The Programme of the Medical Research Council*, London, HMSO, 1975.

Thomson, R. *The Pelican History of Psychology*, Harmondsworth, Pelican, 1968.

Titmuss, R. *Problems of Social Policy: History of the Second World War*, London, HMSO, 1950.

Treacher, A. and Wright, P. (eds) *The Problem of Medical Knowledge: Examining the Social Construction of Medicine*, Edinburgh, Edinburgh University Press, 1982.

Trudgill, E. *Madonnas and Magdalens: The Origins and Development of Victorian Sexual Attitudes*, London, Heinemann, 1976.

Turner, B. *Medical Power and Social Knowledge*, London, Sage, 1987.

Vertinsky, E. *The Eternally Wounded Woman: Women, Exercise and the Doctors in the Late Nineteenth Century*, Cambridge, Cambridge University Press, 1990.

Vicinus, M. *The Industrial Muse: A Study of Nineteenth Century British Working Class Literature*, London, Croom Helm, 1974.

Vicinus, M. *Independent Women: Work and Community for Single Women 1850–1920*, Chicago, University of Chicago Press, 1985.

Vicinus, M. and Bea Nergard (eds) *Ever Yours, Florence Nightingale: Selected Letters*, London, Virago, 1989.

Waddington, I. *The Medical Profession in the Industrial Revolution*, Dublin, Gill and Macmillan, 1984.

Watson, F. *Dawson of Penn*, London, Chatto and Windus, 1950.

Wear, A., Geyer-Kordesh, J. and French, R. (eds) *Doctors and Ethics: The Earlier Historical Setting of Professional Ethics*, vol. 24, Clio Medica, Amsterdam, Rodopi, 1993.

Webster, C. *The Great Instauration: Science, Medicine and Reform 1626–1660*, London, Duckworth, 1975.

Webster, C. *Problems of Health Care: The National Health Service before 1957*, London, HMSO, 1988.

Webster, C. *Aneurin Bevan on the National Health Service*, Oxford, Wellcome Unit for the History of Medicine, 1991.

Wersky, G. *The Visible College*, London, Allen Lane, 1978.

White, R. *Social Change and the Development of the Nursing Profession: A Study of the Poor Law Nursing Service 1848–1948*, London, Henry Kimpton, 1978.

White, R. *The Effect of the National Health Service upon the Nursing Profession 1948–1960*, Oxford, Oxford University Press, 1988.

Widdowson, F. *Explorations in Feminism: Going Up to the Next Class: Women and Elementary School Teaching, 1840–1914*, London, WRRC, 1980.

Williams, E. and Palmer, H. (eds) *Dictionary of National Biography*, Oxford, Oxford University Press, 1971.

Williams, E. and Nicholls, C. (eds) *Dictionary of National Biography 1961–70*, Oxford, Oxford University Press, 1981.

Williams, R. *Culture and Society 1780–1950*, London, Chatto and Windus, 1958.

Witz, A. *Professions and Patriarchy*, London, Routledge, 1992.

Woodward, J. *To Do the Sick No Harm: A Study of the British Voluntary Hospital System to 1875*, London, Routledge and Kegan Paul, 1974.

Wooldridge, A. *Measuring the Mind: Education and Psychology, c.1860–1990*, Cambridge, Cambridge University Press, 1994.

Later articles

Adams, W. 'Lloyd George and the Labour Movement', *Past and Present*, 1953, vol. 3, pp. 55–64.

Alba, R. and Kadushin, C. 'The Intersection of Social Circles: A New Measure of Social Proximity on Networks', *Sociological Methods and Research*, 1976, vol. 5, pp. 77–103.

Allen, G. 'The Transformation of a Science: T.H. Morgan and the Emergence of the a New American Biology', in A. Oleson and J. Voss (eds), *The Organization of Knowledge in Modern America, 1860–1920*, Baltimore, Johns Hopkins University Press, 1979, pp. 173–210.

Allen, S. 'Gender Inequality and Class Formation', in A. Giddens and G. MacKenzie (eds), *Social Class and the Division of Labour: Essays in Honour of Ilya Neustadt*, Cambridge, Cambridge University Press, 1982, pp. 137–47

Armeny, S. 'Organised Nurses and Women Philanthropists, and the Intellectual Bases for Co-operation among Women', in E. Condliffe Lagemann (ed.), *Nursing History: New Perspectives, New Possibilities*, New York, Teachers College Press, 1983, pp. 13–45.

Arton, M. 'The Caretaker Council of the General Nursing Council and Sick Children's Nursing, 1920–23', *Bulletin of the History of Nursing Group*, 1987, vol. 2, p. 1.

Arton, M. 'The Chapple Amendment: Parliamentary Intervention and the General Nursing Council', *History of Nursing Journal*, 1992/3, vol. 4, pp. 178–83.

Atkinson, P. and Delamont, S. 'Professions and Powerlesness', *Sociological Review*, 1990, vol. 38, pp. 90–110.

Baly, M. 'The Nightingale Nurses and Hospital Architecture', *Bulletin of the History of Nursing Group*, 1986, vol. 2, pp. 1–6.

Baly, M. 'The Nightingale Nurses: The Myth and the Reality', in C. Maggs (ed.), *Nursing History: The State of the Art*, London, Croom Helm, 1987, pp. 33–59.

Baly, M. 'Profiles of Pioneers: Florence Lees', *Hist. Nursing. Soc. Journal*, 1990, vol. 2, pp. 79–84.

Barfoot, M. 'Brunonionism Under the Bed: An Alternative to University Medicine in the 1780's', *Medical History*, 1988, Supplement no. 8, p. 22.

Baron, G. 'The Teachers' Registration Movement', *British Journal of Educational Studies*, 1954, vol. 2, pp. 133–44.

Beck, A. 'The British Medical Council and British Medical Education in the Nineteenth Century', *Bulletin of the History of Medicine*, 1956, vol. xx, pp. 150–3.

Booth, C. 'Clinical Research', in J. Austoker and L. Bryder (eds), *Historical Perspectives on the Role of the MRC*, Oxford, Oxford University Press, 1989, pp. 205–6.

Briggs, A. 'The Language of Class in Early Nineteenth Century England', in

A. Briggs and J. Saville (eds), *Essays in Labour History in Memory of G.D.H. Cole*, London, Macmillan, 1960, pp. 43–73.

Bullough, V. and Bullough, B. 'Achievements of Eminent American Nurses of the Past: A Prosopographical Study', *Nursing Research*, 1992, vol. 75, pp. 120–4.

Burstyn, J. 'Brain and Intellect: Science Applied to a Social Issue 1876–1885', *Actes xiie Congres International D'Histoire des Sciences, Paris, Histoire Des Sciences Des Hommes*, 1971, vol. 9, pp. 13–16.

Burstyn, J. 'Education and Sex: The Medical and Religious Case against Higher Education for Women in England 1870–1900', *Proceedings of the American Philosophical Society*, 1974, vol. iii, pp. 79–89.

Burstyn, J. 'Educator's Response to Scientific and Medical Studies of Women in England 1860–1900', in S. Acker and D. Warren Piper (eds), *Is Higher Education Fair to Women?*, Guildford, Warren Piper, 1984, pp. 65–78.

Campbell, F. 'Latin and the Elite Tradition in Education', in P. Musgrove (ed.), *Sociology, Education and History*, London, Methuen, 1970, pp. 249–64.

Carpenter, M. 'The Subordination of Nurses in Health Care', in E. Riska and K. Wegar (eds), *Gender, Work and Medicine: Women and the Medical Division of Labour*, London, Sage, 1992, pp. 95–130.

Cassell, R. 'Lessons in Medical Politics: Thomas Wakely and the Irish Medical Charities, 1827–39', *Medical History*, 1990, vol. 34, pp. 412–23.

Chambers, D. 'Does Distance Tyrannize Science?', in R. Home and S. Kohlstedt (eds), *International Science and National Scientific Identity*, London, Kluwer Academic, 1991, pp. 19–38.

Christy, T. 'Equal Rights for Women', *American Journal of Nursing*, 1971, vol. 71, pp. 288–93.

Cook, B. 'A Utopian Female Support Network: The Case of the Henry St Settlement', in R. Rohrlich and E. Hoffman Baruch (eds), *Women in Search of Utopia*, New York, Schocken Books, 1984, pp. 109–16.

Cooter, R. 'The Power of the Body in the Early Nineteenth Century', in B. Barnes and S. Shapin (eds), *Natural Order: Historical Studies of Scientific Culture*, London, Sage, 1979, pp. 73–96.

Davidoff, L. and Hall, C. '"The Hidden Investment": Women and the Enterprise', in L. Davidoff and C. Hall, *Family Fortunes: Men and Women of the English Middle Class 1780–1850*, London, Hutchinson, 1987, pp. 272–315.

Davidoff, L. and Hall, C. '"The Nursery of Virtue": Domestic Ideology and the Middle Class', in L. Davidoff and C. Hall, *Family Fortunes: Men and Women of the English Middle Class 1780–1850*, London, Hutchinson, 1987, pp. 149–92.

Davidoff, L. and Westover, B. 'From Queen Victoria to the Jazz Age: Women's World in England 1880–1939', in L. Davidoff and B. Westover (eds), *Our Work, Our Lives, Our Words: Women's History and Women's Work 1880–1939*, Basingstoke, Macmillan, 1986, pp. 1–36.

Davies, C. 'Experience of dependency and control in work: the case of nurses', *Journal of Advanced Nursing*, 1976, vol. 1, pp. 273–83.

Davies, C. 'A Constant Casualty: Nurse Education in Britain and the USA to

1939', in C. Davies (ed.), *Rewriting Nursing History*, London, Croom Helm, 1980, pp. 102–22.

Davies, C. 'Making Sense of the Census', *Sociological Review*, 1980, vol. 28, pp. 595–609.

Davies, C. 'Professionals in Bureaucracies: The Conflict Thesis Revisited', in R. Dingwall and P. Lewis (eds), *The Sociology of the Professions*, London, Macmillan, 1983, pp. 177–94.

Davies, C. 'Professionalising Strategies as Time and Culture-bound: American and British Nursing circa 1893', in E. Condliffe Lagemann (ed.), *Nursing History: New Perspectives, New Possibilities*, New York, Teachers College Press, 1983, pp. 47–64.

Davin, A. 'Imperialism and Motherhood', *History Workshop*, 1978, vol. 5, pp. 9–66.

Dean, M. and Bolton, G. 'The Administration of Poverty and the Development of Nursing Practice in Nineteenth Century England', in C. Davies (ed.), *Rewriting Nursing History*, London, Croom Helm, 1981, pp. 76–101.

Digby, A. 'Women's Biological Straitjacket', in S. Mendus and J. Rendall (eds), *Sexuality and Subordination: Interdisciplinary Studies of Gender in the Nineteenth Century*, London, Routledge, 1989, pp. 192–220.

Dingwall, R. 'Men in Nursing', in M. College and D. Jones (eds), *Readings in Nursing*, Edinburgh, Churchill Livingstone, 1979, pp. 199–209.

Duffin, L. 'Prisoners of Progress', in S. Delamont and L. Duffin (eds), *The Nineteenth Century Woman: Her Physical and Cultural World*, London, Croom Helm, 1978, pp. 57–91.

Dyhouse, C. 'Social Darwinistic Ideas and the Development of Women's Education in England, 1880–1920', *History of Education*, 1976, vol. 5, pp. 41–50.

Dyhouse, C. 'Towards a "Feminine" Curriculum for English Schoolgirls: The Demands of Ideology 1870–1963', *Women's Studies Quarterly*, 1978, vol. 1, pp. 298–9.

Dyhouse, C. 'Working Class Mothers and Infant Mortality in England, 1895–1914', in C. Webster (ed.), *Biology, Medicine, and Society 1840–1940*, Cambridge, Cambridge University Press, 1981, pp. 73–98.

Dyhouse, C. 'Storming the Citadel or Storm in a Teacup?: The Entry of Women into Higher Education 1860–1920', in S. Acker and D. Warren Piper (eds), *Is Higher Education Fair to Women?*, Guildford, Warren Piper, 1984, pp. 51–64.

Emden, C. 'Ways of Knowing in Nursing', in G. Gray and R. Pratt (eds), *Towards a Discipline of Nursing*, Edinburgh, Churchill Livingstone, 1991, pp. 11–30.

Fee, E. 'Nineteenth Century Craniology: The Study of the Female Skull', *Bulletin of the History of Medicine*, 1979, vol. 53, pp. 415–33.

Feld, S. 'The Focused Organisation of Social Ties', *American. Journal of Sociology*, 1981, vol. 86, pp. 1015–34.

Fox, D. 'The National Health Service and the Second World War: The Elaboration of Consensus', in H. Smith (ed.), *War and Social Change: British Society in the Second World War*, Manchester, Manchester University Press, 1986, pp. 32–57.

Gamarnikov, E. 'Nurse or Woman: Gender and Professionalism in Reformed

Nursing 1860–1923', in P. Holden and J. Littlewood (eds), *Anthropology and Nursing*, London, Routledge, 1991, pp. 110–29.

Goffman, E. 'The Nature of Deference and Demeanour', *American Anthropologist*, 1956, vol. 58, pp. 473–512.

Gomersall, E. 'Ideals and Realities: The Education of Working-class Girls, 1800–1870', *History of Education*, 1988, vol. 17, pp. 37–53.

Gosh, P. 'Style and Substance in Disraelian Social Reform c. 1860–80', in P. Waller (ed.), *Politics and Social Change in Modern Britain*, Brighton, Harvester, 1987.

Granshaw, L. 'Fame and Fortune by means of Bricks and Mortar: The Medical Profession and Specialisation in Britain 1800–1948,' in L. Granshaw and R. Porter (eds), *The Hospital in History*, London, Routledge, 1989, pp. 199–220.

Gray, A.M. 'The NHS and the History of Nurses' Pay', *Bulletin of the History of Nursing Group*, 1989, vol. 2, pp. 15–29.

Greene, J. 'Men in Nursing and the Royal College of Nursing', *History of Nursing Journal*, 1992/3, vol. 4, pp. 3–8.

Hall, C. 'The Early Formation of Victorian Domestic Ideology', in S. Burman (ed.), *Fit Work for Women*, London, Croom Helm, 1979, pp. 15–32.

Harrison, B. 'State Intervention and Moral Reform', in P. Hollis (ed.), *Pressure from Without in Early Victorian England*, London, Arnold, 1974, pp. 289–322.

Hektor, L. 'Florence Nightingale and the Women's Movement', *Nursing Inquiry*, 1995, vol. 1, pp. 38–45.

Helmstadter, C. 'The First Training Institution for Nurses: St John's House and 19th Century Nursing Reform Part II', *History of Nursing Journal*, 1994/5, vol. 5, pp. 3–18.

Horn, P. 'The Education and Employment of Working-class Girls, 1870–1914', *History of Education*, 1988, vol. 17, pp. 71–82.

Howarth, J. 'Introduction', in E. Davies, *The Higher Education of Women: A Classic Victorian Argument for the Equal Education of Women (1866)*, London, Hambleton, 1988, pp. vii–liii.

Hugman, R. *Power in Caring Professions*, London, Macmillan, 1991.

James, J. 'Writing and Rewriting Nursing History: A Review Essay', *Bulletin of the History of Medicine*, 1982, vol. 58, pp. 568–84.

Johnson, R. 'Education Policy and Social Control in Early Victorian England', *Past and Present*, 1970, vol. 49, pp. 96–119.

Johnson, T., Larkin, G. and Saks, M. (eds) *Health Professions and the State in Europe*, London, Routledge, 1995

Jordonova, L. 'Natural Facts: A Historical Perspective on Science and Sexuality', in C. MacCormack and M. Strathern (eds), *Nature, Culture and Gender*, Cambridge, Cambridge University Press, 1983, pp. 42–69.

Jordonova, L. 'The Social Construction of Medical Knowledge', *Social History of Medicine*, 1995, vol. 8, pp. 361–82.

Klein, R. 'Policy-making in the British National Health Service', *Political Science*, 1974, vol. 22, pp. 1–14.

Lowe, R. 'Hours of Labour: Negotiating Industrial Legislation in Britain 1919–1939', *Economic History Review*, 1982, vol. 35, pp. 254–71.

Maggs, C. 'The Register of Nurses in the Scottish Poor Law Service 1885–1919', *Nursing Times*, 1981, vol. 77, pp. 129–32.

Maggs, C. 'Profit and Loss and the Hospital Nurse', in C. Maggs (ed.), *Nursing History: The State of the Art*, London, Croom Helm, 1987, pp. 176–89.

Maggs, C. 'Ethel Manson and Henry Burdett: Two Great Minds Not Thinking Alike', *Bulletin of the History of Nursing Group*, 1989, vol. 2, pp. 1–6.

Manthorpe, C. 'Science or Domestic Science?: The Struggle to Define an Appropriate Science Education for Girls in the Early Twentieth Century', *History of Education*, 1986, vol. 15, pp. 195–213.

Morgan, D. 'Woman Suffrage in Britain and America', in C. Emsley (ed.), *Essays in Comparative History: Economy, Politics and Society in Britain and America, 1850–1920*, Milton Keynes, Open University Press, 1984.

Morgan, K. 'Dr Christopher Addison and Social Reform', *Society for the Social History of Medicine Bulletin* 1981, December, p. 23.

Mosedale, S. 'Science Corrupted: Victorian Biologists Consider the Woman Question', *Journal of Hist. Biol*, 1978, vol. ii, pp. 1–56.

Musgrave, P. 'The Definition of Technical Education', in P. Musgrave (ed.), *Sociology, History and Education*, London, Methuen, 1970, pp. 65–74.

Nolan, P. 'Mental Nurse Training in the 1920's', *Bulletin of the History of Nursing Group*, 1986, spring, pp. 15–23.

Norton, B. 'Psychologists and Class', in C. Webster (ed.), *Biology, Medicine and Society 1840–1940*, Cambridge, Cambridge University Press, 1981, pp. 289–314.

Novaks, S. 'Professionalism and Bureaucracy: English Doctors and the Victorian Public Health Administration', *Journal of Social History*, 1973, vol. 6, pp. 440–62.

Oppenheim, J. 'Sir James Crichton-Browne', in *'Shattered Nerves': Doctors, Patients, and Depression in Victorian England*, Oxford, Oxford University Press, 1991, pp. 54–78.

Parr, L. 'The Writings of Eva C.E. Luckes, Matron of the London Hospital 1880–1919', *History of Nursing Bulletin*, 1989, vol. 2, pp. 8–11.

Pelling, M. 'Contagion/Germ Theory/Specificity', in W. Bynum and R. Porter (eds), *Companion Encyclopedia of the History of Medicine*, vol. 1, London, Routledge, pp. 309–34.

Peretz, E. 'A Maternity Service for England and Wales: Local Authority Maternity Care in the Inter-war Period in Oxfordshire and Tottenham', in J. Garcia, R. Kirkpatrick and M. Richards (eds), *The Politics of Maternity Care: Services for Childbearing Women in Twentieth Century Britain*, Oxford, Clarendon Press, 1990, pp. 16–29.

Poslusny, S. 'Feminist Friendship: Isabel Hampton Robb, Lavinia Dock and Mary Adelaide Nutting', *Image*, 1989, vol. xxi, pp. 64–8.

Prochaska, F. 'Body and Soul: Bible Nurses and the Poor in Victorian London', *Historical Research*, 1987, vol. 60, pp. 336–48.

Purvis, J. 'Working-class Women and Adult Education in Nineteenth-century Britain', *History of Education*, 1980, vol. 9, pp. 193–212.

Purvis, J. ' "Women's Life is Essentially Domestic, Public Life being Confined to Men" (Comte): Separate Spheres and Inequality in the Education of

Working Class Women, 1854–1900', *History of Education*, 1981, vol. 10, pp. 227–43.

Rafferty, A.M. 'The Education Policy of the General Nursing Council for England and Wales', *Society for the Social History of Medicine Bulletin*, 1987, Bulletin 41, December, pp. 56–9.

Rafferty, A.M. 'Mrs Bedford Fenwick and Project 2000', *Bulletin of the History of Nursing Group*, 1989, vol. 2, pp. 1–11.

Rafferty, A.M. 'Some Historical Aspects of the International Council of Nurses', in K. Robinson, A.M. Rafferty, G. Bergman, L. Quam and J. Quinlan, *Nursing in the World*, London, Polytechnic of the South Bank, 1989, pp. A11–12.

Rafferty, A.M. 'Nursing Policy and Nationalization of Nursing: The Representation of "Crisis" and "Crisis" of Representation', in J. Robinson, A.M. Gray and R. Elkan (eds), *Policy Issues in Nursing*, Buckingham, Open University Press, 1992, pp. 67–83.

Rafferty, A.M. 'Historical Knowledge', in K. Robinson and B. Vaughan (eds), *Knowledge for Nursing*, London, Butterworth Heinemann, 1992, pp. 25–41.

Rafferty, A.M. 'Art, Science and Social Science in Nursing: Occupational Origins and Disciplinary Idenity', *Nursing Inquiry*, 1995, vol. 2, pp. 141–8.

Rafferty, A.M. 'Internationalising Nursing Education', in P. Weindling (ed.), *International Health Organisations and Movements 1870–1939*, Cambridge, Cambridge University Press, 1995, pp. 275–6.

Reverby, S. 'A Caring Dilemma: Womanhood and Nursing in Historical Perspective', *Nursing Research*, 1987, vol. 36, pp. 13–17.

Robertson, A. 'Children, Teachers and Society: The "Overpressure" Controversy, 1880–1886', *British Journal of Educational Studies*, 1972, vol. xx, pp. 315–23.

Rose, S. 'Gender Antagonism and Class Conflict: Exclusionary Strategies of Male Trade Unionists in Nineteenth Century Britain', *Social History*, 1988, vol. 13, pp. 192–208.

Rosen, G. 'Attitudes of Medical Profession to Specialisation', *Bulletin of the History of Medicine*, 1942, vol. xi, pp. 342–54.

Rosenberg, C. 'Florence Nightingale and Contagion: The Hospital as Moral Universe', in *Explaining Epidemics and Other Studies in the History of Medicine*, Cambridge, Cambridge University Press, 1992, pp. 90–108.

Rosenberg, C. 'Florence Nightingale on Contagion: The Hospital as Moral Universe', in C. Rosenberg (ed.), *Healing and History: Essays for George Rosen*, New York, Dawson, Science History Publications, 1979, pp. 116–36.

Rosenberg, C. 'Towards an Ecology of Knowledge: On Discipline, Context, and History', in A. Olesen and J. Voss (eds), *The Organization of Knowledge in Modern America, 1860–1920*, Baltimore, Johns Hopkins University Press, 1979, pp. 440–55.

Ross, D. 'The Development of the Social Sciences', in A. Oleson and J. Voss (eds), *The Organization of Knowledge in Modern America, 1860–1920*, Baltimore, Johns Hopkins University Press, 1979.

Ross, R. 'American Social Science and the Idea of Progress', in T.L. Haskell (ed.), *The Authority of Experts: Essays in History and Theory*, Bloomington, Indiana University Press, 1978, pp. 157–75.

Rossiter, M. 'The Organization of the Agricultural Sciences', in A. Oleson and J. Voss (eds), *The Organization of Knowledge in Modern America, 1860–1920*, Baltimore, Johns Hopkins University Press, 1979.

Rustin, M. 'William Cobbett and the Invention of Popular Radical Journalism', *Soundings*, 1995, vol. 1, autumn, pp. 139–56.

Salvage, J. 'The New Nursing: Empowering Patients or Empowering Nurses?', in J. Robinson, A. Gray and R. Elkan (eds), *Policy Issues in Nursing*, Milton Keynes, Open University Press, 1992, pp. 9–23.

Shapin, S. 'Homo Phrenologicus: Anthropological Perspectives on an Historical Problem', in B. Barnes and S. Shapin (eds), *Natural Order: Historical Studies of Scientific Culture*, London, Sage, 1979, pp. 41–72.

Shaw, B. 'The Diffusion of Innovation in Clinical Equipment', in R. Loveridge and K. Starkey (eds), *Continuity and Crisis in the NHS*, Milton Keynes, Open University Press, 1992, pp. 101–17.

Showalter, E. 'Florence Nightingale's Feminist Complaint: Women, Religion and *Suggestions for Thought*', *Signs*, 1981, vol. 6, pp. 395–412.

Silver, H. 'Aspects of Neglect: The Strange Case of Victorian Popular Education', in *Education as History*, London, Methuen, 1983, pp. 17–34.

Simnet, A. 'The Pursuit of Respectability: Women and the Nursing Profession, 1860–1900', in R. White (ed.), *Political Issues in Nursing: Past, Present and Future*, Chichester, John Wiley, 1986, pp. 1–24.

Stevenson, J. 'Planner's Moon?: The Second World War and the Planning Movement', in H. Smith (ed.), *War and Social Change*, Manchester, Manchester University Press, 1986, pp. 58–77.

Summers, A. 'Pride and Prejudice: Ladies and Nurses in the Crimean War', *History Workshop Journal*, 1983, vol. 16, pp. 33–56.

Summers, A. 'The Birth of the VAD: Nursing Reserve Schemes, 1906–14', in *Angels and Citizens: British Women as Military Nurses, 1854–1914*, London, Routledge, 1988, pp. 237–70.

Summers, A. 'The Mysterious Demise of Sarah Gamp: The Domiciliary Nurse and her Detractors', *Victorian Studies*, 1989, vol. 32, pp. 365–86.

Summers, A. 'Ministering Angels', *History Today*, 1989, vol. 39, pp. 31–7.

Summers, A. 'The Costs and Benefits of Caring: Nursing Charities, c.1830–c.1860', in J. Barry and C. Jones (eds), *Medicine and Charity Before the Welfare State*, London, Routledge, 1991, pp. 133–48.

Summers, A. 'Hidden from History?: The Home Care of the Sick in the Nineteenth Century', *History of Nursing Journal*, 1992/3, vol. 4, pp. 227–43.

Sutherland, G. 'Recent Trends in Administrative History', *Victorian Studies*, 1970, vol. xiii, pp. 408–11.

Sutherland, G. 'The Movement for the Higher Education of Women: Its Social and Intellectual Context in England c.1840–80', in P. Waller (ed.), *Politics and Social Change in Modern Britain: Essays Presented to A.F. Thomson*, Brighton, Harvester, 1987, pp. 91–116.

Thom, D. 'The 1944 Education Act: The "Art of the Possible"', in H. Smith (ed.), *War and Social Change*, Manchester, Manchester University Press, pp. 101–28.

Thomas, K. 'The Double Standard', *Journal of the History of Ideas*, 1959, vol. 20, pp. 195–216.

Thompson, E.P. 'Time, Discipline and Industrial Capitalism,' *Past and Present*, 1967, vol. 38, pp. 56–97.

Tomes, N. 'The Silent Battle: Nurse Registration in New York State 1903–1920', in E. Condliffe Lagemann (ed.), *Nursing History: New Perspectives, New Possibilities*, New York, Teacher's College Press, 1983, pp. 107–32.

Veysey, L. 'The Plural Organized Worlds of the Humanities', in A. Oleson and J. Voss (eds), *The Organization of Knowledge in Modern America, 1860–1920*, Baltimore, Johns Hopkins University Press, 1979, pp. 51–106.

Waddington, I. 'The Development of Medical Ethics – a Sociological Analysis,' *Medical History*, 1975, vol. 19, pp. 36–51.

Watt, K. 'The Civil Nursing Services in War-time', in C. Dunn (ed.), *The Emergency Medical Services*, London, HMSO, 1952.

Webster, C. 'Historiography of Medicine', in P. Corsi and P. Weindling (eds), *Information Sources in the History of Science, Medicine and Technology*, London, Butterworth Scientific, 1983, pp. 29–43.

Webster, C. 'Nursing and the Crisis of the Early Health Service', *Bulletin of the History of Nursing Group*, 1985, vol. 2, pp. 4–12.

Webster, C. 'Conflict and Consensus: Explaining the British Health Service', *Twentieth Century British History*, 1991, vol. 1, pp. 115–51.

Weindling, P. 'Theories of the Cell State in Imperial Germany', in C. Webster (ed.), *Biology, Medicine and Society 1840–1940*, Cambridge, Cambridge University Press, 1981, pp. 96–156.

White, R. 'Some Political Influences Surrounding the Nurses' Registration Act 1919', *Journal of Advanced Nursing*, 1976, vol. 1, pp. 209–17.

White, R. 'The Nurses Act 1949', *Nursing Times*, Occasional Papers, 1982, vol. 78, no. 3, 27 January, and no. 4, 3 February.

Whittaker, E. and Olesen, V. 'The Faces of Florence Nightingale: Functions of the Heroine Legend in an Occupational Sub-culture', *Human Organisation*, 1964, vol. 23, pp. 123–30.

Wilding, P. 'The Genesis of the Ministry of Health', *Public Administration*, 1967, vol. 45, pp. 149–68

Wilkinson, R. 'The Gentleman Ideal and the Maintenance of a Political Elite. Two Case-Studies: Confucian Education in the Tang, Sung, Ming and Ching Dynasties and the Late Victorian Public Schools 1870–1914', in P. Musgrove (ed.), *Sociology, History and Education*, London, Methuen, 1970, pp. 126–42.

Williams, K. 'From Sarah Gamp to Florence Nightingale: A Critical Study of Hospital Nursing Systems from 1840–1897', in C. Davies (ed.), *Rewriting Nursing History*, London, Croom Helm, 1980, pp. 41–75.

Witz, A. 'Gender and Medical Professionalisation', in *Professions and Patriarchy*, London, Routledge, 1992, pp. 73–103.

Index